Just a Little Prick

This book is dedicated to the late Dr Robert Reisinger.

Just a Little Prick

Peter and
Hilary Butler

Published by the Robert Reisinger Memorial Trust

ISBN 0-473-10844-5

Copies of this book are available on request from the Publisher.
Email: butler@watchdog.net.nz

Designed and typeset by Egan Reid Ltd, Auckland
www.eganreid.co.nz

Contents

Acknowledgements

THE LATE DR ROBERT REISINGER for enabling this book to be published. His work on gut flora, endotoxemia, SIDS, and the crucial role of mammalian milk in the healthy foundation of infant-raising in any species, has been steadfastly ignored. He felt this work was a crucial part of the puzzle in vaccine and drug reactions, and the medical profession's failure to understand this, has been to the detriment of parents who were denied this knowledge, and their children whose lives have been blighted as a result. His only desire when alive, was that mothers somehow, be shown the whole picture, and the place of breastfeeding and life-long balanced gut flora in that puzzle.

ALL THE PARENTS AND CHILDREN who allowed their stories to be told, and all the ones who would have liked to, but who were put in a position where the constraints of "society" didn't allow them to feel free to do so.

THE LATE DR ROBERT MENDELSOHN, for being an encouraging beacon at a time when they were few and far between.

DR J. ANTHONY MORRIS, for being a mentor and friend, and for his insistence on scientific rigour and logic; and being a rare example of honesty in the scientific community to his long-term cost.

DR ARCHIE KALOKERINOS whose books showed that people exist whose heart shines from the page. His courage in the face of peer aggression and oppression may one day show him to be the Oliver Wendel Holmes of the 1900's. If someone is brave enough or honest enough to write history accurately.

PANEL OF MEDICAL READERS, whose tireless suggestions and input tightened the focus of this book.

A BRITISH MUM, whose constant harassment about loose use of language ensured that most ambiguous pronouns were clarified in the first draft.

To A LAWYER, who forced me to realise that honesty is irrelevant in the world of defamation.

MARY EGAN and GERARD REID and their staff, particularly BELINDA and LISA, who put up with, helped educate publishing greenhorns, and probably rolled their eyes every time they heard the word "But . . ."

TWO EDITORS whose contributions showed us that it's not what you write that matters, but how people interpret what you say.

EVERYONE ELSE involved in bringing this book to fruition, who wouldn't want to be named, but should be acknowledged.

To some in THE MEDICAL SYSTEM (so dependent upon the vested interests that prop them up), for providing a litany of strangely dogmatic examples from their own history, statistics, literature, research, zealousness in their behaviour, and actions in the media, thus providing the context for this book. However, having made such a statement we must be fair and acknowledge with gratitude those with whom we have had personal dealings who have supported us in achieving the type of medical advice and assistance acceptable to us.

Welcome to
Just a Little Prick

For over twenty years the authors' lifestyles have been determined by choices, which have become strongly held convictions. They make no apology for telling their story in the way they have done. They have chosen to be unconventional, and when necessary to buck the systems that so often try to tell us how we should think and live.

They have chosen to use a range of styles when writing the chapters of this book – serious or tongue-in-cheek; profound or light hearted; seemingly irrelevant; maybe even irreverent; repetitive; subtle or glaringly obvious; philosophical and personal.

Some readers may feel distracted or even threatened by the style, the format, or the personal details and opinions included in the telling of the story.

Exercising choice can alienate.

This is a risk of which the authors are well aware.

However, the book can be read in several ways to accommodate the dictates of mood, time available, or the degree of concentration and thinking required. It is your choice. Above the footnote line is easier reading, but below the footnote line are more complex explanations where this was felt to be necessary. And of course, there are two voices, which provide options as to how and when you read them.

Peter and Hilary Butler
April 2006

Peter

Hi there. I'm Peter.

With hindsight, this book has probably been written because of a disaster that occurred on 28 November 1979, when an Air New Zealand DC10 crashed into Mt Erebus in the Antarctica, killing all 257 people on board. One of those was my wife of 22 years.

This disaster changed the course of my life.

And also of Hilary's.

In June 1980 she and I were married.

From that marriage have come two sons.

And a unique lifestyle.

Something of that lifestyle will be reflected in this book. The stories being enacted on "the stage" are recounted by Hilary but every now and then as the curtain falls, and before it rises again, I would like to share with you a few snippets from that lifestyle which we chose – perhaps unknowingly at the time – over 25 years ago.

In August 1980 we moved from the northern Bay of Plenty to a small country school at Waipipi, five miles north of Waiuku, on the Awhitu Peninsula. About 30 minutes' travelling time away was the largish town of Pukekohe, famed for its market gardening – especially its production of onions and potatoes – and its motor racing circuit.

Another 11 kilometres further south is the small town of Tuakau with a population of approximately 3300 people.

Auckland lies roughly north of the three towns mentioned – about 50 minutes' drive away.

Equipped with such a precise description you should be able to locate where events we refer to took place. If all else fails, use the index in a book of maps!

Between 1983 and 1985 our lifestyle began to take on real form and substance.

We made decisions which set us apart as being "different".

We began to stick our necks out, and that's always dangerous. For some strange reason it seems to threaten other people's security.

It's always much easier to go with the flow.

To be a conformist.

To be compliant.

We questioned the systems and their representatives!

We had a home birth!

We decided to home-educate our children!

We bought a housebus!

After 35 years I resigned from teaching in the State education system, with 7 years to go before we would be eligible for superannuation, and no school house to live in!!

Where would we go?

How would we earn a living?

Hilary

This is actually the second book I have written.

My first, a more technical work on vaccines, remains unpublished. The book review panel soon let me know that after 23 years of learning chemistry, physiology, immunology and everything else that is necessary to understand the literature, I needed to bring the issue down to size, and tell it how it is. I'd concentrated too hard on getting every detail right. As things got tough, someone said, "Why don't you just write what happened, how it affected you, and how you feel about it all?" And suddenly an outline sprang into shape.

The first question anyone who picks up this book will ask is, "Who is she anyway?"

While I had no formal training in anything to do with the medical profession, my clinical experience came with the territory as a mother and friend and helper to many people with seriously ill children. Many times those children had problems for which most in the medical profession had nothing to offer. Watching other doctors prepared to step outside the square clinically and succeed with these children has taught me that there is another world of medical reality that many people within the hospital system have yet to understand. Some of those doctors cast their eagle eye over the technical and medical aspects of this book.

I was born in Scotland, on the Isle of Cumbrae in the Firth of

Clyde, where my father worked as a Marine biologist. We came to New Zealand just as I turned seven.

My father had been appointed by the New Zealand Government after he replied to an advertisement for a marine biologist to research problems with crayfish, oysters and crabs, and what might be required to establish a mussel industry. In 1961 we arrived in New Zealand on a ship called the *Ruahine*.

My mother was a teacher, with an interest in gardening. My father also had a huge interest in the environment, and as a child I spent some time in the marine laboratory, looking at drops of water full of things that turned into amazing creatures under magnification, and other wonders in the huge tanks set up there.

Although my father gave me a good understanding of how robust an ecosystem could be, he also talked about how little it might take to destroy something which you thought was robust. He illustrated all the scientific papers he wrote with intensely detailed dot drawings, and did wonderful water-colours and oils which emphasised light and dark.

My father's passion in his work taught me, from an early age, that it's often the things you don't think about that can have huge repercussions in the long run.

There was much discussion at home about Rachel Carson's *Silent Spring*[1] when it was published, because in all Dad's research years he had seen many a marine ecosystem change, often for the worse, through man's unthinking stupidity. His other childhood passions were birds and snakes. Before we came to New Zealand, he along with others had seen how bird's eggs had become fragile, and how some species in the UK were not thriving as they should. It was only later that people understood that DDT and other sprays could seriously weaken raptor[2] eggshell and chick genes. So even at a very young age, I couldn't help but be tuned into ecosystem analysis and critical thinking.

When I was young, my doctor encouraged me to go to medical school. Unfortunately, in the year I would have sat the Bursary exam, I landed up in bed with glandular fever from February to September. Then I came down with "serum" hepatitis, a common result of phlebotomists using re-usable needles, and in those days serum hepatitis[3] barred you from any medical training for seven years.

1 A book about DDT and other sprays.
2 Raptor = hawks, falcons, eagles, etc.
3 Serum hepatitis now known as Hepatitis B.

My two main interests have always been world history and medical issues. That year, as I became allergic to antibiotics, my interest in medical matters increased, because when you lie in bed for a long time, there is plenty of time for thinking through how it feels to be sick. The usual question that arises is "Why me?" My mother had gone back to England during that time, so my father took sabbatical leave from university to look after me, and in that year Dad often challenged my thinking on issues which on the surface seem straightforward.

The following year, with my main interests cut out from underneath me, I did a secretarial course, with business practice, shorthand and typing, as a stop-gap measure which I did not enjoy. The business studies were interesting enough, but the rest was a major grind, and I knew I was marking time. Towards the end of the year, the business studies tutor, who was also a journalist, encouraged me to go for an interview for an international journalism scholarship.

Thinking that I had totally bombed my chances with my somewhat radical answers to questions on world politics, I left the interview assuming the possibilities were zero. We were all told not to expect an answer for months, because being an international scholarship, other countries would also be canvassed. After some months spent working as a typist in the Police Department, I finally received a letter saying that I had won the journalism scholarship. Unfortunately, I couldn't raise the peripheral finances to take it up. I could literally feel the energy draining away, and within a month was back in bed with a glandular fever relapse with much worse blood test results than the first time. Most of that time was spent in our Waikanae house.

Our doctor there, Dr Frater, was a lovely older doctor, an ex-missionary with great compassion and understanding. He was also very widely read, and musical, and often called in on me after work. Sometimes he'd stay for a talk, if I needed to talk. My mother was back in England by this stage. My father looked after me in the evenings, but travelled to Wellington each day to work. It was dawning on me that illness isn't a simple matter of a bug causing a disease. While lying there, I reviewed my two episodes with glandular fever, and the doctor and I had several talks about why people get ill. As a missionary doctor, he saw this issue and the answer to it in a slightly different light to most other people.

With tensions between my parents, my childhood hadn't been ideal. Looking back on the conflict in our family, which reached enormous levels of stress when I was 12 and continued after that, patterns relating to sickness became obvious. Both times that I had come down with glandular fever had been times when I felt totally boxed in emotionally, as if the ground had been completely cut from underneath me with no one to talk to. I was starting to see that sometimes the events surrounding our lives have a huge bearing on why or whether we become sick. How we cope with them and adapt will sometimes be the thing that determines how quickly we become well.

This doctor also lent me books from his library showing how, in times of war, desperation and huge stress, the personal, social and political dynamics can lay the foundations for infectious disease epidemics and chronic illness patterns. I started to understand that, from my point of view, to get well I had to take control of my life for the first time, which wasn't going to be easy. My mother's influence on what I ate, wore, studied, thought and looked like, had been very strong from the start, and she didn't relinquish control readily. Up-front conflict wasn't my forté.

When I worked out a plan which gave me positive focus, my blood tests started to improve rapidly as if my body was saying "Yes, let's get going." I was up and running in six weeks.

The doctor and I had identified exactly what the real problem was, and I knew that I needed a job where I'd be on the move constantly, to have space away from destructive family dynamics, so I chose dairy herd-testing.

In one sense it was a great job, because herd-testers stayed in a different house every night, and every day revolved around milking cows, and testing milk. Cow-shit is green, smelly, liquid, and washes off. So what you see, is mostly what you get. I experienced other families, other dynamics, and sat back and watched them. I met some great families, and some not so great families, which enabled me to put some of my home experiences into a wider context.

By the end of the season I was feeling mentally at rock bottom. I knew that herd-testing wasn't what I wanted to do either, and that there was no future in it. I went back to Wellington, to the doctor of my childhood, who might have some idea of the best way to resolve the problems I now faced.

I walked into his office and said, "If I can't go somewhere and deal with these things, I can't see how I can move forward at all." He agreed, and sent me to Ashburn Hall in the south of the South Island, for 10 months.

Ashburn Hall was chosen for two reasons. First, one of the symptoms that betrayed problems was an eating disorder, and Ashburn Hall had a referral unit that specialized in eating disorders and the dynamics that can lead up to that. In my teens, as a reaction to feeling powerless and having no control at home, I had developed bulimia. Because my weight was normal, bulimia was the one thing the doctor had never suspected. The second reason Ashburn Hall was chosen was that it was as far away from my mother as I could get.

Ashburn Hall was an amazing place, catering for a vast variety of patients, most voluntary. I didn't talk with anyone there who didn't know the need to be there, though none of us might have wanted to be. Everyone had a focus on future wellness. The director of the hospital lived across the road, and his house and grounds were open to patients on request or invitation. I had never seen a garden like it, and it was to become a place where I could go to think things through. The hospital grounds were huge with rhododendrons, large trees, lawns, and a free-range hen area. Ashburn Hall was also surrounded by farmland, hills, cows and plenty of open space.

It was a difficult 10 months. Laying your life, events and thoughts bare is never easy, and, having a brain that wouldn't shut down, I was lucky to get three hours sleep a night. Many nights were spent down in the staff room talking to a Polish night sister, called Sister Sipoetz, who ran a menagerie of animals on a country block nearby. She had come out of Auschwitz and we often talked over issues that perhaps we shouldn't have, if you obey the rules. Not just my life, but also Auschwitz, history, and why it is that people do what they do. In retrospect, it was those nightly illegal sessions that probably did me more good than anything else.

Gradually, as her life was spun out in front of me, my troubles started to look like nothing. If someone could go through all that as a child, who was I to think my childhood had been so bad?

My mother is now dead. I wish that I had been able to talk to her about her childhood, and to try to understand her problems and how they affected her, but right through her life she was never able to communicate in that sense. As a mother, she had to be right. We were always children to her, even as adults. How much we differed from her was how she measured how stupid we were.

After Ashburn Hall, I looked at people with completely different eyes, and knew that I had to start from scratch, work out who I really was, and what I wanted to be. Medicine was still not an option because of hepatitis, so it was stop-gap work until I decided. People became all-important to me, but after three years as a tele-typesetter, doing photo-mechanical transfer[4] during the day, and a waitress at night, I felt I was in a rut, and wanted a job with more challenge. I applied for a position as the Personal Assistant to the Chief of Naval Staff knowing that it required top-level security clearance, which meant I had to sign over rights for them to see all my medical files, to interview all my doctors, and the staff at Ashburn Hall, and five personal referees. I was interested to see what the Defence Department was going to feel about that, because in those days, people could be very narrow-minded about certain parts of your *curriculum vitae*.

Security clearance took months, as there were a lot of applicants. We were spread around Defence Department typing pools during that time, and surprisingly to me in spite of the social stigma I had received from having been in Ashburn Hall, I got through all the interviews and was told I had the job. Only when I had the job, and realized what it was all about, did I see what a bad decision I had made. After Ashburn Hall, manipulation had become the worst possible dirty word to me.

If I had something to say, I wanted to say it, not hold my breath and say nothing, as I had in the past, while wondering what havoc would be wrought if I really spoke my mind. A civilian who hasn't come through the ranks can find work in the Navy a bit of a shock. In the Navy, at times, success is all about position, manoeuvring and power games, not to mention preconceived sexist ideas. I didn't want to fit that mould.

The first couple of months had been very interesting, because we had American ships in harbour, so much of my work was related to that, and I didn't see what normal naval life really was. After the Americans left, there was a promotion board meeting where people wanting to move up a rank were interviewed. We all had to attend Friday Mess, which was where the fronts came down, and prejudices came up. I felt smothered, and wanted to be in a more honest, open environment that had more respect for women. Ironically, my boss

4 Photomechanical transfer = Turning a photograph into a dot picture for newspapers.

was just the best and when I resigned he wasn't happy, but he knew that I felt I would never really fit in.

I went back herd-testing for another year. I had broken up with my long-time boyfriend and had unfinished business in my head. I was nearing the end of my seven-year bar from anything medical and wanted to get fit, spend some time thinking, and see if perhaps I had the courage to go back to school in 1980 to complete the subjects I needed in order to study medicine.

At the end of the herd-testing season I took a job with a mining company, with really good pay. I was considering my longer-term options when an airplane carrying sightseers to Antarctica flew through white-out into the side of Mt Erebus. It was the disaster in which my husband's first wife was killed. Naturally, the community got behind Peter at that time, and he and I spent a few afternoons talking, and walking along muddy estuaries and pulling out errant mangrove seedlings threatening to choke small waterways. The following year, we married and shifted to a rural school where we could have space and time to start a new life together.

Obviously, the question of children came up. To begin with, we agreed not to have children. He already had three, but the real reason was that I was too scared, and still felt I was too scarred. The thought of becoming a mother was more than frightening. Parents could make or break a person's life, and though I knew what sort of parent I didn't like, I didn't know how to be the parent I wanted to be.

I cannot praise my husband highly enough, and if I did he would be embarrassed. But as time went on we talked out all my fears and worries, and he made me see that he did want to have a family with me and he would always be there to help me through all that. And he has been true to his word. He has never left me in a situation where I couldn't cope and he taught me that we just have to deal with each circumstance as it arises, to step out, to think ahead, and to put ourselves in our children's position and always parent, asking what we would want said or done, for or to us.

I can't say I've been a perfect mother. I've made many mistakes, and have said or done things I wished I hadn't. It's given me an appreciation of my mother that I never had before. She was partly a product of her time, and she, too, had to deal with whatever her fears were, in whatever way she was able.

Looking back, I realise that in a roundabout way, the ride I had as a child fitted me out for my life now, in a way that nothing else could have. Adversity can become a positive force, and now I can truly be thankful for my childhood, because it has so greatly enriched my adulthood.

As to this book, perhaps you should just blame Peter. After all, I'd never have had to think through all this if we had never had children! Fortunately Peter's love for me, and the trust I knew I could have in him, overcame my doubts, and I'm so glad that we have two lovely sons now.

This is the personal foundation upon which this book is based. It has led to my interest in medical issues, and my years of reading in medical libraries. Most of this book looks at the issue of immunization from personal experiences that illustrate what it's like to be dissident parents dealing with new issues for the first time, and the people you meet and the situations you get into. But we wanted to provide an opportunity for a few of the hundreds of people we've met, to tell you about their lives, their children, vaccine reactions and resultant issues they have had with the medical profession. It is a raw, personal look at the challenges we all faced as a result.

To write this sort of book is hard. To understand some issues in this book, it's necessary to have some dry stuff, which I hope will be tolerated.

Science isn't all there is to the vaccination issue. A bug isn't all there is to a sickness issue. Sometimes the greatest barrier people can come up against when dealing with the medical profession, isn't science. It's attitudes. Dismissal. Particularly if medical people are only interested in compliance, and can't relate to any other option than the choice they would make.

I was lucky right through my childhood to be looked after by an older generation of doctors who had been through all the major epidemics, but who also had a balanced view on life which saw the world as a whole, not as pasteurian one for which drug companies have the only solution.

Peter and I were brought up at a time when our parents' generation was the first to see antibiotics and vaccines as the ultimate magic bullets that would rid the world of all plagues. The doctors from my childhood were trained just before the vaccine era. They saw sickness and treated some of the serious diseases for which we have vaccines, like diphtheria and polio, but I feel they also had a better perspective of people as people, and the actual impact of disease on the community as a whole.

When you listen to vaccinationists now, you would think whole schools, whole communities, were completely wiped out by polio, diphtheria and whooping cough, and that without vaccines, the world would empty rapidly. If you sit down with older people and actually ask them how many people they knew who were laid low by diphtheria or polio, it isn't that many. Just as there are some communities and schools in this area that have never seen a case of meningococcal disease in the past, and probably never will in the future, even without a vaccine. They might, however, be immune to the many types of bacteria that are implicated in meningococcal disease.

This book tells of the events, places, incidents and disasters that forced me to re-evaluate my own mindsets. It talks about issues that I hadn't realized were an issue before I became a parent. This book is personal, and emotional, and I make no apology for that, because when you boil it down, the real issues are human ones. This coin as Peter and I see it, has three sides. Heads, tails, and the outer rim.

This book is about the outer rim.

1 Will "Justice" Be Done?

Imagine a courtroom.

For those not familiar with legal proceedings there always seems a certain foreboding about such a place. Maybe it's just imagination. After all, it is here that justice will be done, isn't it?

There is always some member of the public who attends the sittings out of curiosity, or for fun. Their interest is impersonal and casual. Others are there because of personal involvement – very personal in fact. Maybe they are victims of one sort or another.

In a sense, the courtroom is like a theatre – a drama is to be acted out. All eyes and ears are on the players.

The accused. The prosecution. The defence. And of course, the Judge.

On this particular occasion the prosecution and defence seemed engrossed in last-minute reading of their files. It is difficult to tell how the accused feels. He is being charged with failing to give due regard to the public good; of behaving in an irresponsible manner, and of failing to give due regard to the recommendations of those in high places. To the uninitiated it all sounds terribly serious and intimidating.

Such a person must surely be a criminal.

The Judge – what about him? What awesome responsibility rests on his shoulders! After all, he must weigh up the evidence from both sides. He must be fair. He must be ***seen*** *to be fair. To uphold the finest traditions of the judicial system of the country. To ensure that the accused is treated as innocent until proved guilty. Proved guilty beyond all reasonable doubt.*

The trial begins.

The prosecution states its case.

The first witness is called and the evidence presented.

The defence counsel rises to cross-examine.

"Objection Your Honour!" calls the Prosecution.

"Objection sustained," says the Judge.

Spectators begin to look interested.

Another witness is called. Obviously they're all experts in their field.

Again the defence rises to cross-examine.

"Objection Your Honour," drones the Prosecution.

"Sustained," intones the Judge.

More witnesses come to the stand and in response to more attempts at cross-examination objections by the prosecution are sustained.

The defence counsel slumps in his seat looking more bewildered with each rebuff. His feelings of frustration and anger at such treatment are only slightly mollified by his determination to make the case of the defence succeed. To allow every witness he would call and to expose to the full the weakness of the prosecution's evidence.

At last the prosecution rests its case.

The Judge clears his throat.

The defence counsel gets to his feet in anticipation. Now the alleged facts can be challenged and indisputable evidence presented.

The Judge speaks.

"I find the accused guilty."

A stunned silence fills the courtroom. Nobody moves – people everywhere seem transfixed by what they have just heard. Surely they must be dreaming. Why, the accused hadn't even had the chance to have a say – to put the other side.

Such a trial makes a mockery of fair play and no doubt we would all be loud in our condemnation of such treatment of the accused.

"Shocking! Unbelievable! Words fail me . . .! It couldn't happen here though!"

Couldn't it?

Let's go back to that imaginary courtroom, and identify the main characters.

The accused: *Concerned, thinking, questioning parents, wanting the facts.*

The prosecution: *The conditioned medical advisers, politicians, Health Department officials. The vested interests of drug companies.*

The defence: *The unimpaired immune system of the human body. Researchers, parents who don't like what they are finding out.*

The Judge: YOU?

2 What Does Any Parent Want?

We want healthy, genetically strong children who will guarantee the integrity of future generations.

We like to think that if our children get married, they will marry a healthy, sensible person, and they will both go on to have healthy children. How many of the children you look at today are really healthy? If you listen to older doctors just retired, or about to retire, they will talk about how children now, are so . . . so . . . well . . . unhealthy. When they were young, there was not the high level of asthma, allergy, atopy and chronic disorders we see today.

Doctors then saw many cases of measles, chickenpox and mumps, most of which were mild; but there were never more than a handful of serious cases of diphtheria, polio or meningitis in any one practice. You can get a feel for that by asking your doctor how many cases of meningitis they have seen in their general practice. The majority of children were strong, robust, sleek, with good dental arches, and lots of energy, who rarely got seriously ill. And if you look at the early history of the Maori from Health Department records, one thing that stood out for me was that until the 1940s, the physical health of the Maori and resistance to many diseases, especially diphtheria was, in many respects, (with the exception of typhoid) superior to that of the Europeans here.

Now the story is rapidly becoming different for all races. If all children in a class lined up the drugs they were on, there wouldn't be too many desk-tops with nothing on them. Asthma inhalers would be one of the most common. Ritalin, and other controlling drugs would come high up the list as well.

All the blame for that obviously can't be laid at the doorstep of vaccination. Some is the result of a lack of understanding in modern times of real preventive medicine, which sounds ironic. What do doctors consider to be real preventive medicine? What do parents understand about how to bring up healthy children? How much are my parents, your parents and the tenets of this doctor-orientated magic bullet, pharmaceuticals based culture to blame for the loss of good, old-fashioned common sense in caring for children?

If I broke my leg, or arm, or had reason for a definitive diagnosis I would go to a doctor, or a hospital. They have valuable services to offer in many areas, so long as the decision making is left in the hands of the consumer.

It bothers me just how far medical science is prepared to go. It's almost as if what is done, is done because they can, rather than because they should. Some doctors don't just hand out antibiotics for everything viral, but others do. Some doctors are quite happy with a mindset that works by the "Find a diagnosis, look up a drug in a book and prescribe it" method, but others aren't. There is always a line between what should be done and what could be done. What is even more important is why and when, and who should be the one to decide.

A doctor prescribing antibiotics for a simple cold presents the patient with an opportunity to ask "Why?" Antibiotics are antibacterials only, and are therefore useless for a viral cold, so in this case, the prescribing of antibiotics is wrong. Asking why will give the doctor an opportunity to justify their thinking, or question their own prescription practices.

Parents should feel able to ask, "Are there other alternatives? What other options can you suggest?"

Simply prescribing antibiotics takes very little time, which doesn't usually involve much discussion or educating parents about the actual problem. A prescription gives the illusion that doctors have been useful, and many parents might think that the doctor has fixed the cold with his drugs, when in fact the cold fixed itself, and possibly not quite as soon as it would have done without any drugs in the first place. This type of medical practice reinforces dependency on the doctor, and creates a drug-linked mentality.

One day, I decided to make good use of my time at the doctor's. I had a condition I wanted to talk about, so I read which drugs they used, what side effects and problems they had. Then I looked at what alternative medicine had to say. When my appointment time came, I had a pad and a pen, and, knowing that there would be some time to wait before the doctor got round to seeing me, went around the room looking for everything provided by drug companies that had brand names, or company names on them. When I'm not concentrating on something, I often don't see those sorts of things, and to my surprise, my pad was full very quickly.

After the doctor went through my questions and we agreed upon a "non-conventional" treatment plan, I handed him the pharmaceutical freebie list. Even he was surprised, but he made the interesting observation that he was rarely offered expenses-paid conferences or large volumes of samples because his preference for non-drug treatment and scepticism of drug-rep patter had long before tagged him as a non-conformist. Yet his knowledge of drugs and their problems was extensive. It wasn't until he left his practice that I appreciated what a dissident he was.

One year he put on free evening discussions for his patients every two weeks, and always had a dedicated core group of people attending. But the few people who came were the already converted.

Some doctors are trying to practise medicine in a different way, but in doing so, their actions mark them as misfits, renegades and traitors to the cause in the minds of the establishment.

These dissident doctors face three main hurdles.

The general population is often conditioned to want only quick-fix magic bullet solutions. Because of this, dissident doctors' practices have become a self-selected clientele mostly of people prepared to travel to someone who isn't primarily an extension of a prescription pad. Some still have patients who want a text message answer, and a pill to fix it. These doctors talk with frustration about patients who consider that a doctor has failed in his or her job to fix their problem if they don't prescribe a drug.

The second hurdle these doctors face is any colleague who views them and their patients as drop-out jokesters.

The third hurdle is the food corporate entities and pharmaceutical companies. Doctors who wish to establish a partnership-with-patients practice where their use of pharmaceutical drugs is minimal, are considered "useless eaters" by drug reps reluctant to wait in the waiting room to show their wares, knowing that there won't be much profit put in their company's bank-balance afterwards.

Dissident doctors also don't fit into the new corporate Health Department, where your worth as a practitioner is determined by whether every woman has smear tests, and whether you adhere to routinely prescribed protocols which might bypass the individual's right of choice.

Doctors who really hear you are few and far between, which means parents may be forced to register with a doctor who might not be their choice. If you are lucky, accommodation of a truce-type can be found, so long as your family can be buried amongst the morass of the conformed, and doesn't affect the overall compliance figures, especially for ideal vaccination percentages. This is particularly true in countries like Great Britain, where how much money a practice is gifted from the government depends on a doctor having large numbers of vaccinated children on the books.

When you become a pregnant parent, what is the first thing that can happen?

Even with a midwife for a primary care giver it is possible that you will begin a feeling-out process, to try to find a balance between the mother's ideals and a professional's need to be in control. Depending on the care provider, there might be regular Glucose tolerance testing, and ultrasounds every month. All in the name of being diligent. But do you need all this?

At first, we don't see the control aspects of routine ultrasounds and other tests, because we're excited and optimistic. We might feel slightly uncomfortable about being pushed around a bit but to begin with the odd test seems okay, because it's new. But as we move on we can find ourselves at a crossroads. Do we take the road that most people follow, and do as we are told, or do we find out what we need to know ourselves, to continue in a way that leaves us with a sense of identity and control?

For years now, I've watched people run over by the system, myself included. The mindsets and tactics of people not used to working by consensus rarely change. When confronted with authority, we can lose the ability to question, analyse or think. It's much easier to transfer decision making and the responsibility to someone we have been led to believe is the only one who can keep our children safe.

In 1997, Rose Daley, a TV3 reporter, interviewed a doctor about the safety of the MMR vaccine. He didn't supply her with information. He simply said: ***"Parents should just trust us".*** It was a doctor's job to decide these issues for the good of one of their children. Whose children? As medicine appears to be becoming more complicated, and technology-centred (technocentric) in approach, parents are intimidated into feeling that the solutions to health problems can be understood only by trained experts.

Doctors have also had their views shaped by four years of classroom lectures, being courted constantly by drug companies, and then two exhausting years as underpaid, overworked house surgeons. They too, can fall into a rut. Many don't question the pharmaceutical company representatives' carefully crafted words because they believe that if anything the pharmaceutical companies said was wrong, surely the AMA, the FDA, the IOM, the WHO, the NZMA, would have told them so.

Ignorance is bliss. Except for the poor parent of the child at the receiving end of the ignorance, not to mention the child.

Take the use of drugs and side effects. How much do people know? Adolescents were being given antidepressants like Zoloft and Paxil but most parents didn't know these drugs can cause serious problems and be addictive.

What about the Vioxx, Celebrex and Bextra controversy? Hopefully, most readers will have heard about these issues and will just nod their heads.

But as a quick discussion point, lets look at Zoloft, an antidepressant, otherwise known as Lustral, Cipramil, Cipralex and Faverin. In December 2003, these drugs were banned for use in children after authorities were forced to review over ten years' data which showed that more children[1] became suicidal on these drugs than when given nothing. Prozac was not added to this list, but doctors were warned that Prozac might help only one in ten children.

The problems were made public after a very long battle, taken on by parents who believed that their children became hooked on the drugs and became uncharacteristically violent, or committed suicide under

1 Boseley, S. 2003. "Rules on medicines 'need big shake-up'. Anti-depressant ban for children reveals flaws in system, says Mind." Retrieved on 13 December, 2003 from <http://www.guardian.co.uk/medicine/story/0,11381,1104470,00.html>

the influence of these drugs.[2] For years, pharmaceutical companies, with the help of government agencies, refused to show the parents the relevant information, and the FDA attempted to silence doctors who wanted parents to know this information.[3] The last paragraph of this report noted that the FDA had instituted criminal proceedings to find out who leaked the information the *British Medical Journal* had just published.

So now, because of parents who wouldn't be silenced, we know that these drugs are dangerous.

The drug companies can afford to remove Zoloft from the market, because they've already banked billions in profits from all the brand names; the patent has nearly run out, and they will have some new exclusive product ready to replace Zoloft until maybe other parents find out something about that drug too.

The *Observer* also reported that a secret report had come out in which the manufacturer wanted to market Seroxat widely as "a cure for a raft of less serious mental conditions".[4]

Unlike Zoloft, immunization is not a niche market where if one vaccine keels over, drug companies can replace it with another. If something goes wrong, and confidence is lost in any vaccine, that can affect all vaccines, and also the stock market. The information stakes

2 Barron, C. 2004. "Big Pharma Snared by Net". Retrieved on 26 September, 2004 from <http://www.guardian.co.uk/print/0,3858,5024634-110418,00.html> "The web has helped consumers turn tables on drug giants . . ." ". . . a group of about two dozen American parents sued GlaxoSmithKline (GSK), seeking refunds for treatment of their children with the drug . . . The GSK suit created the tipping point in the pharmas' change of fortune and has revealed the force behind it. The formal complaint drew heavily on research by public health campaigners and consumer advocates about the hazards of antidepressant use. These activists had toiled in deepest obscurity – some of them, for a decade – until their discoveries were featured on a Panorama programme, *Secrets of Seroxat*, in Autumn 2002."

3 Lenzer, J. 2004 "Secret US report surfaces on antidepressants in children." *British Medical Journal*, 329:307 "'The FDA . . . attempted to silence Dr Mosholder [but] repeatedly claimed to 'support his concern' for the safety of children," added Professor Hoffman, "but this apparently didn't extend to supporting his desire to express that concern publicly. That may be the most dangerous aspect of this entire affair.'"

4 Doward, J. and McKie, R. 2004. "Revealed: secret plan to push 'happy' pills". Retrieved on 7 November, 2004 from <http://observer.guardian.co.uk/uk_news/story/0,6903,1345512,00.html> "The contents of the 250-page document have alarmed health campaigners who accuse the firm, GlaxoSmithKline (GSK), of putting profit before the therapeutic needs of patients by attempting to broaden the market for the drug which has been linked to a spate of suicides . . . What this document makes clear is that a number of different forms of anxiety were being targeted in a systematic way. 'The thrust was to move sales beyond the $1-billion to $2-billion mark by pushing it to people who were not clinically depressed,' said Professor David Healy, a psycho-pharmacologist at Cardiff University, who has given evidence to the House of Commons Health Select Committee."

are huge when it comes to vaccines. Vaccines are targeted to a captive world-wide market; potentially billions of people of every age in the world, who all add up to a multi-trillion dollar industry.

Healthy people who can be injected with ever-increasing numbers of vaccines which, within about 20 years, could total more than 250 per person, with all their primary schedules and regular boosters. Think about it.

Having such a cradle-to-grave healthy pincushion would be any drug company's dream come true, so long as they don't have to foot any liability issues. If you can persuade every healthy person on this planet to become so scared of everything around them, that they take lots of vaccines for lots of diseases that most likely they will never catch, just to reassure themselves that they won't be one of the very few who might have died from one name on that long list of diseases, you have it made – so long as the vaccines don't get a bad name by being proven to cause problems that reduce a person's quality of life.

Better still to convince doctors to make politicians pass laws making vaccines compulsory, so people have to have them all!

The problems start when something happens in peoples' lives that doesn't match up with what they were told. When people start to think it through and realize they weren't told the whole truth, that is when some people wake up.

For example, think about the carefully cultured perception that vaccines are the major discovery that historically saved more babies' lives than anything else ever has. Really?

Quinquennial average death rates of infants under 1 year of age per 1,000 live-births

Period	Epidemic Diseases	Tuberculosis	Infantile Convulsions	Respiratory Diseases	Gastric and Intestinal Diseases	Malformations	Early Infancy	Other Causes	Totals
1872–1876	13.5	5.5	9.7	12.9	24.2	1.2	25.0	17.3	109.3
1877–1881	10.2	5.2	7.5	12.3	19.8	1.4	21.9	15.3	93.6
1882–1886	9.3	4.7	7.9	11.8	19.1	1.2	25.5	12.3	91.8
1887–1891	8.9	3.7	6.3	10.5	18.5	1.3	24.7	8.8	82.7
1892–1896	9.8	3.3	6.6	11.0	16.6	1.4	24.9	11.2	84.8
1897–1901	6.1	2.6	5.6	10.0	17.2	1.5	26.2	9.7	78.9
1902–1906	5.5	1.5	4.1	9.7	15.3	1.3	27.6	7.9	72.9
1907–1911	5.9	1.3	3.3	7.6	15.5	1.9	26.7	6.3	68.5
1912–1916	3.6	0.6	2.2	5.1	7.4	3.9	26.2	3.5	52.5
1917–1921	3.2	0.5	1.9	4.7	4.5	4.3	26.1	2.9	48.1
1922–1926	1.8	0.4	1.3	4.3	2.8	4.8	22.4	3.3	41.1
1927–1931	1.5	0.3	0.5	3.7	1.7	5.0	19.4	3.1	35.2
1932–1936	1.5	0.2	0.6	3.3	1.2	5.0	17.5	2.4	31.7
1937–1941	1.4	0.2	0.2	3.1	1.3	5.5	17.4	2.5	31.6
1942–1946	1.1	0.1	0.1	2.9	1.2	4.6	16.1	2.6	28.7
1947–1951	0.6	0.1	0.1	2.3	0.8	3.8	13.6	2.0	23.3

Source: New Zealand Official Year Book (1953) p. 73.

3 The Wake-Up Call

I was just an average, normal mother, who had asked a few questions. We had thought about a home birth, but the doctors were far too nervous about such an idea. We were too far away, or so we thought, from the home-birth areas. The doctors felt there was a perfectly good little country obstetric unit, which should meet everyone's needs. That's where you had nice, normal births, so I agreed with them.

But that was not to be how, or where, our son would be born.

I had had leaking membranes since I was 32 weeks pregnant, but it was nothing more than mild dampness. I had talked to an obstetrician from Holland who said it was no big deal. He advised me not to stick anything up there and told me that in Holland doctors just left it alone. So when at 37 weeks' pregnancy my doctor wanted to do an internal I explained to him why I didn't want him to. Expecting a shrug and the same calm reaction I had had from the Dutch obstetrician, I was taken aback when the doctor got very upset and wanted me in hospital immediately.

I managed to talk him into two days' grace, but he was convinced that in that time, something terrible would happen, and if I waited the baby would die. Because we had prepared for birth in a country hospital, the idea of being sent to a large teaching hospital was frightening, and something I felt we needed to talk over.

There is no doubt that I felt blackmailed by the statement that leaking membranes can kill a baby. Why did the Dutch obstetrician not climb all over me with this sort of doom and gloom? Once we had reluctantly agreed to an induction, the doctor was very upbeat and happy about it saying it would take about eight hours, that the hospital was a nice place, and that he'd see us back in the country hospital the next morning. Hanging onto that comment, we went to "do the best for our child".

We arrived at 4 o'clock in the afternoon with a letter that asked medical staff not to do the enema or episiotomy unless absolutely necessary. In those days, these things were standard procedures, and we had arranged with the country hospital to skip them. But the first person we met was a harried, annoyed ward sister who had no time for us or the letter, and snapped "What? . . . we lost a baby yesterday because of a fruit-loop like you."

It didn't feel like a good start.

I was taken to an examination room, and an obstetrician came in, and went over what had gone before. I told him what the Dutch obstetrician had said, that it was just a hind leak, and he asked to examine me. The next thing I knew there was excruciating pain and suddenly water was everywhere. I was upset and asked what he had done, and he said "Oh, well, since I was in there, I thought I might as well do the job properly, and get things going, don't you think?" In walked the staff sister with a drip and a thing called *Synto* ". . . just to get you going dearie." I was told I was going to be induced.

Just like that! Everything was rigged up, the drip inserted, and contractual tsunamis came immediately, at spaces of four minutes. A young paediatrician came in with sad eyes. I don't think he liked what was going on, and he could see I was upset. He talked to me about his wife, and his baby, and tried to put me at ease. But nothing could have, because I felt set adrift in a whirlwind that wasn't under my control, and emotionally, I had lost it inside. From the outside I looked quiet, but inside, nothing made sense in my brain.

This wasn't how it was supposed to be. By 8 pm that night, I had refused pethidine twice. They would come in, offer it to ease the pain, and when I said no, they would leave. They didn't suggest any of the methods discussed at antenatal classes or offer their time or emotional comfort.

Feeling deserted with no midwifery support, I called a close friend, and ask her to come in, which really annoyed the staff because she was a home-birth midwife. But I felt I needed better female emotional support, and to talk through what was going on, which wasn't happening with the hospital staff. I felt like a number and part of a process, and that something wasn't right. The body language of the staff was sullen, and sometimes angry, and I felt as if information was being withheld. I said to my friend: "I don't know what is going on, but something is. I can feel it. I can't put my finger on it, and I feel totally helpless." She replied, "Now, Hilary. . . I don't think anything is going on. Let's just work through this together, huh?"

Sometimes all the tricks antenatal classes suggest, like playing cards or Scrabble, just don't work during labour. I wasn't in the mood for that. By 10 pm, things were pretty uncomfortable, when a new nurse walked in, took one look at the syntocinon chart and said "My God, who put this up, so high and so fast?" The next thing we knew everything was turned off, and my contractions stopped as quickly as they had started.

A female obstetrician came in, and said that the induction was going "wrong" and they wanted to put me in theatre, put in a spinal anaesthetic (epidural), restart the induction and see how that went. They also wanted to put a strap around my stomach to monitor my contractions and put a monitor on the baby's head. I asked what it was, and she said "It's a small monitor we screw into the scalp." I was horrified. "Will it hurt?" I said. She said it wouldn't. She screwed it into the baby's head, and he proceeded to kick the daylights out of my ribs, which hurt for the rest of labour and beyond.

I remember lying there and thinking that this is what it feels like to be a sausage in a sausage factory, to be processed, talked over and still I felt that things were not as they seemed, but didn't know why or how.

An epidural was inserted into my spine which dropped my already low blood pressure even lower, so sometimes my head swam. The syntocinon drip was in my left arm, so a constant blood pressure monitor was put on my right arm. Then they decided to catheterize me, to save me from having to go to the toilet. The last decoration was the (tachodynomometer[1]) around my stomach.

I was told to stay on my back, and exactly what else can you do when you are a cross between a beached whale and a stranded upside-down fly on a window-sill? I tried to lift my head, and was told not to

1 Tachodynomometer = Monitor to record the intensity of uterine contractions onto a strip of paper.

do that as I would get a spinal headache later. I asked as a follow-on from that, whether I would be able to get up and squat later, to get the baby out and was told that I would. At the time I didn't compute how illogical that statement was.

Then they disappeared and left my husband, me, and my friend alone for two hours. But very quickly, the baby really started to squirm, and my friend suggested that being on my left side would be a lot more comfortable and it was. After an hour, my friend went, because there was no point in her staying. Events had gone beyond the point where she could be of any help, and this was no longer our labour, but something being done to us.

At some point, a buzzer went and they came back and topped up the epidural and there was some discussion. They wanted to monitor me flat on my back. The minute they put me like that, the baby got agitated again, started to move a lot, and I got very uncomfortable. A short while later, the doctors came and said that his heart rate was much too high and that he was in distress. I said that I was too, and that the baby had started to get upset when they put me on my back, so I turned over onto my left side, which immediately felt better again. They put me back on my back, which restarted the baby's kicking, and made me more distressed.

They began talking about prepping me for a Caesarean which started to upset me, but just at that point an older nurse in her forties came in, and said, "I'm the new midwife, replacing someone who had gone off sick . . ." She walked up to the monitor and said, "What are you using Abigail for? You know it doesn't work . . ."

"Abigail? . . ." I asked . . . "Oh, just our name for the monitor . . ." she said, then placed her hand on my stomach . . .

"Why not use Abigail?" I asked. My brains started to turn over as I heard the reply . . .

"Oh, Abigail has a malfunction, and doesn't register contractions properly, but yours are rumbling along very nicely . . ."

Near to tears I said, "Just before you walked in, they were saying they needed to do a Caesar on the basis of Abigail's printout."

Not a word was said, and no-one moved. You could hear the silence as I said, "And they were monitoring me flat on my back, which hurts and is making the baby kick a lot."

She opened her mouth, shut it, and looked at me in astonishment.

"And to begin with the synto was set up too fast and too high . . ."

More silence. "And I can feel contractions in two spots on my tummy, and nowhere else." . . . She started to move away. "Please don't go," I said quietly. "Okay . . . I'll stay," she said and for the first time in that hospital, I felt as if I had a friend.

She went off to get a cup of tea just before six o'clock the next morning. Not long after that I wanted to push, but the young nurse said that wasn't possible, because not long before, I'd still only been a couple of centimeters dilated. Just then, my older nurse friend returned with cup of tea, to tell me she wanted to leave at seven o'clock. I asked her if she could possibly stay until Ian was born, because I felt she was the only one I could trust . . . and I told her I wanted to push. She examined me, and sure enough, the baby's head was right there. But there was a problem. He wasn't presenting correctly, and had his forehead upward, not his crown. By this time, the obstetrician had arrived and wanted to use forceps, picked them up and put them on something at the end of the bed.

I suddenly got angry and kicked everything off the bed and said I didn't want that, and she wasn't even giving me a chance. She looked at me, and said she was going to scrub up and I had "40 minutes to get the baby out" and if I couldn't in that time, they would take the baby out. When she left, I asked my friend if she thought I could manage, and she said yes, because my contractions were good and strong. Trouble was, I couldn't feel them.

When the obstetrician came back, I asked if I could squat because I'd practised that, and felt I couldn't do anything on my back. She said no, that it would give me a headache. When I said, "But when I asked earlier you said I could squat and push . . . you . . . lied." She replied, "You are too difficult to tell the truth to . . ."

She then said, "Take a deep breath and push." With full lungs, I couldn't hold a push. It felt pathetic, and while I was thinking about that, she told me that that push was hopeless. But I realized that you can't push like that, and wondered if she had even had children and tried it herself. Next contraction, I took that deep breath, but let most of it out, and used my abdomen muscles as if imagining a set of hands pushing down and out which was very effective. The obstetrician wanted to do a double episiotomy, and I refused. The baby was right down in two pushes, but then, just as the next one was starting, and

I was starting to push, the midwife stifled a "NO!"

The obstetrician had cut an episiotomy anyway, but did not support it, so it ripped a long way up, as Ian had been pushed out quickly and steadily.

He was alert, but floppy, quiet and wide-eyed. As they turned on all the theatre lights I became aware of a whole room full of people, yet I had specifically asked not to have anyone in there for the birth. I was not happy.

While they stitched up the torn episiotomy, Ian latched on almost straight away and was happily helping himself, when the doctor came in and very angrily said that he wasn't supposed to be feeding; that they had wanted to do other tests on him first. That was news to us. Just at that point, the nurse said that they needed me to get up straight away and use the bed-pan. I had been catheterized, but they hadn't been able to get anything out for a while, and she thought my bladder would be full. They took the baby while I filled one-and-a-half bedpans. During that time, Ian cried out, and in asking what they had done, they said they had given him vitamin K. They also said something about wanting to do other tests, but we said, "No".

They left us alone while Peter floated Ian in a warm bath. He stretched his arms, poked his tongue out and looked around inquisitively. I felt as if I had been run over by a truck. Peter dried him, did the necessaries and got him ready for our journey to the second floor, where we hoped that we would have peace and quiet. I just wanted to go home.

From the moment we arrive upstairs, nurses kept on coming in and piling blankets on Ian as if the colder temperature outside was inside. He started to feel hot so I would take them off and he would cool down again. Nurses would come back in and pile them back on, and I began to wonder what on earth was wrong with these people, with hospitals kept so claustrophobically hot anyway.

Five hours later the door swung open and we were confronted by what I will call the Cavalry, which consisted of three doctors and four nurses. You could have cut the air with a knife. The doctor that appeared to be in charge of the group leaned on the window sill and casually questioned a scar on my left breast. I told him what it was. Then suddenly they told us that Ian had spinal meningitis, and was running a temperature, seriously ill, and if they didn't take him away and do the tests they had wanted to do he might die.

Well, what do you do? The fear that sort of statement puts in first-time parents leads to only one thing in the absence of knowledge and that is helplessness. We asked them what they wanted to do and they told us. We didn't like it, but didn't feel we had any options, and we complied.

They took our baby away.

We had to wait five hours until a nurse came in. Though I was upset with the waiting, the nurse was really upset. She had come to take us to see him, but warned us on the way to ICU, that they had done eleven needle insertions into his spine to get a sample and he hadn't liked it, and that we weren't going to like what we saw.

In front of us lay a swollen-faced, puffy-eyed, rigid baby, with fists tightly clenched, looking shocked and locked away. Apparently he had screamed for three hours. He wouldn't respond to us.

The kingpin of the Cavalry arrived at that point, and asked us to leave, saying Ian would be fed formula at night, and I was not to be there between 8 pm and 8.30 am.

I told him that if so much as a teaspoon of formula got into my baby, he would be hearing from a lawyer, and that if he cried I was to be sent for immediately to feed him at any time including night time. I wanted it written in the records, and him to sign it. One of the nurses behind him winked at me and gave me the thumbs up, which surprised me. During that shift, she was great. Not like the head nurse on the next shift who was a formula lady, and had no time for breastfeeding.

I didn't sleep very well that night, and the next morning when I had a shower, large clots and a mess like raw lambs-fry dropped into the shower base. The nurses got all upset, and thought I should have a curette.[2] There had been a lot of pushing on my stomach and pulling on the cord, after Ian was born, but I didn't connect the two until the nurses suggested "retained placenta bits". I refused to consider a curette, and just as they were going to argue with me about it, I knew by instinct I had to be down in ICU. Grabbing my dressing gown, I set off, with people parting to let me through, not realizing where I was going. The lift had an *out of order* sign but I didn't have time to wait for it anyway even if it hadn't, so I rocketed down the stairs two at a

2 A curette is a spoon-like device that is inserted into the uterus and is used to scrape the lining to get anything else left in there, out. Sometimes called a D&C (dilation and curette).

time. The nurses following were upset and were saying that patients must use the lift, not the stairs.

As I crashed through the doors to Ian's ICU room, a nurse was holding my screaming son and a doctor was about to stick a needle somewhere. I erupted, "What the hell do you think you are doing?" They both flinched in fright, and the next part went in slow motion. Ian twisted his head around, pulled up his feet, planted them on the nurse's chest and pushed for all he was worth. He popped right out of her hands, and as I instinctively caught him in the air, I remember thinking a mix of "are babies able to do that?" and "I've had enough!"

The Cavalry arrived again, strenuously objecting to the blood on the floor, me being down there at times prohibited by the rules, that X, Y and Z needed to be done, that I should have taken the lift . . . but I was past listening to all that. First I pointed out that you can't take a lift with an *out of order* sign on it.

Forty-eight hours before, I might have been a stupid ignorant fool, but now I had had time to think. I no longer trusted what they were saying to me, and I have to admit, I let rip. Experts say they know best, and would never do anything except in the best interests of a baby, but so many things had happened that didn't sit well with me that I decided to trust my instincts. A lot of things had been bothering me. There was no eye contact between the senior staff and myself, some of the junior staff avoided me, and every time I asked a question they evaded answering it. Body language was either evasive or aggressive.

"Where are these test results showing that my baby has spinal meningitis? I want to see them please," I asked. My request was met with silence. "Well???" I persisted.

"They are at the lab," the head of the Cavalry said. "Why are they not in his notes? I want to see them right now," I said. No-one moved. It was surreal, and I started wondering if I was dreaming, and said, "You are all lying to me. The more I think about it, the more I feel there is not one of you here who has not lied to me." I leaned against the door, holding Ian, so that they were trapped in the room.

"Prove it," said the head of the Cavalry . . .

"You know I can't, because you have all the power. Well, I'm sorry, but that won't work now." I walked over to my son's chart, picked up a pen, and wrote on the cover sheet that all tests consented to previously and all treatments were now cancelled. I said that my baby was not only NOT to be touched by anyone there, but that he was to be up in my room by the half hour at the latest, or else I would sign both of us out of the hospital.

I read out what I had written, whereupon Cavalry head announced that they could bring in the police. "I've worked for the police," I said. "Please do . . . maybe they will be able to find me the test results."

I placed Ian in the bassinet, tucked him up, and went back to my room to clean up a huge mess, have a fast wash, get dressed and pack my small bag.

Almost exactly on the half hour in swept the bassinet and baby, and they left just like that. I just wished Peter had been there because I needed him, but he wasn't due until 4 pm. I hoped they'd leave me alone for a while, but no. The Cavalry again: always the same seven. I was told that I would be allowed to keep Ian there, but he must have two injections of high potency antibiotics around the clock every eight hours.

The Cavalry head then said that he didn't think with a front as small as mine that I'd be able to feed my son. I told him my milk had already come in, and he looked at me as if I was a liar, so I lifted my T-shirt and squirted his white coat. One of the nurses tried not to choke with laughter. I didn't see how I could refuse the antibiotics, and had no way to get home anyway. So I said yes. Peter arrived at four o'clock. After we had talked, he sat and held Ian while I slept. Ian was safe while Peter was here. That night, I jammed Ian in the corner by the window heater and put the bed diagonally between him and the door. I would never have slept otherwise.

At six o'clock the next night the Cavalry head arrived on his own quite suddenly, but the body language was quite different. He was holding U-bags which are urine collectors for little boys. There was still no eye contact, but I didn't feel threatened. I asked what the problem was and he told me about a seriously ill baby downstairs who required breastmilk only, and that the nurses had assured him that I was correct and my milk had come in. "According to the nurses," he said, "you are the only one in two floors breastfeeding. So I wanted to ask if we could have some of your excess please."

"Yes, but how?" I asked, as he moved around the side of the bed. "Well, I'll show you if you'll pull up your T-shirt." I did and he showed me the sticky edges of the U-bags and told me how to attach them either side of the nipple. "Once the milk starts flowing, press on the side of the breast with your upper arm." He handed me my baby who was waking anyway, and I followed his instructions. His neutral face changed to astonishment as the U-bag filled up so fast that he had to move quickly, to swap over to an empty one, then left with one and a half bags of milk from one side.

At ten o'clock that night, the nurses came for the next lot of injections, and also armed with more U-bags. One of them told me, while smiling from ear to ear, that he had tried to send them up the first time, but they had refused to come, on the basis that he had given me such a rough time, that he should go and ask me himself.

The next morning, the staff handed me the BCG vaccination consent form, which I refused to sign. I couldn't see the point in giving another injection to a sick baby.

But about two hours later, the doors flew open again, and the Cavalry arrived with accusations that we were compromising national TB immunity and being irresponsible towards our child and society.

I asked the head of the Cavalry what the vaccine was made of and he started to say, "It's a bacterial vaccine . . ." I didn't hear the rest really. I blurted out, "Why do you want to give this to my baby, who you said to me two days ago, was dying of spinal meningitis? You have him on potent antibiotics to kill those bacteria so why would you want to give him a live bacterial vaccine? That doesn't make sense to me." His bleeper went . . . they left, and didn't come back.

Next day, the nurse who had held the baby for the lumbar puncture came in and wanted to talk privately. She was feeling bad about me being isolated from other patients, which I hadn't realized was the case as I was too busy. She told me that I was considered a trouble-maker, and that everyone in the hospital knew what was going on except me. My instincts had been right, and I was being lied to. She told me that Ian did not have meningitis. The little BCG slip of yesterday was proof of that because the TB vaccine is never given to sick babies. In my room they were caught in the dilemma of either admitting they had lied, or admitting you don't give a sick baby a TB vaccine.

I was aghast. She told me the problem was now my assertiveness; that they had lost a baby the day before I came in, because that baby's mother wouldn't listen at all. Even worse for my head, she told me that there had been a meeting in ICU with the doctors before the induction where a Caesarean was decided on right from the start, with the induction managed with that in mind, so that our baby could immediately be transferred to ICU. All because of someone else the day before? It didn't make sense to me.

Our conversation became even more unbelievable when she told me that the test results from the lumbar puncture and swabs had been in the file and if I'd picked up the file and opened it, I would have seen for myself that they were normal. After I had left, they had been put through the shredder, and another one was constructed, to show raised levels of white cells, to indicate an unspecified infection.

I was gutted, and angry with myself for being stupid enough for not thinking to look through the file when I had the chance. I told her that I couldn't understand why anyone would do that. It made no sense, and thought it was downright cruel, but it also confirmed in me the feelings I'd had from the start that I was having the wool pulled over my eyes.

I was in tears, and the nurse was in tears too. I asked her what prompted her to come and tell me, and she said that it was when they did the eleven needle insertions she had thought about telling me, and when I had fought on the second day, and had said I didn't believe them, she felt I deserved to know what she saw and heard.

On day five, the Cavalry head decided that our baby was jaundiced, and suggested another trip to ICU to have him under the lights. He was checking Ian's hips while talking, when suddenly, Ian not only fountained him, but covered him in bright yellow omelette. It was the only satisfying justice Ian could mete out.

I said, "No," and he looked daggers at me. I glared at him, saying, "Over my dead body. And what are you going to do about it?"

"Then, I will discharge you tomorrow," he said, and that was the last I saw of him.

That night, just after midnight, when all sane people are supposed to be asleep, I sneaked down the corridor, and removed my file from a wooden slot stand, took it back to my room and had a good read. The comments astounded me. I noted down some from coloured pieces of paper, with their allocation numbers.

When we got home, we sent a letter to the legal section of the hospital board, asking for access to my files in front of the superintendent. For various bureaucratic reasons, this process took over 12 months. One afternoon, we arrived at the superintendent's office, to find a very efficient-looking man, with military-shined shoes, and small round glasses sitting at his desk. He suddenly said, "Seeing your records isn't possible, Mrs Butler, since we don't know your, or your baby's number . . ." I handed him over a piece of paper with both numbers on, and he picked it up and walked out. Thirty minutes passed before he came back, during which time my heart dropped. It doesn't take that long to find records.

He dropped the file down on the table in front of us. Instead of opening it, I flicked through the pages looking for certain colours. They had gone, but on removing the paper fastener in the corner, all the coloured corners fell out.

I asked, "What happened to the rest of these pieces of paper?" and he shrugged, then looking hard at me, volunteered . . . "Well, you know, space is a premium in this place . . ." I pushed the point, and got angry, whereupon he exploded with, ". . . we know how to deal with the likes of you. Take us to court if you wish. We will string it out until you run out of both money and energy. You have no proof of anything."

To have said that, he must have known the significance of those file notes. I later found out that everyone in the hospital had known what was going on; almost down to the staff in the Post Office, which then had a branch in the hospital.

For the first three months we had a baby who didn't do much except scream and want to be carried. So long as we did that, he would relax and quieten down. We rarely saw any smiles. I had a front pack and a rocking chair, both of which were heavily used. I got fit from walking miles, and read a lot.

At the six-week visit I told the doctor I wanted to postpone the 3-month vaccinations but he said, "Don't wait too long; after all, if you don't vaccinate, he could get sick and die." He assured me that in his extensive nine months of practice, he had never seen a vaccine reaction; vaccines were wonderful and safe . . . and I should just do it.

I couldn't help thinking about being berated for not signing the BCG form. This was the third time I'd been told if I didn't do something my baby might die. This line of reasoning was starting to become an irritant, because what I wanted was fact, not emotional blackmail.

Ian started to emerge from his world, like a startled rabbit, open to the rest of the world, for once, but very fragile emotionally. He could not be put down when distressed, and would work himself into a lather. For months after birth, his face would become distressed, showing outrage, abandonment, betrayal and frantic panic if I so much as went out of his sight. He lived on my front, his father's back, in the bouncer, or in our bed and so long as we were there, he was fine. Anyone in a white coat, even the vet, reduced him to a sobbing wreck on sight.

4 The Key

The key to our unique lifestyle was unquestionably our decision to home-school our children.

I spent a large chunk of my life being a teaching principal as well as holding appointments in other teaching positions involving responsibility within the school system.

Home-schooling offers an opportunity for a totally integrated "lifestyle-related" curriculum. It **will** be unique. It cannot be anything else.

But to succeed in this option, at least two elements are necessary.

The first is a solid conviction that this is right for your lifestyle. Back in the 1980s there were plenty of obstacles in the road to discourage you.

The second is commitment. Education does not occur in a few hours a day as it does in a specifically designed educational environment – a compartment within the day labelled "school". Because the teaching and learning should ideally involve the whole family as much as possible and takes place in the home with all its security and natural opportunities, every waking moment has the potential to provide meaningful learning opportunities.

As I would be responsible for meeting the requirements of the

Certificate of Exemption from having the children enrolled in a registered school, that was a commitment of at least 15 years!

I was also prepared to share that commitment with other families if they wanted advice and practical help.

In 1983 CHESM (Christian Home Education Support Ministries) was born.

Ian was just over one year old. It would be a year before David appeared on the scene.

I started writing material which would be helpful to others and over the years this has amounted to several sizeable volumes.

All the typing has been done by Hilary. Bless her.

Leaving behind the school system, the questions of where to live and how to provide the necessities of daily living were resolved in miraculous ways.

On 29 August 1985, we moved to Tuakau.

For the next six-and-a-half years, a number of part-time jobs allowed us the flexibility for the lifestyle we had chosen and which was beginning to unfold in more detail.

One of the main projects to be undertaken was to write a curriculum which set out the integrated lifestyle approach.

Living Beyond Conformity, in four parts, was the result.

***Home-schooling was the key that opened the door for Hilary to be who she is today.** It provided her with the opportunities to write, to research, to speak, and to be available to others. While I taught the children, her knowledge and experience grew. Her list of contacts increased. Many educational experiences for the children could be combined with her trips to the Auckland Medical Library, or going to other towns when she was invited to speak at meetings.*

The children were certainly exposed to a wide range of social situations, especially when parents who came to talk to Hilary brought their children with them; or when TV crews set up their cameras in our sitting room.

5 Obstacles and Impossibilities

Looking back, I had assumed that I had known enough, but one week in hospital had shown me that I didn't know nearly enough to be able to protect my child. I was also getting a sense that the prejudices, motives, and other agendas of some doctors were a risk to both me and my child. My GP was young, not long in practice, and still ever the bouncy enthusiast.

The first example of assumptions showed itself very quickly. The catheterization had caused a urinary tract infection, considered serious enough to warrant trying an antibiotic not on the list of antibiotics I'm allergic to. After three doses, I was a lot worse, Ian was screaming harder, and his faeces changed colour to a horrible purple green. When I returned to the doctor to tell him why I had stopped taking the antibiotic, I asked to borrow his obstetrics textbook.

So long as I looked up everything I didn't know in a medical dictionary, I understood every word in it. At my next visit, I asked some questions I'd written down while reading. The answers the doctor gave me exactly described what had happened to me in hospital, but the answers I read out from his book, which were supposedly best practice, were very different. The doctor was somewhat uncomfortable and confessed that he had never read the textbook from cover to cover. He said he was far too busy getting practical experience on the ward, and listening to his teachers to read his textbook. I wondered out loud if his teachers had only listened to their teachers as well?

At the six-week check he was horrified at the episiotomy which was a painful knot which objected every time I sat down. The doctor offered the opportunity to go back to hospital and have it redone, but I didn't fancy the idea.

At the three-month baby visit, the subject of vaccinations came up. Again.

I had initially been prepared for Ian to have his shots, if the doctor could prove to me that there were no side effects, and that the vaccines were proven to work. He handed me two sheets of paper saying what the shots were, and the ages they should be given.

I looked at him directly in the eye and said, "That's not good enough. Given that I have been consistently misled about his birth, and a whole raft of related things, do you expect me to make a decision based on these two pieces of paper?"

His eyes flew open, as he said, "But the Health Department wouldn't recommend them if they weren't safe and the right thing to do."

"Ah," I pondered. "You mean like no-one could possibly have a mismanaged induction either?" He winced. I went on, "I think I will take a trip to the medical library and find out the information for myself."

Ten months later I returned with a stack of information and we resumed the conversation. At least, I did. He had been continually nagging me about it before that, so when I arrived in his office with a box filled with medical articles, I said to him, "Let's do a trade. You read these, I will read whatever you now have and then we can discuss it." Then came the most amazing answer. "I'm not interested."

He agreed to a truce, after I said, "Then if you won't read your own medical literature and discuss with me some concerns, neither should you continue to pressure me to vaccinate my son."

I had mistakenly assumed that doctors would know about, or at least be interested in knowing about the jabs they gave or recommended.

Where does the average mother go to fill in informational black holes? When I first became pregnant and was sitting there looking at the doctor at the first visit, he asked, "What do you want to know?" But if you don't know what there is to know, how can you know what questions to ask? Immunization and other health issues are the same. You can't ask questions, if you don't know some of what there is to know. Also, you don't know what the doctor knows, and what he or she doesn't know.

My first chance to find out what my doctor knew and what he didn't, was when our son developed eczema at three months, which had started on his face, and within a few weeks had spread to patches scattered between his face and knees. The doctor prescribed a steroid cream. When I filled the prescription I thought, "What do I know about this cream? What have I been told?" I knew nothing and had been told nothing, but when I asked, the chemist showed me the pharmacopoeia. I didn't like what I read there.

Knowing nothing about eczema either, I went to the local library, then the medical library and read what was there with one eye, and translated it using a dictionary with the other. I looked at all the pharmaceutical options, which weren't many. The questions which arose from that were, "Why would you want to use a potentially dangerous steroid cream, which did nothing to get to any root cause of eczema, and which will only suppress the problem, by suppressing the immune response?" And, "In order for your baby to have the *appearance* of being normal, why would you want to use steroid cream all the time, given the possible side effects?"

This seemed a stupid first option to try, so I took the cream and the information back to the doctor and explained that I had decided to go and see a homoeopath and why. He asked me if I knew anything about homoeopathy and homoeopaths and since my answer was "no", proceeded to infer that they had nothing to offer and would most likely make things a lot worse.

By then, I didn't feel I had too much to lose apart from money. After an hour-long consultation with the homoeopath, I was handed a remedy which I was to take myself. Apparently the problem was me, and the remedy would go through to the baby via breastmilk. None of it made sense, but given that the reading I had done had led me to understand that homoeopathic remedies were not toxic and didn't suppress the immune system, it made sense to try it before anything else.

So I took one dose as instructed: that's all. Three days later, the skin on Ian's knees started to soften, and within a month all the eczema had gone. Even more interesting, all my warts and the verrucae on my feet disappeared. I had tried everything and more to get rid of them in the past, and they had stubbornly remained. How nice to pumice the feet and not have to avoid certain painful areas.

Once the children grew up, if the eczema came back, I would give them one dose of this remedy in their mouths, and the eczema would go away. When my verucas came back, one dose, and they'd be gone in days.

When the doctor saw my son a few weeks after the first appointment, he had nothing to say. What could he say? Far from making things worse, the homoeopathic remedy had fixed two problems, not one.

The next piece of clinical education I received was even more interesting. The doctor failed to recognize rubella (German measles) when my son contracted it, and assumed he had a rash caused by a virus. Our Plunket nurse recognized it, and showed me the glands at the back of the neck and explained the different measles rashes. She thought that since the doctor hadn't been a GP long, he might not have seen it before. There were a couple more missed diagnoses of various problems.

I became pregnant again, but the thought of another labour and delivery didn't thrill me. My confidence in our doctor wasn't very high, so I talked to friends about other options. We were told about a doctor called Dr John Hilton whose practice was two hours' away. He agreed to do shared care with our GP. He was also prepared to do a home birth, and because of what had happened the first time, asked us to work with Joan Donley.

In preparing for this birth, the Home Birth Library was my first real proof that I was truly ignorant. The information was quite different to what was in the local library, and was exactly what I needed. After reading the contents of their library in about six weeks flat, I wrote overseas for more information on two subjects: birth and immunization.

Birth was the more urgent topic in my mind. As we wanted to give birth as we had wanted the first time, we needed to know how to be prepared to avoid the same mistakes. I needed to read more widely about natural birth, but also needed books which discussed the system and why the system worked the way it did. If I had to go to hospital again, I wanted to be more prepared.

There were a few problems in the second labour, which happened because of the interference in the first labour, but Joan Donley had the skills to work through them with me. She had attended enough second labours after traumatic first ones to have a good idea how, why and where people hang up. David was a home birth, alert, with a strength that the older son hadn't had. Nothing could prepare us for the difference in babies, quite aside from personality. On day three, when Joan came and I said he was asleep in the pram, she went in and found him raised up onto clenched fists, looking over the pram edge.

Every day, Dr Hilton took him for tours of the house holding him, one hand under his bottom, the other under his armpits and across his chest, telling him about the pictures. John had a soft spot for David, because as he put David on my stomach he had given John such a huge full-face smile, that he had fallen in love with him straight away. Or perhaps it was because he had just emptied both his bladder and bowels all over me that he was so happy? It was another few weeks before I was to be given such a smile.

What hit me most was a feeling that I had more than betrayed our older son. What he had gone through so contrasted with the way David was born. It came home to me how ignorant I had been, what I had deprived my older son of, and how it could have been so different, if I had known more, had more backbone, and had protected him.

Since the birth of our first son I have been an avid collector of medical books of all sorts. As we realized that there was a whole world of knowledge out there that we are never told about, Peter and I started to do some serious thinking about incidents in the past when we had been told certain things, and had believed them, yet had mental question marks; or where explanations just didn't seem to ring true.

The more we read, the more questions came to mind. For example, my bilateral carpal tunnel problems and arthralgia which had started after a rubella vaccine, and had been blamed on my being a gymnast and my job, which involved a lot of twisting of flasks as a dairy herd tester. That had progressed to full-blown arthritis from which I only got relief during pregnancy or in the two hottest summer months.

We then looked at aspects of my husband's medical history. He had only ever had two vaccine types in his life, and both vaccinations were followed by problems of a different nature. As a teaching principal at Otangiwai, he had been given all the Salk vaccines and paraded as an example to his students of how much the little pricks weren't going to hurt. Then he was later expected to show how easy it was to drink the little pink oral polio ones as well, though he never questioned why it was that the Salk ones weren't good enough, and he was expected to have seven polio vaccines altogether. In those days, you just did as you were told.

Not long after the polio vaccinations had been completed, his lower back started to ache with pain through the legs, and standing was very painful. He bought a special high chair so that he could sit at a lectern and teach. The muscles in his back were also constantly sore and tired. A doctor in Taumarunui prescribed aspirin. After shifting to Whangamata, his back problems continued and the doctors there prescribed pills of a pink or reddish colour, which were supposed to do something but didn't. A colleague of Peter's suggested he should see a chiropractor, but first was referred to an orthopoedic specialist in Tauranga who explained three possible options – a waist-to-armpits cast for approximately three months; bed rest on a firm mattress for approximately three months, or surgery. Interestingly, there was no diagnosis.

Not liking those options, on his way home Peter visited a chiropractor who took X-rays, and so began weekly treatments which continued for about two years. This gave him temporary relief until some activity would cause another bad spell. Eventually a couple of treatments from an osteopath proved to be much more effective.

Peter had also been given some tetanus vaccines when teaching in Otangiwai, and after each one he would get such bad tonsillitis that he was treated with the usual courses of penicillin. After the third shot, and third lot of tonsillitis, Amoxicillin was prescribed. He had a nasty reaction to this, so he stopped using both antibiotics and vaccines. Given the fact that the only time Peter has had serious health problems has been following those two vaccination series, the connection of the problem with the vaccines isn't likely to be coincidental. Accepting there are still limitations as to how and what activities his back will tolerate, Peter since then has enjoyed over 30 years of a relatively trouble-free active lifestyle.

But in 1984, as the information was collected, we both felt there needed to be serious discussions about a thing called informed consent, because when it came to vaccinations, and even medical practice in general, we were both beginning to realize that informed consent was an illusion.

6 The Quest for Information

"Modern medicine can't survive without our faith, because modern medicine is neither an art nor a science. It's a religion." [1]

I wanted information. Where better to get it than from a paediatrician of the standing of Robert Mendelsohn? With a CV the envy of most paediatricians in USA, his colleagues probably had an emotional tornado when he turned his critical eye to vaccines. Standing in a queue to buy a money order for a subscription to his newsletter *The People's Doctor*, I was greeted with the news that the Reserve Bank had devalued the dollar that morning to 40 US cents/$1.00 NZ. No matter. The information was more important than the cost, because coming from a paediatrician, it would give me clues as to where else to look, and what to look for.

No one in this country was talking or even thinking about vaccination at that time. As far as the media were concerned, immunization was like a bar of soap. Everyone uses soap, so what else was there to say or ask?

I'd just read Dr Mendelsohn's 1979 book *Confessions of a Medical Heretic*. Dr Mendelsohn's newsletter, *The People's Doctor*, started

1 Mendelsohn, R.S. 1979. *Confessions of a Medical Heretic*. Chicago: Contemporary Books. ISBN: 0809277263.

arriving, and helped me learn another way of thinking. As time went on and I became familiar with Auckland's Philson Medical Library, and was able to source material elsewhere in the world, the habit of sending Dr Mendelsohn copies of interesting "gems" became well established.

The Home Birth Association in Hamilton invited me to do a talk on 2 November 1985 for which I wrote a paper called "Immunization: A Dissenting View". Someone from the meeting gave a reporter a copy of the paper. The reporter decided that perhaps vaccination wasn't as simple as *"a bar of soap"*, and wrote an article[2] which was published on 1 February 1986.

Suddenly our phone started ringing, and it seemed as if New Zealand was instantly filled with parents of children who had had problems after vaccinations. These parents thought that they were the only ones who had ever had problems after vaccines, but the intriguing common feature of their stories was that the medical profession told them all, not only that the problems were very rare, but also that the problems were completely coincidental.

Parents with slightly more educated doctors were told that serious vaccine reactions were the one in a million minuscule price someone had to pay for protecting society. Given the population of the country, their child would probably be the only one around anyway. These children were essentially being called collateral damage.[3] Sad, and rare, but vital to the cause.

One paediatrician told four sets of parents (two of whom I knew at the time) in his own practice over a period of three years, that each of their vaccine-injured children was the one in a million. At that time, the country didn't even have four million people in it. When these parents eventually connected with each other and shared notes, they were not impressed.

Parents who accepted the medical slant, who shut up and got on

2 Warner, K. 1986 "Is vaccination more risky than the disease?" *New Zealand Herald*, 1 February.

3 Walters, L.B. 1979. Retrieved on 18 September, 2005 from <http://www.909shot.com/Articles/gnsvaxin.htm> Center for Bioethics, Washington. "In mandatory immunization programs, a system of conscription is employed to recruit soldiers for this anti-disease campaign. Most of the recruits in the war on infectious disease are children . . . As in all wars, some soldiers are injured . . . At present, the draftees who are injured in the war on infectious diseases are in effect told by the conscripting authorities, 'Thank you for your contribution to the war effort, and best of success in coping with your disability.' In the military context, such treatment of wounded soldiers and their families would be unthinkable."

with life, continued to be accepted by the medical profession. Most felt isolated, believing they were the only ones, and didn't have any option. Most didn't know about applying for compensation from the Accident Compensation Corporation[4] because it wasn't something doctors talked about.

No one who read the article in the *New Zealand Herald* had forgotten about their children's responses to vaccines, and now they all wanted to talk. As time went by, where people were near each other, I linked them up. The article was like opening up a Pandora's box for those who read it, and if you assume, on the basis of the then small *Herald* readership, that the majority of New Zealanders did not read it, then the total numbers of parents harbouring such stories can only be guessed at.

I'm glad the readership wasn't the whole of the country, for had it been so, I doubt we would have survived as a family. As it was, survival was a thin thread for some weeks and my husband nearly divorced the phone. Most parents just wanted to talk. All of them lived very hard lives, and their children, being different, left them worried and exhausted, and many of them wondered what might happen to their children when they grew up. None could see any other avenue to pursue, and neither could I, since I didn't know how the system worked.

The extent of the problems out there that no one knew existed was mind-blowing. I was contacted by some older Intellectually Handicapped staff, and listened as they told me that once, most children came to them at an older age, but as the shots were given at a younger age, the children who came to them got younger as well. All of them suspected vaccines in many cases, and one said there was even mention of the problem in one of the IHC handbooks.

Then, into my life, walked Amelia.[5] When Amelia's infant son John died, the death certificate said he was a victim of SIDS (Sudden Infant Death Syndrome). But when Amelia recounted his whole medical

---

4 ACC is a "no fault" apology for a compensation system which protects doctors from being sued for medical misadventure, but means that parents can get miserly compensation, if they are very lucky, and are able to prove causality to the satisfaction of the assessors. The reality is that the bureaucratic roadblocks put in one's way and the logistics of the exercise make it similar to scaling an almost insuperable mountain.

5 "Amelia". Although the parents were happy for names to be used, all names have been changed in this book at the suggestion of our defamation lawyer in order to avoid identification of medical personnel and to reduce the risk of medical people suing anyone.

history, it was clear that after his second DPT he had stopped putting on weight, and a month after that, had whooping cough. After being given the run-around, Amelia finally had whooping cough diagnosed privately, but remarkably, her doctor still wanted John to have the third DPT, though he still wasn't well.

She refused, but two weeks later was told that if she didn't bring him in for it to be done, they would come to her. She gave in. Within two weeks, John was dead. While the attending doctor signed the death certificate SIDS, there were aspects of this case that were clearly not, and had never been, related to SIDS. When Amelia described John's face, the whites of his eyes, the froth from his nose and mouth and the colour of his lips and face, I felt he had died from a seizure. She did too. She was an epileptic. Whenever confronted with the physical evidence, members of the medical profession denied it repeatedly, but were very evasive about letting Amelia or her lawyer see relevant files. Some doctors privately admitted that John's death did not fit the criteria for SIDS, but they would not go on the record to say so.

Later, when Amelia was again pregnant, her specialist refused to let her have a breathing monitor because he said she was not at risk. And at no point did the medical profession face up to the glaring fact that, in the year John supposedly died of SIDS, there was a notoriously hot batch[6] of DPT vaccine in use, and there were a record number of such deaths that year. When an overseas immunization expert wrote a report to be tabled at the coroner's inquest in which he implicated the vaccine, it was put to one side on the basis that an overseas expert isn't an expert on what is happening in this country.

I could not help wondering at the time how many SIDS deaths were an incorrect label attached to keep a national immunization record free of blemish and controversy.

A few years later, Amelia's sad story had a sequel. Amelia's cousin Jane had her healthy five-week premature baby, Mary, vaccinated with DPT and Hib. Jane hadn't hesitated to vaccinate her first three children, but had a gut feeling not to do so with Mary but allowed the doctor to talk her around. But she was so upset about it, that she had to leave the room, and left the nurse and doctor to do it themselves.

On the way home, she noticed that Mary was very quiet, and at

6 Hot Batch = a batch that has more reactions than normally seen.

home, almost non-responsive and pale. Thinking she was sleepy she put her to bed, but was puzzled because she had been due a feed just after the jab and had refused it. Mary slept for five-and-a-half hours, and then woke up. After a few sucks, she went back to sleep, then suddenly woke up screaming. She was inconsolable, and back arching. The next day was a mix of lethargy, paleness, screaming, long sleeping spells and refusal to feed properly, then she literally collapsed into sleep at 10 o'clock that night. At 5.45 am, the mother found Mary arching, eyes all over the place, and frothing from the eyes and nose. The baby's face was purple, she had blue lips and was choking. Jane's husband took the baby while she called an ambulance, which arrived very fast, quickly resuscitated the baby, and took them to hospital.

The parents told the hospital staff everything that had happened, including the fact she had been vaccinated, and had been fine before that. To their astonishment, she was diagnosed as having gastric reflux, and prescribed an indigestion drug, which did . . . nothing. Only after much insistence on Jane's part did another paediatrician reassess the case, and diagnose the convulsions the baby was having as a vaccine reaction.

Later, Jane's two fully vaccinated primary school children got whooping cough, only to have doctors insist that it couldn't possibly be whooping cough. After all, the children had been vaccinated. They were put on asthma drugs which made no difference. Unfortunately Jane's baby caught whooping cough from the older children, and the seizures increased, so she had to be hospitalized again. Jane's older children were reassessed, and found to have whooping cough as well.

While in hospital the second time, one event really distressed Jane. A mother came in with a baby with identical symptoms to those Mary had, following her DPTH.[7]

She sat and listened to the mother tell the whole familiar story only to hear the paediatrician diagnose this baby with gastric reflux and prescribe the same indigestion drug. Yet while she watched, that baby had the exact same tiny convulsions that her baby had started off having.

After considerable bureaucratic obstruction, Jane was finally

7 DTPH = Diphtheria, Tetanus, Pertussis, Haemophilus B vaccine.

granted Accident Compensation, and ongoing medical costs on the basis of a severe vaccine reaction.

But what about the other baby? And what about the other babies of whom we know nothing?

Or are we honestly supposed to believe that these are the only two babies ever diagnosed as having gastric reflux after a severe vaccine reaction? Even one nurse I discussed this with admitted to me that she wondered why it was that so often babies who had fed perfectly well until six weeks, suddenly got reflux after their first lot of vaccines.

Maybe it was reflux. But sometimes, maybe it wasn't.

7 Invalidating the Warranty

He was a master of design and manufacture.

He specialized in original creations and his workmanship was of the highest order.

His greatest masterpiece was a unique machine, which had worldwide distribution.

Like all his products of excellence this machine was supplied with a comprehensive instruction manual as well as the maker's own personal guarantee.

This guarantee is valid only because of, and under, the following conditions:

- that the machine is precision made and no two machines are exactly alike;
- that it will give a lifetime of reliable service, as long as it is not abused;
- that any "maintenance" must use materials named in the maker's manual;
- that no unauthorized persons or organizations shall interfere with, or modify the machine;
- that the manual be strictly followed in all situations;

- *that any questions and advice will be dealt with personally by the manufacturer on the international toll-free telephone number, operating twenty-four hours every day of the year;*
- *that all genuine machines carry their own individual identification mark and seal of quality and this shall be retained throughout the life of the machine.*

Just above the maker's personal signature on the guarantee were four very important words – a promise – YOU CAN TRUST ME.

How often I have read in an advertisement the words, "We are only a phone call away", or "We are as close as your telephone". When I make a phone call, I may not see a face, but I can talk to a person (although these days you may have to run the gauntlet of computer-generated voices and menus).

But however convenient a direct free phone line may be, there will always be some who will ignore it, or bypass it. The same is true of guarantees. They can be ignored and other choices substituted, even though by doing this people expose themselves to serious risks, which may turn out to be very costly.

In the world in which we live there are people who are always looking for opportunities to capitalize on what they see as business opportunities. So the performance record of this worldwide machine soon attracted attention. One of the first things the experts set out to do was to discover all they could about the machine.

How did it work?

What was it capable of?

What did the parts look like?

How were all the bits and pieces integrated?

Could it be copied?

Could anything be done to enhance its performance?

And so on.

Because these machines were everywhere (in fact, everyone owned one), it was galling that all maintenance and repairs should be in the hands of one person.

Gradually the research, the experiments, the "new" ideas and the lure of profits began to gather momentum.

When you have something to sell, you advertise. Advertising is often couched in extravagant and emotive language which can be misleading. So in a very short time vested interests were driving a number of new products that this machine needed, and if you could persuade and convince the market that this was for everyone's benefit then you had it made.

Insurance schemes were devised.

Parts from expired machines were organized for re-use.

All sorts of formulations that could be added to the fluids so necessary for smooth and continuous functioning were prepared in eye-catching containers.

Various concoctions were invented which could be injected into the machine to provide all sorts of safeguards – or so the blurb said.

Technology enabled the internal workings of the machine to be observed. Printouts from a range of testing procedures and scans, could be obtained and evaluated with suitable tune-up packages recommended, which, if not heeded, could have dire consequences for the machine.

But it was the consultancies that proved so very popular. By making an appointment with these General Providers and Specialists, the responsibility for the machine's maintenance could be handed over to others. With such a range of sophisticated services and "expert advice" available, did the machine maker's guarantee conditions really matter? Depending totally on the designer and creator of the machine for everything, was risky too, wasn't it? Where were the "authorized persons" anyway? The fact that counterfeiters might be lining their own pockets at the expense of the machines' health and well-being didn't seem to be a concern. With such an array of visible services supported by the latest hi-tech gadgetry and scientific discoveries, how could you possibly go wrong? Especially when so much printed material was available to allay any fears. The message from *all quarters clearly said:*

"YOU CAN TRUST US."

Who is worthy of that **trust**?

Is it the designer, creator and manufacturer who knows each unique machine so intimately and whose guarantee offers such protection?

Or is it those who are still learning (often from their mistakes), and experimenting, and offering no guarantees?

It is vital that the right choice should be made.

That unique machine is my body.

I will let you into a secret.

My trust in that toll free number and the maker's promise has never failed me.

8 What Causes Sickness?

"If they can get you asking the wrong questions, the answers don't matter."[1]

Why, in your opinion, do you get sick?

Different cultures think about causes and treatment of sickness in many ways. These could be described as spiritual, old wives tales, their traditional methods, such as Ayurvedic medicine, acupuncture, or whatever their culture uses. Then there is the current pharmaceutical medical way which says that you find the microbe or condition causing the problem and kill or fix it with a drug, and the newer gene research which consists of concepts so lofty that most of us have no understanding of them at all.

Generally speaking, in the sickness sense, the word "germ" means "something small and bad" that can make you sick or cause problems. But what is your mental picture of a germ? Did you sit in primary school surrounded by posters showing a toothbrush chasing "Bertie germ"?

As we get older, we learn that there are microbes (which include bacteria, fungi and viruses) and protists (which include algae and amoebas, slime moulds and protozoa).

---

1 Pynchon, T. 1995. *Gravity's Rainbow*. Penguin Books; Reprint edition ISBN: 0140188592.

If your teachers were really fancy they might have taught you about archaea. Some archaeans have genes that aren't found in anything else, and live in boiling water, volcanoes or acidic deep water so are sometimes called extremophiles.

All of these microbes can, under certain circumstances, cause sickness.

What are those circumstances that might allow microbes to make you sick?

Again, your mother probably told you that if you went outside, got wet and cold,[2] you'd probably catch a chill. Scientists now know that is true. So you knew that certain things you did could cause illness.

Things that can help make you sick could be environmental things, like pollution. For instance, we know that soldiers who witnessed nuclear experiments were exposed to radiation which caused diseases later in their lives, and changed the genes in their sperm, so some of those problems were handed down to their children.

We know that bad diet can do several things. Eating the wrong foods, and too much, can result in obesity which puts strain on your pancreas and heart. This in turn can cause diabetes and heart attacks. A diet which doesn't contain enough of the right minerals and vitamins can switch off your immune system. So if you don't have enough vitamin A, and you get measles, you can become very, very sick. If you eat a good diet, and have enough vitamins and minerals, particularly selenium, in your body, viruses like influenza and Hepatitis stay dormant, and do nothing.

How much of this people understand depends on whether they were interested in it at school, and how much they have read and understood since then.

We have grown up in a world where the medical profession tells us vaccines are necessary. But they tell us what they want us to know. Here is an example.[3]

The aim of this pamphlet is to impress in your mind the words

"Brain damage, heart defects, blindness and deafness".

2 Reuters. 2005. "Chilly feet can cause a cold, say researchers." *New Zealand Herald*, 17 November: A5.

3 Public Health Commision (1995) Code 4172.

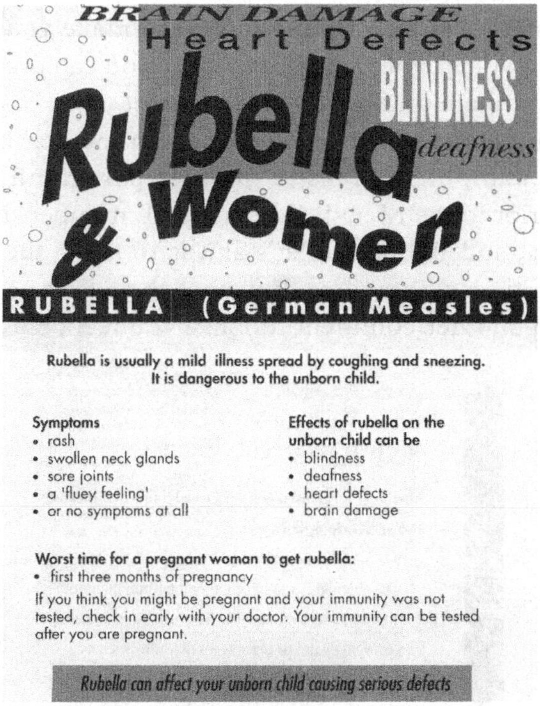

Another pamphlet[4] uses a different strategy:

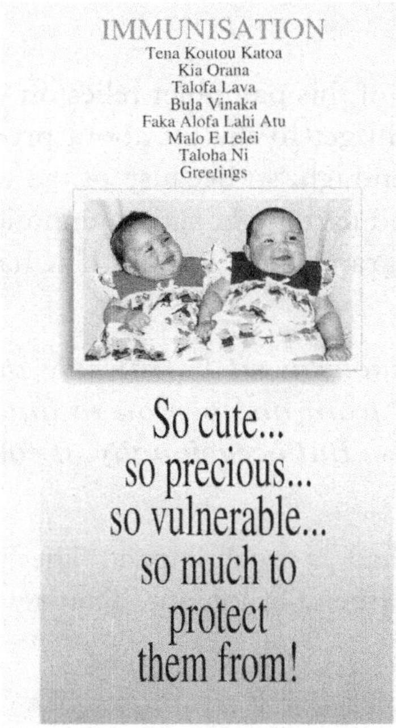

4 North Health, no date.

The words on the cover are chosen to make you feel that your babies are so vulnerable that the only way you can protect them is by doing what you are told inside the pamphlet.

But information changes, depending on the era. Compare these meningitis pamphlets. This is the first paragraph from a 1996[5] pamphlet prior to the MenzB. Meningitis B numbers had been rising for six years, and the pamphlet's aim is to make the parent realize that meningitis can be serious. But since there isn't a vaccine yet, the authors add another comment to make you feel better. If you get to read it.

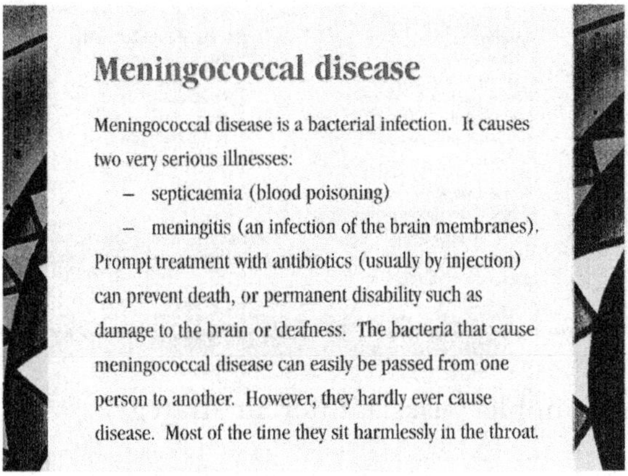

Meningococcal disease

Meningococcal disease is a bacterial infection. It causes two very serious illnesses:

- septicaemia (blood poisoning)
- meningitis (an infection of the brain membranes).

Prompt treatment with antibiotics (usually by injection) can prevent death, or permanent disability such as damage to the brain or deafness. The bacteria that cause meningococcal disease can easily be passed from one person to another. However, they hardly ever cause disease. Most of the time they sit harmlessly in the throat.

The main impact of this pamphlet relies on you not reading very far. Most parents will get to the bit about prompt treatment, and will have absorbed enough, so because of the way the paragraph is structured, the second part might slip by unnoticed.

Would this paragraph have impact if it had started with this information?:

> ***Meningococcal bacteria sit harmlessly in the throat, can easily be passed from one person to another and hardly ever cause disease. But occasionally, it can cause two very serious illnesses . . .***

It wouldn't have had as much impact. The first thing you read is often the thing you remember longest. That's why papers dramatize

5 Ministry of Health *Meningococcal Disease* (1996, June). Code 7024.(also August 1997).

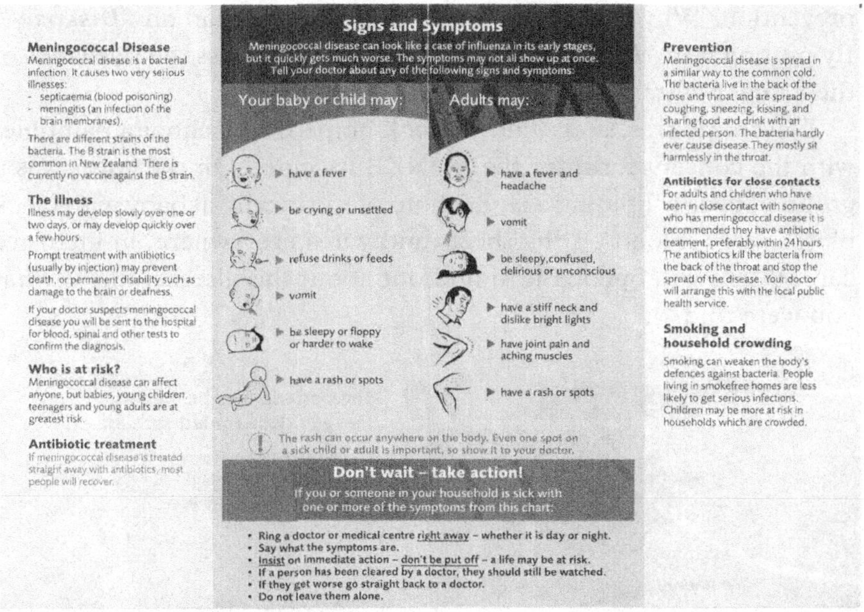

Meningococcal Disease
Meningococcal disease is a bacterial infection. It causes two very serious illnesses:
- septicaemia (blood poisoning)
- meningitis (an infection of the brain membranes).

There are different strains of the bacteria. The B strain is the most common in New Zealand. There is currently no vaccine against the B strain.

The illness
Illness may develop slowly over one or two days, or may develop quickly over a few hours.

Prompt treatment with antibiotics (usually by injection) may prevent death, or permanent disability such as damage to the brain or deafness.

If your doctor suspects meningococcal disease you will be sent to the hospital for blood, spinal and other tests to confirm the diagnosis.

Who is at risk?
Meningococcal disease can affect anyone, but babies, young children, teenagers and young adults are at greatest risk.

Antibiotic treatment
If meningococcal disease is treated straight away with antibiotics, most people will recover.

Signs and Symptoms
Meningococcal disease can look like a case of influenza in its early stages, but it quickly gets much worse. The symptoms may not all show up at once. Tell your doctor about any of the following signs and symptoms:

Your baby or child may:
- have a fever
- be crying or unsettled
- refuse drinks or feeds
- vomit
- be sleepy or floppy or harder to wake
- have a rash or spots

Adults may:
- have a fever and headache
- vomit
- be sleepy, confused, delirious or unconscious
- have a stiff neck and dislike bright lights
- have joint pain and aching muscles
- have a rash or spots

The rash can occur anywhere on the body. Even one spot on a sick child or adult is important, so show it to your doctor.

Don't wait – take action!
If you or someone in your household is sick with one or more of the symptoms from this chart:
- Ring a doctor or medical centre right away – whether it is day or night.
- Say what the symptoms are.
- Insist on immediate action – don't be put off – a life may be at risk.
- If a person has been cleared by a doctor, they should still be watched.
- If they get worse go straight back to a doctor.
- Do not leave them alone.

Prevention
Meningococcal disease is spread in a similar way to the common cold. The bacteria live in the back of the nose and throat and are spread by coughing, sneezing, kissing, and sharing food and drink with an infected person. The bacteria hardly ever cause disease. They mostly sit harmlessly in the throat.

Antibiotics for close contacts
For adults and children who have been in close contact with someone who has meningococcal disease it is recommended they have antibiotic treatment, preferably within 24 hours. The antibiotics kill the bacteria from the back of the throat and stop the spread of the disease. Your doctor will arrange this with the local public health service.

Smoking and household crowding
Smoking can weaken the body's defences against bacteria. People living in smokefree homes are less likely to get serious infections. Children may be more at risk in households which are crowded.

headlines. Watching television is different, since the last thing you hear is usually what you remember.

When you open the March 2003[6] pamphlet you see this:

Meningococcal Disease
Meningococcal disease is a bacterial infection. It causes two very serious illnesses:
- septicaemia (blood poisoning)
- meningitis (an infection of the brain membranes).

There are different strains of the bacteria. The B strain is the most common in New Zealand. There is currently no vaccine against the B strain.

So on the left-hand side you see some information on Meningococcal disease. Here there is no mention that *"The bacteria hardly ever cause disease."*

BUT . . .

On the top right-hand side of the pamphlet, Under Prevention – in the place you'd least expect to see it – is written *"The bacteria hardly ever cause disease. They mostly sit harmlessly in the throat."*

Prevention
Meningococcal disease is spread in a similar way to the common cold. The bacteria live in the back of the nose and throat and are spread by coughing, sneezing, kissing, and sharing food and drink with an infected person. The bacteria hardly ever cause disease. They mostly sit harmlessly in the throat.

Exactly WHAT has this got to do with

6 Ministry of Health, "*Meningococcal Disease*" March 2003, Code 1303. (also printed in October 2002)

prevention? Why is it not included in the information on *"Disease"?* By putting it in *"Prevention"*, will most people miss the relevance of the actual point?

Eleven months later children took home from school a pamphlet with the consent form for the MeNZB vaccine.[7] On the cover was a group of people holding a large photo of a critically ill baby with black blotchy legs, blood on the sheets and wires everywhere, in intensive care. When you opened it to find out about the disease, this is what you were told.

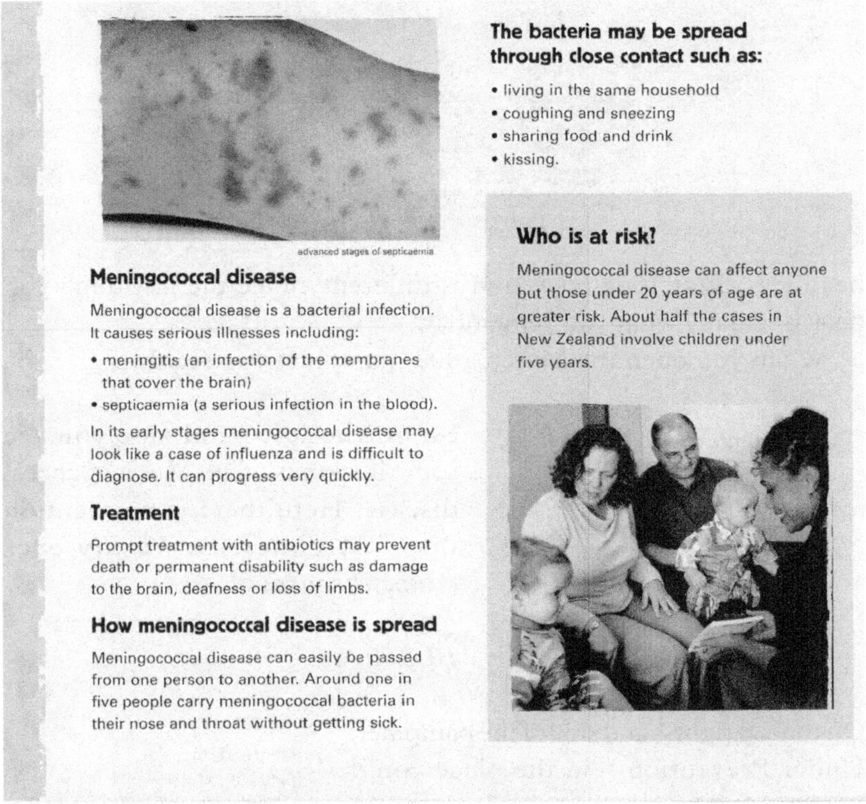

advanced stages of septicaemia

Meningococcal disease

Meningococcal disease is a bacterial infection. It causes serious illnesses including:

- meningitis (an infection of the membranes that cover the brain)
- septicaemia (a serious infection in the blood).

In its early stages meningococcal disease may look like a case of influenza and is difficult to diagnose. It can progress very quickly.

Treatment

Prompt treatment with antibiotics may prevent death or permanent disability such as damage to the brain, deafness or loss of limbs.

How meningococcal disease is spread

Meningococcal disease can easily be passed from one person to another. Around one in five people carry meningococcal bacteria in their nose and throat without getting sick.

The bacteria may be spread through close contact such as:

- living in the same household
- coughing and sneezing
- sharing food and drink
- kissing.

Who is at risk?

Meningococcal disease can affect anyone but those under 20 years of age are at greater risk. About half the cases in New Zealand involve children under five years.

Instead of being told that the bacteria rarely cause disease, under *"Who is at risk?"* we are told that the disease can affect anyone. And under *"How meningococcal disease is spread"* they said:

7 Ministry of Health, April 2004, code MVA0401.

"one in five people carry meningococcal bacteria in their nose and throat without getting sick."

Is this message designed to be translated in the average reader's brain to mean that the other four out of the five who carry meningococcal bacteria in their nose and throat *will* get sick, and 4 out of 5 people is 80% of the population, which means I don't have much chance of *not* getting sick and dying?

So . . . eleven months after telling you that *"the bacteria hardly ever cause disease"*, the Health Ministry seems to be promoting the message which implies that anyone/most people will get sick and possibly die. Are you now really scared? If the vaccine consent form had told you that the bacteria hardly ever causes disease, as they stated in previous brochures would you have been scared enough to immediately agree to letting the doctor or nurse vaccinate your child?

When we make choices about vaccines, it appears that the only questions we are supposed to consider are what the Health Department wants us to know about what they say are the consequences of these diseases, but even that changes depending on how they want you to respond. Vaccine pamphlets are designed to achieve a behavioural outcome, not to inform people. Discussing this very subject, the Otago Medical School website[8] says:

"If parents have no fear of vaccine, but fear of disease, the argument in favour of vaccination is clear-cut. If they have no fear of vaccine, but also no fear of disease, there may be inertia. When they have no fear of disease, but fear of vaccines, parents are likely to refuse immunization."

The people who implemented the vaccination programme were quite clear. They said that the last 14 years has

"provided many with close experience of its unpredictable occurrence and often terrifying severity. Fear of the disease, together with parochial support for a local initiative are likely to enhance vaccine uptake . . ."[9]

8 Salisbury, D. Retrieved on 19 November, 2005 from <http://immunet.otago.ac.nz/vactopic.htm>

9 Thomas, M. 2004. "Prevention of Group B meningococcal disease by vaccination: a difficult task." *New Zealand Medical Journal*, 117, No. 1200: 117–1200 and 1016.

However, in 1994 the low uptake of the MMR vaccine during a mumps outbreak was explained[10] in this way: *"**ESR believe uptake may have been low because publicity about mumps was fairly low key and couched in reasonably conservative terms.**"* What that means is they told the truth.

To have no fear of a vaccine, but fear of the disease, is not an argument in favour of vaccines, or a way to make a choice. It is an emotion called fear, which determines the action taken in order to stop the sweat running down the fearful person's face. The question is, is the fear-induced sweat justified, or a medically induced malady?

Yes, the disease could be serious, and it might kill you, but how likely is that? What is it that the Health Department isn't telling you?

Who are the people in the community in whom these infections are most likely to be serious? Are the answers to questions about who is most at risk not on brochures because they want to lead you to their desired outcome?

Parents will soon have to consider new vaccines some of which are chickenpox, meningitis C and Pneumococcus (PREVNAR is the vaccine's name). Nikki Turner says[11] that these new vaccines show excellent safety profiles and give good disease control, and that assessing new vaccines also requires consideration of the disease and its impact in New Zealand. Why does a vaccine's mere existence seemingly eliminate a parent's right of choice?

Let's think about chickenpox.

A pamphlet I was given by a practice nurse, called *Childhood Infections and Immunization. Everything you should know*[12] has this section in it:

COMMON CHILDHOOD INFECTIOUS DISEASES

	SIGNS AND SYMPTOMS	INCUBATION PERIOD	INFECTIOUS PERIOD	NURSING AND TREATMENT	SPECIAL POINTS
CHICKENPOX	May start with a cold, headache or sickness. High temperature. Small red pimples (first on body then on face and limbs) which turn to yellow blisters, then break.	2-3 Weeks	From 1-2 days before rash emerges until rash dries up, about 7 days later.	Bed rest. Relieve itching with calamine lotion. Try to stop child scratching (little ones may need cotton mittens) to prevent further infection and scars (pockmarks). Keep child's nails short and clean.	One attack usually gives immunity for life. As harmful complications are rare, no vaccination is necessary.

Note the Special Points which says: "*. . . **no vaccination is necessary***".

10 St John, P. 1994. "Low key GP response to Mumps epidemic." *New Zealand Doctor*, 15 September, p. 14.

11 Turner, N. 2005. (Letter to the Editor) "Chickenpox Vaccine". *New Zealand Herald* 15 November, p. A12.

12 No date. Published and distributed through practices by Sterling Winthrop (NZ) Ltd, Auckland, and featuring large advertisements for Panadol.

I will be interested to see how dangerous chickenpox will be made out to be in the new chickenpox vaccine pamphlets in order to make parents fearful of it.

We don't know very much about any Pneumococcus epidemic in this country, though there is this information.[13]

SPECIAL POINTS

One attack usually gives immunity for life.
As harmful complications are rare, no vaccination is necessary.

"Dr Grant also leads a study on Auckland's rate of childhood pneumonia, which is 5 to 10 times higher than in the United States. The high rate of such diseases was due partly to increasingly overcrowded houses in the past 10 to 15 years, and variable access to family doctors, he said. But it now seemed that illness also stemmed partly from poor diet."

It would also appear that in New Zealand[14] abuse of antibiotics is a possible reason for the increase of *Streptococcus* pneumoniae, and increases the carriage of *S.* pneumoniae in children by two to seven times.

Interestingly, there is no recent document on the Public Health Surveillance website[15] that tracks the figures of any type of childhood pneumonia, or yearly totals for the pneumococcus types in the Prevnar vaccine. So where does the data for ***"5 to 10 times higher than in the US"*** come from? Which groups are at risk? Where is the evidence? And what is causing the increase in the first place? All of those factors will affect who is at risk, and the possible consequences of the disease for that person. In the meantime, the reason you've probably not heard about Pneumococcus is that you're probably already immune to it even though you've never had the disease.

Most information reads similar to this news item which says: ***"The bacterium is carried by many healthy people but develops into potentially fatal illness in only a small minority of cases."***

---

13 Collins, S. 2005. "Vitamin lacking in 1 of 10 toddlers". *New Zealand Herald*, 10 January. Retrieved on 18 September, 2005 from <http://www.nzherald.co.nz/index.cfm?c_id=1&ObjectID=9006061>

14 Leathart, C. 1999. "Focus: Antibiotic resistance and the GP: when less is more". Retrieved on 18 September, 2005 from <http://www.rnzcgp.org.nz/news/nzfp/June1999/focuscl.htm> Children who have recently had antibiotics are two to seven times more likely to subsequently carry resistant strains of *S.* pneumoniae as commensals (normally carried bacteria in the throat which do nothing). Among patients with invasive disease due to *S.* pneumoniae, recent antibiotic use has been identified as a risk factor for infection with strains resistant to multiple drugs.

15 Retrieved on 18 September, 2005 from <http://www.surv.esr.cri.nz/>

Smokers[16] ***are "four times as likely to catch Streptococcus pneumoniae as non-smokers and passive smokers are two and a half times more likely to catch it than people who are not passive smokers".***

Which overseas babies/children does the medical literature show are most likely to get serious pneumococcus invasive disease? In Finland, Alaska and the USA,[17] the children most at risk from serious disease had previous antibiotic use, were in day-care (environment and stress), and had underlying illness (hereditary and/or immune system). What was the one thing parents could do to protect their children? The article stated that ***"there is ample opportunity for prevention of invasive pneumococcal disease by increased breastfeeding."***

The same information probably applies here but I doubt that any of it will be in any pamphlet promoting a vaccine. If it were published in a pamphlet, you could know that, because your child doesn't go to day-care, or have an underlying illness, because you've never used antibiotics, you breastfeed, and your children have a good diet, you will be far less likely to think a vaccine is necessary. The truth might not make you fear the disease.

The article[17] assumed that the only factor in increasing the incidence of illness in day-care was greater numbers of bacteria spread amongst children. But is invasive pneumococcus just a matter of ***"bacteria causes disease"***? Or does something else cause the disease? Like stress? Day-care is very stressful for children, particularly those who don't like being away from their mothers and being with lots of other children and adults.

When it comes to acute disease, the medical profession says little on preventable risk factors. Stress is usually only talked about in terms of heart disease or strokes.

Over the last few years, the media have been publishing many articles saying things like ***"Bad genes cause disease"***. After researching

---

16 "Smokers 'need' pneumonia bug jab". 2000. *BBC News*: Friday 10 March. Retrieved on 9 March, 2006) from <http://news.bbc.co.uk/1/hi/health/671602.stm>

17 Levine, O.S., Farley, M., Harrison, L.H., Lefkowitz, L., McGreer, A. and Schwartz, B. 1999. "Risk Factors for Invasive Pneumococcal Disease in Children. A Population-based Case-Control Study in North America." *Pediatrics*, Vol 103(3): p. e28. ". . . the findings of this study highlight the importance of day-care, underlying illness (27% of cases), and recent antibiotic use as risk factors for invasive pneumococcal disease in children, and the protective effects of breastfeeding." <http://pediatrics.aappublications.org/cgi/content/full/103/3/e28?ijkey=EWr0xTyWSRNX2&keytype=ref&siteid=aapjournals#B11> Accessed on 18 September, 2005.

genes for a long time, suddenly geneticists have changed their minds. They are now saying that the important part of the gene theory is now Epigenetics. What does this mean?

"Epigenetics[18] means, 'What we eat, how we live and love, alters how our Genes behave'"

Actually, the correct way to define epigenetics is:

"the lousy diet, the stress, the toxins, lack of sleep, lack of exercise, and the behaviours that we shouldn't do, can alter the way our genes behave, and can cause disease."

So why do most people not get a disease? Dr Gadjusek says that the reason is "genetically predetermined":

"In most infections only a rare individual becomes ill or suffers rare complications, and that individual may be genetically predetermined . . . For example, HTLV-1 infects 1–2 million Japanese, but only one in over a thousand gets adult advanced T cell leukemia over 40 years, and fortunately only about one in a thousand gets HAM, HTLV-1 associated myelopathy. Those unfortunate rare individuals are the problem, not the problem of the innocuous, or carriers, the other one thousand who die without ever knowing they had it, and having no ill effect. The same can be said of poliomyelitis, where it takes 1,000 infected cases in order to induce a paralysis, the others don't know they were infected;"[19]

---

18 Duke University Medical Center, 2005 "'Epigenetics' Means What We Eat, How We Live and Love, Alters How Our Genes Behave". Retrieved on 18 September, 2005 from <http://www.dukemednews.org/news/article.php?id=9322> "'We can no longer argue whether genes or environment has a greater impact on our health and development, because both are inextricably linked Each nutrient, each interaction, each experience can manifest itself through biochemical changes that ultimately dictate gene expression, whether at birth or 40 years down the road . . .' '. . . Even the lowest detectable limits of a chemical can have dire effects on a living organism,' . . . Atrizine is a prime example. Less than one part per billion of this widely used corn herbicide de-masculinizes developing frogs or causes dual male-female genitalia. Yet often the Environmental Protection Agency's instrumentation doesn't record such minute levels of chemical exposure . . . 'If Atrizine is having this effect in animals, we question its effect on humans,' said Schlesinger . . . 'Epigenetics . . . explains why individuals respond differently to environmental cues . . . provides the missing link between the environment and the development of diseases that goes beyond many of the subtle changes in DNA that explain only a fraction of the diseases (that) humans develop.'"

19 Gadjusek's, C. 1999. "Scientific Responsibility", in *Human Genome and Research and Society Proceedings of the Second International Bioethics Seminar*, 20–21 March, in Fukui,

Here is another statement from medical literature:

> ***Contrary to widely held beliefs, most 10-year-old children with negative or unknown chickenpox histories are actually immune to varicella, according to a report by Canadian investigators . . . the current findings[20] indicate that nearly two thirds of children without a positive history are actually immune.***[21]

So, how was it that these two-thirds of children, who never saw pox became immune?

How was it that the 999 who got polio, never knew it, but the one person paralysed did? How is it that the majority of people today have carried Pneumococcus in their throats regularly, as well as neisseria meningitidis, haemophilus, and many other bacteria, and all they got was immunity? Was that genetically predetermined too?

Everywhere around us are the real examples of why people get sick. ***"Worry can make strokes fatal"***,[22] ***"Chasing deadlines can be deadly"***,[23] ***"Stress lowers immune function"***.[24] Anyone who knows something about stress hormones knows that cortisol and adrenalin suppress the immune system. Stress isn't just caused by work, or going to school. Stress can also be any situation where what is happening bothers you to the extent that you don't want to be there most of the time. You cannot classify what stress is, because what is stress for one person may be fun for another.

Here's something really simple. Sleep. Using a vaccine trial, researchers[25] found that those who were sleep-deprived didn't have a good immune response to the vaccine in the first month. Their last sentence was ***"our findings support the concept that adequate amounts of sleep are needed for optimal resistance to infectious***

---

pp. 205–210 Retrieved on 9 March, 2006 from <http://www2.unescobkk.org/eubios/HGR/HGRCG.htm>

20 Boulianne, N. et al. 2001. "Most ten-year-old children with negative or unknown histories of chickenpox are immune". *Pediatr Infect Dis J.* 20(11) 1087–8. PMID 11734718.

21 Retrieved on 18 September, 2005 from <http://id.medscape.com/reuters/prof/2001/12/12.17/20011214clin008.html>

22 Reuters. 2002. "Worry can make strokes fatal". *New Zealand Herald*, 7 January: A11.

23 Bloomberg. 2004. "Chasing deadlines can be deadly, researchers find". *New Zealand Herald*, 18 December: A13.

24 AFP. 1999. "Stress 'lowers immune function'". *The Dominion*, 29 July.

25 Spiegel, K. et al. 2002 "Effect of sleep deprivation on Response to Immunization". *JAMA*, Sep 25; 288(12): 1471–2. PMID: 12243633.

challenge". How many children who come down with serious infections are sleep-deprived?

In 1991–1994, when fully vaccinated Cuba experienced an epidemic of sickness which looked similar to polio they called it epidemic neuropathy. CDC[26] researchers went to Cuba to help look for a causative virus. For a long time they found nothing and though the reports mentioned smoking and homebrew, CDC said the cause was unknown. The authors of this article commented that the remaining team would ***"focus on the role of . . . dietary insufficiencies, ingested toxins, pesticide exposure . . ."*** A doctor not associated with the CDC, found that the disease resolved when Vitamin B supplements[27] were given to those sick.

Researchers subsequently found viruses antigenically related to viruses known as the Coxsackie virus group in the spinal fluid of patients. Coxsackie viruses are capable of causing acute flaccid paralysis, which looks identical to polio. They said: ***"although it was demonstrated that the illness was associated with toxic and nutritional risk factors, it has not been possible to identify a specific etiology for the symptoms observed."***[28]

Another group of researchers looked at why there were no signs of illness in the Cuban region of Guantanamo, even though the same virus was also found there, and people there also smoked and drank alcohol. They found that the foods people ate protected them from the disease.[29] Ironically, years before, a Dr George Boines[30] detailed his treatment of paralytic polio based on a total overhaul of diet with all sugar prohibited, as well as supplementing B-vitamins, vitamin C and hesperidin, which was more successful than the standard treatment. That eating the right foods prevents many diseases, both acute and chronic, isn't a surprise to some of us. Another study[31] has found that:

---

26 Centre for Disease Control, Atlanta, Georgia, USA.

27 1994. From the Centers for Disease Control and Prevention. "Epidemic neuropathy—Cuba, 1991–1994". *JAMA*, 271(15): 1154–1156. PMID: 8151865.

28 Lago, P.M. et al. 2001. "Mechanism of enterovirus involvement in epidemic neuropathy: hypothesis regarding pathophysiology". *Med Hypotheses*. Mar: 56(3): 339–47 PMID: 11359357.

29 Barnouin, J. et al, 2001. "Nutritional and food protection against epidemic emerging neuropathy. Epidemiological findings in the unique disease-free urban area of Cuba". *Int J Vitam Nutr Res* Sep: 71(5): 274–85. PMID: 11725692 "Riboflavin, carotenoid and selenium contents and specific antioxidants substances (indoleamines, capsaicin), the foods more consumed in Guantanamo could be considered as EN protective factors".

30 1956. *Virginia Medical Monthly*, June. Detailed in: 1960 "Nutrition as a treatment for polio victims". *Prevention*, November, p. 43.

31 Broome, C.S. et al. 2004. "An increase in selenium intake improves immune function

"An increase in selenium intake improves immune function and poliovirus handling in adults with marginal selenium status."

The research showed that those people in Cuba who got epidemic neuropathy which looked like polio, were eating a diet low in selenium, B-vitamins and other nutrients, which was why they got sick. The people in Guantanamo did not get sick, because their diet kept their immune system working properly, and detoxified the body better. Ironically the treatment for Vitamin C deficient guinea pigs suffering lameness from poliovirus is vitamins in their drinking water.[32]

Polio scientists know that there is a whole lot more to polio than they tell us, which is why one Expanded Programme of Immunization newsletter[33] on polio said this:

"Studies will also be presented regarding other causes of acute flaccid paralysis,[34] such as intoxication by Karwinskia or pesticides, AIDS, traumatic neuritis, etc."

In France a study found skeletal muscle disorders manifested by muscle pain, fatigue, proximal weakness in patients with selenium deficiency.[35] A study in China, supplementing a province with selenium[36] showed that the selenium protected the people against viral hepatitis and liver cancer. Another Chinese study[37] pointed out that:

"Epidemiological studies have demonstrated that a low grain Se content is associated with a high regional incidence of hepatitis B virus infections."

---

and poliovirus handling in adults with marginal selenium status". *Am J Clin Nutr*, Jul: 80(1): 154–62. PMID: 15213043.

32 Hansen, A.K. 1997. "A serological indication of the existence of a guinea pig poliovirus". *Lab Anim*, Jul:31(3): 212–3. PMID: 9230501.

33 1992. "Differential diagnosis of cases of acute flaccid paralysis". *EPI Newsletter*, August: XIV(4): 6.

34 "Acute Flaccid Paralysis" is another term for diseases that look like polio. Until around 1950, everything that included flaccid paralysis was called polio. Once it was realized that other viruses cause polio-like diseases, they left "polio" to the polio viruses and everything else is reallocated to other classifications."

35 Chariot, P. et al. 2003. "Skeletal muscle disorders associated with selenium deficiency in humans". *Muscle Nerve*, Jun: 27(6): 662–8. PMID: 12766976.

36 Yu, S.Y. et al. 1997. "Protective role of selenium against hepatitis B Virus and primary liver cancer in Qidong." *Biol Trace Elem Res*, Jan: 56(1): 117–124. PMID: 9152515.

37 Yu, S.Y. et al. 1989. "Chemoprevention trial of human hepatitis with selenium supplementation in China." *Biol Trace Elem Res*. Apr–May: 20(1–2): 15–22. PMID: 2484394

Given that New Zealand is chronically selenium deficient, and these trials began long before New Zealand opted for a Hepatitis B vaccine, I wonder why selenium hasn't been tried here. Not only does selenium and other minerals help the body deal with stresses in general, the selenium status of a person also determines whether and how badly they get influenza.[38] Selenium is protective against prostate[39] and other cancers,[40] so wouldn't you think the New Zealand Health Department would want to kill lots of birds with one stone?

Forget the word epigenetics. It's a barrier to common sense, and has only been coined because geneticists have been forced to acknowledge that what you eat, how you live, toxic pollutants, and the environment are more important than genes in determining your health, or when you die.

> ***"Good nutrition starting in the womb can go a long way towards preventing adult illnesses such as hypertension and heart disease" we are told.***

The article[41] discusses research by Dr Chris Kuzawa, a visiting biological anthropologist who said, ***"Traditionally, hereditary and lifestyle influences were believed to cause disease."*** He talks about how environmental factors subtly alter the way our genes express their function even while in the womb, and mothers who don't eat correctly force their babies to change their hormones, which alters how they respond to stress and will have effects that linger until adulthood.

Liggins Institute director Professor Peter Gluckman said medical science was just beginning to understanding this ***"novel, revolutionary idea."***

That's a very strange thing to say. Even in my tradition, and the way I ate during my pregnancy, I was aware of, and followed a diet which was traditionally enriched to give the baby the best possible chance. It is certainly not a novel concept to me. I did however, refuse some

38 Nelson, H.K. et al. 2001. "Host nutritional selenium status as a driving force for influenza virus mutations". *FASEB J*, Aug: 15(10): 1846–8. PMID: 11481250.

39 Chan, J.M. et al. 2005. "Role of diet in prostate cancer development and progression". *J Clin Oncol*, Nov: 23(32): 8152–60. PMID: 16278466.

40 Combs, G.F. Jr. et al. 1998. "Chemopreventive agents: selenium". *Pharmacol Ther*, Sep; 79(3): 179–92. PMID: 9776375.

41 King, E. 2005. "Good nutrition 'should start in the womb". *New Zealand Herald*, 27 July: A8.

of the ideas some well-meaning oriental friends were keen for me to try. Somehow, sea-slugs just . . . didn't appeal.

My doctor at the time, thought my nutritional enrichment approach and attitudes, along with those of other home-birthing nutters, were plainly ridiculous and unsupported by science.

It seems that science might be catching on but the question is, ***Have they yet got the right end of the stick?*** Shouldn't they be talking to the experts, like obstetrician Dr Tom Brewer, and those parents who, for years, have proved a point that doctors today appear to have missed? A recent study in Ecuador[42] found that women exposed to floral pesticides during pregnancy gave birth to children with lasting neurotoxic damage even when biomarker results were not increased beyond ranges considered normal. They talked about how the blood brain barrier is open until 6 months after birth and provides no protection during development. However, I'm sure such arguments won't be relevant to toxic metals in minute quantities in vaccines when they want to give them to pregnant women or babies. The Equadorian study yet again, underscores the impact of minute environmental toxicities during pregnancy. The study also points out that pesticide exposure in childhood also causes problems, of a slightly different nature. It has long been proven that bad nutrition and environmental toxicities can be the cause of a malfunctioning immune and endocrine system that radically affects how the body responds to acute illness, and lays the foundation for all health, and is the major player in the so-called field of epigenetics. It's all there in the medical literature.

The problem is, many pregnant women, if not most, have lost that connection with their tradition and rely on doctors, most of whom have yet to grasp the concept. Doctors rarely see those who still know those traditions, which might be why this seems such a novel, revolutionary idea to them.

The emphasis of the article was that Dr Kuzawa wanted to work at developing ways to treat adult disease through prevention ***"as early as in neonates"***.

But hang on a minute. Didn't they just infer that hard-wiring was

---

42 Grandjean, P. et al. 2006. "Pesticide Exposure and Stunting as Independent Predictors of Neurobehavioural deficits in Ecuadorian School Children." *PEDIATRICS*, 117(3) March: e546-e556. PMID: 16510633. Retrieved on 18 September, 2005 from <http://pediatrics.aappublications.org/cgi/reprint/117/3/e546>

done in the womb? Yet again, aren't they putting the cart before the horse? I'd prefer that they helped women to get it right in pregnancy, then there might not be very many pieces for them to pick up at the neonatal stage.

A letter to the editor recently stated that even the healthiest, adequately breast-fed child with the perfect diet and best genes in the world can still catch a vaccine-preventable disease and die.[43] That is inferring that every baby as described could die. Do the figures about who is most likely to succumb to infectious diseases in this, or any other country, support that argument?

Back in 1983, when discussing the recipe for long life and good health, we were told[44] that apart from what they ate, the people in Tamysh had, ***"A joy of life, love of work, respect of old age . . . contentment, a well-regulated day's routine, an even temper, an attitude of moderation, subconscious yet strict weight control."*** Staring out at you is a picture of 168-year-old Shirall Mislimov, and on the other page a centenarian astride his saddle on a huge black stallion in the middle of town with a forth generation child in front of him. His 120-year-old wife is leaning out a car window, talking to him.

Professor Nodar Kipshidze, Mislomov's doctor, told me[45] that he rarely saw epidemic disease. In these ***"disgustingly healthy"*** people he has never seen a case of heart failure, stroke, rheumatoid arthritis, diabetes, multiple sclerosis or gallstones. His biggest problem was fires, occasional food poisoning, occasional appendicitis, 100-plus-year-old hunters falling off cliffs, the odd drownings and difficult baby delivery. To fill his 50-plus years there, he studied their diet and life and adopted their ways. The average age of death is 120. The basic key to life on top of their attitudes, is their no-junk-food diet, which is rich in probiotic foods, and the mineral-rich water they drink and use to water their organically grown fruit and vegetables with.

Utopia? Not likely in volatile Abkhazia, ex-Soviet Georgia, but certainly an example of eating right, living right, loving right, to make our genes work right. Geneticists, infectious or chronic disease experts would be out of a job there, but they might learn a thing or two, as did Professor Kipshidze.

---

43 Ram, S. 2005. "Letters to the Editor". *New Zealand Herald,* 21 November: A10.

44 Gris, H. 1983. "Town with the strongest heart in the world". *New Zealand Woman's Weekly,* February 14:20–2.

45 Personal letter answers to questions 14 April, 2002.

9 The Big Disadvantages!

To begin with, Hilary seemed to be learning a foreign language.

No, I don't mean Japanese, though she had a go at that as well.

You could say it is an international "language", which is no comfort to me at all, and it still presents a hurdle for many parents to overcome.

However, I'll be kind and call the problem "a specialist vocabulary".

Or maybe I'm the problem.

Perhaps I'm just a slow learner who responds best to simple and straightforward plain English.

The main disadvantage though, is that no matter how hard I try, I will always be a pretty ignorant lay person struggling to keep up with all the accumulated facts and figures Hilary has amassed.

No doubt Hilary gets frustrated with me because she has to frequently interpret the specialist vocabulary; or she has to remind me who someone is when e-mails come, or what part someone is playing in helping to resolve a case she has undertaken. It can be very confusing and complicated. Flesh-and-blood face-to-face friends are a rare commodity in our lives. Because Hilary's outreach is worldwide, many of our contacts are often hundreds or thousands of miles away and faceless – for me anyway.

However, maybe there is a big plus to all this. Perhaps I can represent the ordinary parent who suffers the same problems that I have, and help all those who may tend to look at Hilary in awe, while feeling that they need to make appropriate noises at what they hope are the appropriate places while they struggle to get their minds around the issues involved.

Hilary is really an ordinary person too. She is well aware of her vulnerability. There will always be people who want to "shoot her down" and who mutter unmentionables about "that woman". She knows her limitations. So in the humanness of our lifestyle I hope we shall continue to complement each other, and that whatever the future brings the disadvantages will be far outweighed by the many pluses of our unique lifestyle.

By the way. How's this for bedtime reading:

> "The immune system has two 'sides'. One is Th1, which is the usual response to diseases caught naturally. A healthy immune system has a 'bias' towards Th1. Th2 is the 'other' side, and people who have allergies, asthma and disease with an autoimmune origin have what is known as a Th2-skewed immune system.
>
> When a mother is pregnant, her pregnancy is controlled by cytokines and requires a predominance of Th2 cytokines in order not to reject the baby because . . ."

No point in going on, is there?

I mean, we all know about this, don't we?

"Elementary, Dear Watson," carefully taking the tongue out of my cheek.

10 Whooping Cough: A "Disease Time-Bomb"?

From 1960 to 1970, the New Zealand whooping cough vaccination schedule was three triple injections at 3, 4, and 5 months of age, but in 1971, the Health Department reduced it to two. In 1981, the schedule for our son was two whooping cough[1] shots at 2 months and 5 months.[2]

We were given a two-sided sheet, less than half an A4-page in size. It was headed up on the inside *"What will happen if we do not immunize? Outbreaks of these diseases will occur."* Nearly half of the inside left-hand side said *"PROTECT your child and the community"*. This message was designed to reinforce an assumption that the whooping cough vaccine had been responsible for wiping out the deaths and outbreaks in the past, and that if you didn't vaccinate, these outbreaks would start up again, and we would go back to the bad old days and have widespread deaths.

Before whooping cough vaccines were even used in USA in the

---

1 Whooping cough, otherwise known as pertussis.

2 "Protect your child . . . Immunize" DPT & Polio – 3 months; DPT & Polio – 5 months; Measles – 12 months; Rubella – Form One; Tetanus Booster – 15 years. Health information series NO 350, issued by New Zealand Department of Health, Code 4344.

1940s, whooping cough deaths had declined 82%[3] as had the incidence.[4] It had even been speculated that it was less severe because the bacteria had changed.[5] Deaths in New Zealand decreased tremendously, but strangely, whereas other countries until recently have boasted huge decreases in incidence and hospitalization because of the vaccines, New Zealand could not.

People said the incidence had disappeared, but because whooping cough was not a reportable disease, statistics on community incidence weren't kept. The statistics that were kept right throughout that time were the hospital discharge rates for whooping cough. That data is best described as it was in a medical journal: ***"the current programme is making little impact on the disease"***.[6]

Our son was 18 months old in 1983 when the pressure really came on to give him the whooping cough vaccine, because there had been an outbreak. I was told that these two shots were vital to prevent my children getting whooping cough. I was also told they would give them immunity *"for life"*. It was inferred that all the children coming down with whooping cough were those who weren't immunized. Peter was a teaching principal, so if our son got whooping cough, we were told, Peter would be dragging the disease up the hill to school, every day, to infect his pupils.

This didn't make sense to me, because what difference would it make to those immunized school children who ostensibly had immunity for life, if my child got whooping cough?

The doctor intoned that Pertussis in our child would be a whopping great cough that could make his eyes go bloodshot, his face would turn purple, and would stop him breathing . . . he would get brain damage, and die.

I managed to track down some of these babies and toddlers with a whopping great cough, and was surprised to find that not only were their eyes not blood-shot, and their faces not purple, but . . . they were

---

3 Mortimer, E. 1978 "Crude mortality rates from pertussis decline 82% between 1900 and 1904 and 1935 and 1939, prior to the widespread use of the pertussis vaccine beginning in the 1940s." *Int Symp. Pert* DHEW Pub No. (NIH) 79–1830.

4 Katz, S.L. 1979. "New thoughts on Pertussis". *Pediatrics*, Jun: 63(6): 942–2. PMID: 36592.

5 Shaw, E.B. 1983. "Pertussis vaccine". *Pediatric Infect Dis J*, May–Jun: 2(3): 264–5. PMID: 6866793.

6 McNeill, C. 1994. "More potent pertussis prevention is necessary". *New Zealand Doctor News*, September: p. 14.

vaccinated. I brought this up with the doctor who told us, "Well, see . . . if they hadn't had the vaccine, THEN they would have died."

This was my first introduction to the view that if vaccines don't prevent illness, they at least make the illness less serious. At the medical libraries, I could find opinion, but I couldn't find studies on this phenomenon perhaps because it undermined the first principle of the time, which was that vaccines meant ***"you can't catch it"***.

When I asked the Health Department about children damaged by vaccines in 1984, they said there had been none. They even stated in a newspaper article[7] that there was no major risk of brain damage from the whooping cough vaccine. That must have struck a chord with a few people, because in reply[8] came an article from a Napier mother responding to the first article, talking about her son Brendon's brain damage after the whooping cough vaccine. Her paediatrician had told her that the numbers of people who died from whooping cough was higher than the number of people who were brain-damaged by the vaccine. The article then went on to quote Dr Frazer from the Kimberley Psychopaedic Training and Nursing Hospital, who admitted that there were a number of patients there with brain damage from the whooping cough vaccine. In discussing the figure of one in 110,000 injections, he made the droll comment that "It was obviously just the tip of the iceberg".

(The statistics for babies dying previous to that year from whooping cough[9] were 2 in 1978, and 1 in 1980.) Brendon's mother clearly wanted something done about the lack of accountability. She said she was powerless; that parents were being kept in the dark, and "some hospitals didn't like it if you asked too many questions". Too true, I thought.

Then in 1988[10] a child named Daniel died. He'd had a reaction in 1983, years of seizures, and major health problems. Years later, I found his number in the CARM register. Interesting.

Neither did the Health Department mention Sophie O'Brien, who in 1982, along with another Wellington girl, had a severe reaction to her 3-month DPT. Both cases were ACC accepted, and both will be

---

7 Parker, C. 1984. "Vaccine babies aren't at risk" *Sun News*, July.

8 Parker, C. 1984. "Napier mother Dawn Simpson and her son Brendon". *Sun News*, 22 July.

9 Checked = Morbidity and mortality yearbooks, appendices to parliamentary journals, medical articles: There was also one death in 1986.

10 Fitzsimons, M. 1988. "Daniel is no statistic." *Zealandia*, 8 April: p. 8.

on ACC and 24-hour care until they die. It seemed that in 1984, it was forbidden to even mention that there could be serious side-effects.

In 1984, like Brendon's mother, most parents were told that vaccine reactions were one in a million, and far less than the brain damage and deaths from the whooping cough. And as I sit here and write this, surrounded by exercise books of people's details, a file box and half a filing cabinet drawer of yet more collateral damage from the last 25 years, I find the fact that none of these parents have ever been given a voice, a fair go, and most of them not even a decent explanation: very depressing. But . . . to be expected.

Today's publicity aimed at persuading parents to vaccinate still relies on the age-old brain-damage from disease message, and *"the vaccine makes it milder"* theme. The most recent example of this occurred in 1999, when Dr Nikki Turner in an effort to persuade parents to vaccinate their children against whooping cough, told the *New Zealand Herald* that outbreaks were directly related to inadequate vaccination coverage, and that these epidemics were inevitable if people didn't vaccinate. She quoted a Swedish study that she said showed brain damage in 4% of hospitalized children, and said that the situation here was the same.[11] If she meant that all 4% were permanently brain damaged (which is what I took her to mean) this wasn't what the study concluded.[12] I faxed the author of the Swedish study and asked him if any of the children had suffered permanent brain damage in that study and he replied to me[13] that:

> ***"there was no long-term follow up done of these patients. Thus, in this study, we cannot say anything about any risk of permanent brain damage after pertussis in Sweden."***

So why did New Zealand's most vocal pro-vaccine doctor incorrectly give readers the impression that the study showed that 4% of hospitalized Swedish children were permanently brain damaged,

11 Rae, B. 1999. "Disease Time Bomb". *New Zealand Herald*, May 8–9: J4.

12 Romanus, V. et al. 1987. "Pertussis in Sweden after the cessation of general immunization in 1979". *Pediatric Infect Dis J*, 6:(4): 364–371. PMID: 3588110. Looked at the years 1980–1985, during which time there had been 36 729 bacteriologically confirmed cases of whooping cough. The study followed 2282 people who had been hospitalized and of those had neurological symptoms (Table 3, p. 369). 11 = Encephalitis. 42 = First time convulsions, encephalitis excluded. Temp <38°C. 20 = First time convulsions, encephalitis excluded. Temp ≥38°C. 1 = convulsions in patients with known epilepsy. 6 = other; ataxia, vertigo. 90 out of 2282 hospitalized patients = 4%.

13 Fax received from Victoria Romanus on 17 August 1999.

and this could happen here too, when this was not the case? Why was the heading *"DISEASE TIME-BOMB"* so emotive?

And why was no clarification published, when the study and the author's comments were sent to the journalist concerned?

Was it also a fluke that the same sound bite appeared as the heading to another article also extensively involving Dr Nikki Turner?:

"Has New Zealand's stance of individual choice on childhood vaccinations led to a disease timebomb?"[14]

14 Dickson, H. 1999. "Has New Zealand's stance of individual choice on childhood vaccinations led to a disease timebomb?" *New Zealand Woman's Weekly*, 17 May: 20–21.

11 House Bus #1

Not only was CHESM born in 1983, but we also bought our first house bus in that year, beginning a strong desire for a mobile, self-contained lifestyle which has continued ever since.

However our original dreams have had to be adjusted as events in our lives have unfolded. We were still at Waipipi living in the school house, and David was not yet born.

At the same time in about July or August, a "For Sale" advertisement appeared in the New Zealand Herald for a mobile home. It was located in Tauranga so we made arrangements to drive down after school and have a look at it. The weather turned wet and darkness set in. We eventually found the house bus parked by the Wairau River, near Bethlehem, and made the acquaintance of long-time gypsy lifestyler, Kim Davy.

We fell in love with the bus straight away. It was an old 1946 Ford, although it had long since lost many of the Ford parts. It had a BMC diesel engine, a Bedford gearbox, a Commer diff and other bits and pieces. It was very comfortably fitted out with plenty of timber lining and turned wooden posts. We agreed to buy it.

During the rest of 1983 we made changes to the house bus so as to accommodate us as a family, and in general put our stamp on the vehicle. Any frequent use of the bus would have to wait until after David's home birth.

Because most of our trips away had to be done during school holidays, there were limits on where we could go. Before leaving Waipipi we travelled to the Dargaville area, but mostly down into the Te Puke region in the Bay of Plenty where at one stage we thought we might be living.

Eventually all the pieces came together in a wonderful way and we bought a house in Tuakau. Unfortunately to assist us with finding the necessary finance we had to sell our mobile home, but we vowed that as soon as possible we would buy another.

Although we never got round to putting a name on Number One, if we had it would have been "Genesis" on the front and "Exodus" on the back, as these names so aptly described what lifestyle changes were taking place

12 Vaccinated Kids Don't Get Whooping Cough?

"The control of pertussis (whooping cough) in New Zealand is not a simple issue yet simplistic solutions are again being offered. The beauty of these is that their failure can be blamed (unfairly) on parents whose children are not vaccinated."[1]

By 1985, the slogan that if your children were immunized they wouldn't catch *"it"*[2] was on all posters and pamphlets. Even though we knew most of the children who caught whooping cough were vaccinated, most doctors never recognized this, or would call it something else.

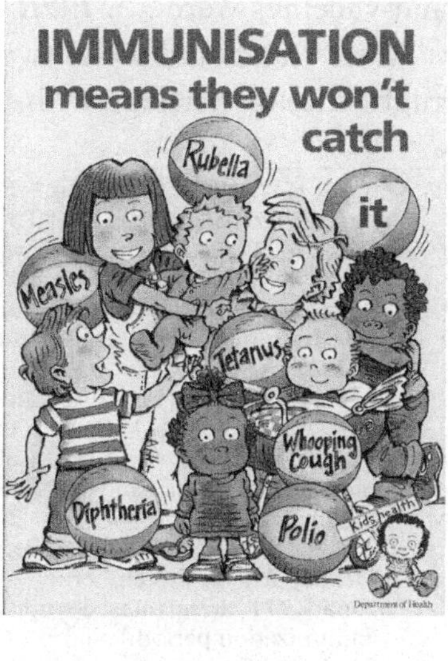

While doctors were still telling parents that their vaccinated babies couldn't catch it, they didn't seem to know that the medical literature was saying the whooping cough

1 Cullen, R. 1996. "Control of Pertussis." *New Zealand Medical Journal*, Mar 22; 109(1018): 107–8. PMID: 8606840.
2 Department of Health (1985). Code 4344 29767E-PT.

vaccine didn't work very well[3] and in other countries even children who had had four shots, got whooping cough and were hospitalized.[4] In New Zealand hospitalized cases had increased since they dropped the schedule from three to two shots, but deaths had continued to decrease.[5] Perhaps doctors didn't think to question why the death numbers had decreased before and after the vaccine, but that hospitalized cases had not. The public was told that decreases in deaths was because of the vaccine.

In 1984, the Health Department put the schedule up to three shots again, but that made no difference either.[6] Still the epidemics came about every fours years,[7] with the 1990 spike even higher than the 1982 epidemic.

In the article mentioned previously[8] parents were told that the **more** children vaccinated against whooping cough, the better, because vaccinated children didn't spread the disease through the community. So naturally, families who didn't vaccinate were accused of infecting everyone else.

Did we vaccinate Ian in 1982? No. On 5 January 1989, both Ian and David were diagnosed as having whooping cough.

In 1990, the Health Department very bravely brought out a new, bolder pamphlet.[9] Yes, the publicity continued to tell parents that being immunized meant you couldn't get it, but now they claimed that vaccines were . . . ***FOR LIFE!***

Well, that could mean two things. If you didn't get vaccinated, you might die, or perhaps with the benefit of hindsight, acknowledging

---

3 Begg, R.C. 1984. "Pertussis – New Zealand 1982/83". *New Zealand Medical Journal*, Jun 27: 97(758) 408–411. "These results indicate a vaccine efficacy of 58% (limits within a 95% confidence level vary between 51.9% and 64.7%)." p. 410.

4 Begg, R.C. 1984. "Pertussis – New Zealand 1982/83". *New Zealand Medical Journal*, Jun 27: 97(758) 408–411. "In a Finnish study (1972–75), 34% of 119 hospitalized pertussis patients had been fully immunized with four doses." p. 410.

5 Begg, R.C. 1984. "Pertussis – New Zealand 1982/83". *New Zealand Medical Journal*, Jun 27: 97(758) 408–411. PMID: 6589532. "Following the change from three injections of plain vaccine to two doses of absorbed vaccine, an increased number of hospital cases in 1974, 1978 and 1982 occurred, but deaths due to pertussis have continued to decline." p. 409.

6 Bandaranayake, D. 1987. "Pertussis in New Zealand". *The Communicable Disease Monthly Report*, December: p. 2. (Dr D. Bandaranayake:) "Except for the period from 1965–1971 these rates do not compare favourably with rates obtained in the pre-immunization period."

7 Clinical Microbiology Unit. 1992. *Communicable Diseases New Zealand*, March: Vol 92(3): 1. Surveillance Summaries, Pertussis in New Zealand.

8 Rae, B. 1999. "Disease Time Bomb". *Weekend Herald*, 8–9 May: J4.

9 Department of Health (1990). Code 4344.

Annual numbers of patients discharged from hospitals from 1914–1996

From 1944–1954 less than 10% of the paediatric population was vaccinated.
From 1955–1959 the whooping cough vaccine was discontinued.

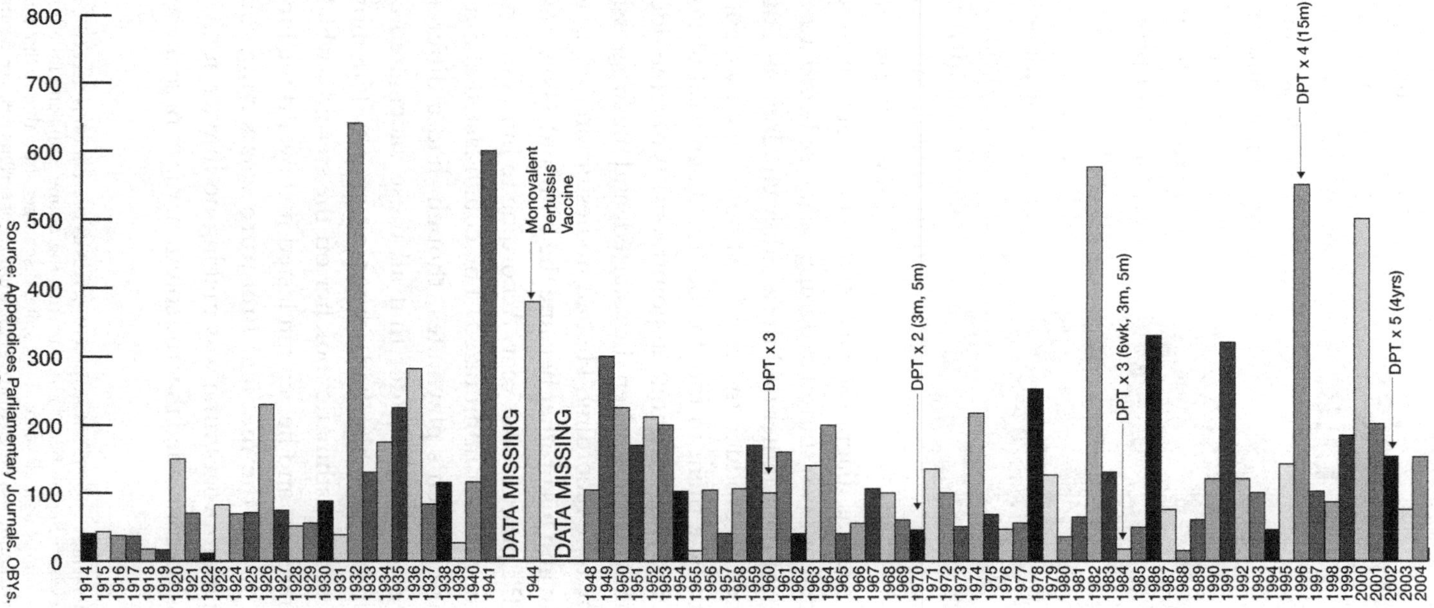

Source: Appendices Parliamentary Journals. OBYs.
Annual Surveillance Summaries

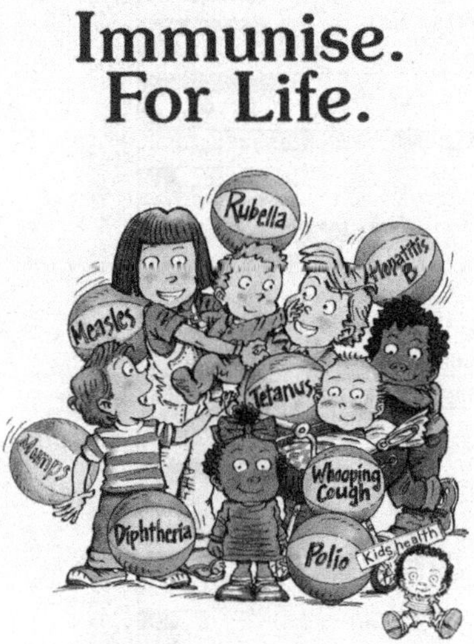

that in the future, your life could be governed by yearly pricks of one sort or another.

As home-schooled children, the boys mainly played with two local families. Their fully vaccinated playmates, who were the same ages, had had prolonged bouts of coughing for some time before our children started their imitations.

One family was told their children had infected bronchitis. The father of another family had come back from Hawaii with a cough that went on forever, and when their daughter got it, she was diagnosed with asthma and put on steroids.

When our two started coughing, what we heard was identical to the coughs of their father and these other children, but our younger son managed to produce the classic whoop, which we got on audiotape. I didn't take them to the doctors for diagnosis but instead rang and made a paying telephone appointment. When the doctor rang I told him the symptoms, when they started, and the progression, and played him the tape recording. He had no hesitation in diagnosing pertussis and Ian and his brother became the 70th and 71st cases of pertussis in our GP's practice that year. According to him, our two were the only two who weren't immunized. The cough lasted about 100 days.

Our children's playmates, though, had a different doctor who refused to even consider that all these vaccinated children in the district who saw him had whooping cough. The mother of the girl diagnosed as asthmatic took her off the steroids, which were making no difference, and her cough lasted just over three months as well.

By 1994, the medical literature was saying that the current vaccination programme was making no impact at all.[10] The medical profession concluded that the solution was to raise the total vaccination

---

10 McNeill, C. 1994. "More potent pertussis prevention is needed". *New Zealand Doctor News*, 15 September. "The current programme is making little impact on the disease . . . for the past 20 years . . . hospital discharges show that in that period the vaccination programme has failed to arrest the number of serious cases or deaths from the disease." p. 14.

rate, and make sure babies got their three jabs on time by five months of age, an explanation that ignored the fact that most cases occurred in babies older than eight months, and young toddlers.

When the 1995 outbreak of pertussis came around, the publicity was the same old stuck record. As before, most of the cases in all ages occurred in fully vaccinated children. In one local school, most of the children who started coughing were sent back to school with a variety of diagnoses, such as infected bronchitis and asthma. But there were four additional labels: adenovirus infection, one-hundred-day cough, bronchoseptica, and the best one? Pseudo whooping cough! Some adults who had had whooping cough as children got it, (though few were diagnosed as having whooping cough) disproving the theory that having had the disease once conferred lifelong immunity.

1995 was the first year that I heard major complaints about children with constant coughs being treated with asthma drugs. Specialists in the country were getting concerned, not that the asthma was whooping cough, for perhaps they couldn't see that, but it was ironic that a Hamilton paediatrician[11] should take doctors to task publicly that year, for prescribing asthma steroids for ***"a whole raft of children with coughing illnesses . . ."*** because these drugs could cause stunted growth, high blood-sugar levels, and premature skin ageing.

The *New Zealand Medical Journal* was now saying that the vaccine was 91% effective,[12] but also that boosters were needed after three shots, so a fourth dose was added. Much later, I found an article which tested the vaccine New Zealand used against newer acellular vaccines in an epidemic situation and found that actually, ours only had an effectiveness of 28.5%.[13] This same article gave the best five-component acellular vaccine a 75.4% effectiveness rate.

The chasm between the propaganda and the reality galvanised a group of local parents affected by the issue to try to do something about the rampant community misdiagnoses. With the assistance of an

11 Young, A. 1995. "Doctors told to take care with children" and "Asthma misdiagnosis worries specialist". *New Zealand Herald,* October: 2–3. Quoting Dr John Gillies on prescription of Betnesol, and Prednisone tablets . . .

12 Lennon, D. 1996. "Control of Pertussis". *New Zealand Medical Journal,* July:109(1026): 283. PMID: 8769055. "Our particular brand of whole-cell vaccine, in a carefully conducted study, had an efficacy of 91% . . . there is no doubt that infants are not fully protected until they have received three doses of the vaccine and then require boosters to maintain immunity."

13 Storsaeter, J. et al. 1998. "Levels of pertussis antibodies related to protection after household exposure to Bordetella Pertussis". *Vaccine,* 16(20): 1907–16. PMID: 9796042.

interested GP, they managed to have eight samples from two families tested.[14] All samples came back positive. The families took the test results to the school and suggested that the other coughing children who their children had caught it from, may have had whooping cough as well, a suggestion which was hotly argued.

The rumpus reached the Health Department, because soon after that a directive was issued that PCR swabs for whooping cough would no longer be accepted from any Auckland doctor. The excuse given was that ***"PCR testing is much too expensive to use on not very sick kids in the community"***.[15]

I think the real reason for the sudden stopping of the tests was that the Health Department didn't want to know what was going on in the community, and certainly didn't want people waving test results around to prove that being vaccinated against whooping cough, means you can still get it.

Browsing through newspaper articles collected over the years, it is interesting to note that most of the children featured in papers had been previously vaccinated. If it was true, as doctors were saying, that the most serious cases always happened in the unvaccinated, why couldn't the papers find all the wan-looking unvaccinated children, whose parents would just love to say that all parents should just vaccinate and save themselves some heartache? If it were true, as we were told all the time, that our whooping cough vaccination rates were worse than abysmal, where were the hundreds of dead or brain-damaged unvaccinated children in New Zealand?

Unvaccinated children don't usually get whooping cough seriously. That is recognized in the literature as well.[16,17] Unvaccinated young

---

14 Two by bacterial swab and six by PCR (polymerase chain reaction). *Auckland Healthcare Laboratory Handbook* (1998). p. 26. PCR is a more reliable test. (8 people tested. Two grandparents who had had whooping cough as children; one parent, fully vaccinated, whooping cough at 13; now at 33, coughing; two children of parents above. Plus family friends; two children, also whooping cough vaccinated, now coughing. One adult of children above.)

15 The explanation given to me directly from two GPs who had tried to get tests done.

16 Cherry, J.D. et al. 1999. "The science and fiction of pertussis vaccine". *Pediatrics*, Dec: 104(6): 1381–3. PMID: 10585991. ". . . a substantial number of B pertussis infections in unvaccinated children are mild and would not meet the case definition."

17 Jenkinson, D. 1995. "Natural course of 500 consecutive cases of whooping cough: a general practice population study." *British Medical Journal* February: Vol. 310: 299–302. PMID: 7866173. Retrieved on 18 September, 2005 from <http://bmj.bmjjournals.com/cgi/content/full/310/6975/299> "Most cases of whooping cough are relatively mild . . . Parents can be reassured that a serious outcome is unlikely . . . publicity . . . has created a widely held perception that the disease is always severe, debilitating and dangerous. Such a perception helps to encourage immunization, but

babies can get very sick if their mothers don't know what they are doing. Yet, according to the medical people of the time, the vaccinated children were all catching it because all the unvaccinated children were spreading it around. During an outbreak in Waikato, the then Medical Officer of Health tried to blame it all on unvaccinated children. In a reply to a query from me, Dr Hood stated that the babies in hospital were unvaccinated, but it turned out that the hospitalized babies were up-to-date with the schedule, but not yet old enough to have had the last injection, and were therefore classified as *"unvaccinated"*.

Medical literature in 1990, had reported widespread silent transmission of whooping cough amongst vaccinated children[18] and one of the more recent articles on the issue admitted that vaccinated children may be the major reservoirs for infection.[19] There is no may about it. But in 1997, such a suggestion was worse than heresy.

A school in Tarras in the South Island with a very high vaccination rate, contacted me one June, after staff and most of the children got whooping cough. I provided them with information on the disease, and testing for it. Three tests were done. In September, the Health Department arrived, with nearby families also being visited by health nurses who wanted not only to re-vaccinate already-vaccinated children, but to fill them with antibiotics as well. In Invercargill the same year, the first case of whooping cough was in a vaccinated child, as was the first reported case in the Hutt Valley that year. Because doctors assumed that pertussis vaccines provide protection, cases of whooping cough were grossly under-reported and under-diagnosed.

In January 2000, the Immunization Awareness Society[20] wrote to Dr Nikki Turner of IMAC to find out how many children with pertussis had had vaccines, and if so, how many injections. The figures

---

if untrue degrades diagnostic accuracy, produces inaccurate epidemiological data and hinders the wise management of those with the disease . . ." This is an excellent article, which is worth reading in its entirety, to dispel even more myths.

18 Long, S.S. et al. 2000. "Widespread silent transmission of pertussis in families: antibody correlates of infection and symptomatology." *J. Infect Dis*, Vol. 161: 480–6. PMID: 2313126.

19 Srugo, I. et al. 2000. "Pertussis Infection in Fully Vaccinated children in Day-Care Centers Israel". *Emerging Infectious Diseases*, Sep–Oct; 6(5): 526–9. PMID: 10998384.

20 Immunization Awareness Society = A group set up to provide extra information and to attempt to ensure that informed choice and compulsory reaction reporting became a reality (an aim which has not been realized).

showed that most children had been vaccinated.[21] Since then, we haven't been able to get this data.

By January 2000, Dr Ossi Mansoor wanted unvaccinated children rounded up, and said the vaccination level was only 70%,[22] while Dr Nikki Turner had said it was 63%.[23] Yet newspapers could still only parade vaccinated children. Strangely though, in a fax sent to Radio New Zealand[24] Nikki Turner quoted vaccination rates of 90.6% in 1996 and 81.2% in 1998. All these sick children were coming from the era of very high vaccination rates. In 2000, there were 4140 notified cases of whooping cough; 2001 – 1334 cases, and 2002 – 1071 cases.

In January 2002, New Zealand added a fifth whooping cough shot to the schedule, to be given at four years of age. Not long after that, Nikki Turner served an interesting side-swipe at non-vaccinating parents:

> ***"You can't snack on health care and say you won't take the vaccine, but that when your child gets sick, and is on a ventilator you want all the tertiary medical services on offer. You have to be consistent."***[25]

An interesting comment, when as far as we could find out, not one child on a ventilator was there because the parent chose not to vaccinate. Is this sort of thing said to people with life-style choice diseases which are such a drain on the health budget?

What are the whooping vaccination rates now? We actually don't know. In 2003, the Counties Manukau area had a vaccination rate of 90%,[26] and local Plunket co-ordinators maintain Franklin levels

---

21 Letter from Dr Nikki Turner of IMAC dated 26 January 2000. Of the total of 913 cases for 1999, 245 were "status unknown". Of those whose status was known, 180 cases had received four immunizations, 275 had received three immunizations, 51 had received two immunization, 50 had received one. BUT that does not tell the IAS the whole story, because we could not find out the age break-down. There had been a lot of cases in babies, so it could well be that the cases didn't occur in people who had not have enough vaccines, but in children who were up-to-date for their age.

22 Langdon, C. 2000. "Poor follow-up blamed for NZ children's disease rate" *The Dominion*, 25 January. Dr Mansoor is quoted as saying: "Home vaccination workers were needed to round up children who were not getting jabs."

23 Rae, B. 1999. "Disease Timebomb". *New Zealand Herald* 8–9 May: J4.

24 Nikki Turner had faxed information to Radio New Zealand News on 7 May 1999 stating a New Zealand rate of 90.6% for 3 DPTH in 1996, and a rate of 81.2% in 1998.

25 Reid, G. 2002. "Immunization debate flares again". *New Zealand Herald*, 22 June. <http://www.nzherald.co.nz/section/story.cfm?c_id=1&objectid=2047971> (accessed 9 March 2006).

26 Walsh, R. 2003. "Jabs monitor boosts baby health". *New Zealand Herald*, 7 May: A7. Quoting Nettie Knetsch from KidzFirst.

are higher, though no data was supplied.[27] What we do know though is that Christchurch boasts a 92.5% vaccination rate[28] and there is a 92.14% rate for the Rotorua district.[29] If you go to the World Health Organization website and look at Immunization Profile – New Zealand, you will see we are right up there at 90% for the primary DPT schedule and have been for years. Or is that a myth?

In a 2002 article[30] Turner argued that ***we needed to get to the Australian rate of 90%, because they are "great now", and had no whooping cough epidemics.*** She had also said the same in 2001.[31] Before publication, I had told the journalist that I had read that Australia's vaccination rate was above 90%, but that as of 2002, they were having the worst outbreak of whooping cough since 1997. The journalist told that to Dr Poutassis (who worked with Dr Nikki Turner at IMAC (Immunization Advisory Centre)) who responded:

> ***"Well, the Aussies don't know they've got an epidemic. I've got their 2002 communicable disease intelligence (CDI) report and they say 'no epidemic occurred in 99–00 and they are not experiencing an epidemic at the moment'."***[32]

I e-mailed the reporter back a copy of the CDI report, which to my mind, said exactly the opposite.[33]

By 2003, Australia reached 95% coverage of full whooping cough immunization in two-year-olds and, as of 2005, Australia reached 95.3% coverage. Here is the Australian whooping cough data. The improved vaccination rate and extra shots don't appear to have

---

27 Personal conversation: "We have the highest rate in the country . . ."

28 Hamilton, M. et al. 2004. "Why do parents choose not to immunize their children?" *New Zealand Medical Journal*, February: 17(1189) (768) Retrieved on 18 September, 2005 from <http://nzma.org.nz/117-1189/768/>

29 Jellyman, T. et al. 2004. "Attitudes to immunization: a survey of health professionals in the Rotorua district". *New Zealand Medical Journal*, February: 17(1189) (769) Retrieved on 18 September, 2005 from <http://nzma.org.nz/117-1189/769/>

30 Reid, G. 2002. "Immunization debate flares again". *New Zealand Herald* 22 June. <http://www.nzherald.co.nz/section/story.cfm?c_id=1&objectid=2047971> (accessed 9 March 2006).

31 Masters, C. 1999. "'Dirt poor' countries top NZ in vaccines". *New Zealand Herald*, 28 September): A5. "This is a major national disgrace that Australia has managed and we haven't."

32 E-mail from Graham Reid dated 22 June 2002, 4.38 pm, and in the article. I replied, with data in next reference that showed that she was wrong in my view, but the *New Zealand Herald* refused to do a follow-up article.

33 "Communicable Diseases Surveillance – Highlights for 4th quarter 2001". 2002. *CDI*, 26(1). Retrieved on 18 September, 2005 from <http://www.health.gov.au/internet/wcms/publishing.nsf/Content/cda-pubs-cdi-2002-cdi2601-cdi2601q.htm> Text, and in particular, Figure 3 which showed the 2001 levels rising to match 1997 levels.

achieved very much:

Cases of Notified Whooping Cough in Australia[34]

Year	Number of cases of notified whooping cough in Australia
1991	323
1992	797
1993	4414
1994	5442
1995	4190
1996	4539
1997	10,749
1998	5672
1999	4359
2000	5985
2001	9504
2002	5405
2003	5101
2004	8731
2005	11,195

Australia also has a four-shot schedule up to four years of age, and in November 2005 approved a booster for 15–17 year-olds, as has America.

Remember when you see these Australian figures that they are only the cases that doctors have admitted are whooping cough. As is the case with New Zealand data, these are likely to be just the tip of an iceberg.

So even in a country with a 95.3% pertussis vaccination rate,[35] based on New Zealand's experience and similar headlines in the USA right now, it comes as no surprise to see a new recent headline saying:

"Whooping cough on the rise".[36]

34 These figures were compiled by going to the Australia Communicable Diseases Intelligence website http://www9.health.gov.au/cda/Source/CDA-index.cmf and using the URL http://www9.health.gov.au/cda/Source/Rpt_5_sel.cfm to obtain the data for each year. (Accessed 24 February, 2006).

35 *Communicable Diseases Intelligence Quarterly report*, Volume 29, Issue no 4, 2005 page 434, Table 8: Retrieved on 18 September, 2005 from <http://www.health.gov.au/internet/wcms/publishing.nsf/Content/cda-cdi2904-pdf-cnt.htm/$FILE/cdi2904.pdf>

36 "Whooping cough on the rise." 2006. *The Advertiser* 23 February. Retrieved on 18 September, 2005 from <http://www.theadvertiser.news.com.au/common/story_page/0,5936,18245776%255E1702,00.html>

The article states that south-east Queensland has had a dramatic increase in whooping cough, and the Health Minister was encouraging all family members to be vaccinated against the highly infectious disease because ***"several babies had been killed since 2001"***. So how many more shots will vaccinated people require before the Health Minister is satisfied? Will he ever be satisfied?

More interesting than that is the total absence in any other Australian papers about even higher rates of whooping cough in New South Wales and South Australia.[37]

Why have we heard almost nothing about the 2004/2005 New Zealand whooping cough epidemic?[38] In 2004 there were 3489 notified pertussis cases, and in 2005 there were 2852 cases.[39] Perhaps one reason we didn't hear about this two-year whooping cough epidemic might have been that the medical focus was diverted by the Meningitis B vaccination programme.

The other reason for silence might have been that the new whooping cough vaccine that has been used since 2001, which had been promoted as the most effective yet, could have an ***"effective vaccination"*** ***". . . as low as 33%"***.[40,41] That's the first time I've read the term: ***"effective vaccination"***. There was however one significant change in the figures in 2004. The number of notified cases in school children markedly increased, which could either reflect the effect of five shots before four years of age, or a new realization that whooping cough in vaccinated children has gone on for decades. Or both.

To justify any more whooping cough boosters in the future, the

---

37 *National Notification Diseases*, 2006. 38 January–10 February, page 3: Retrieved on 18 September, 2005 from <http://www.health.gov.au/internet/wcms/publishing.nsf/Content/C1D433012F16F39ACA256F1900039364/$File/NNDSSreport.pdf>

38 Public Health Service Staff. 2005. *ESR Monthly Surveillance Report*, February: p. 3 of 6, Figure 1. Available from: <http://www.surv.esr.cri.nz/surveillance/monthly_surveillance.php?we_objectID=598>

39 Public Health Service Staff. 2006. *ESR Monthly Surveillance Report* January: p. 6 of 7. Available from: <http://www.surv.esr.cri.nz/surveillance/monthly_surveillance.php?we_objectID=979>

40 Editorial. 2004. *New Zealand Public Health Surveillance Report*, p. 2. Retrieved on 18 September, 2005 from <http://www.surv.esr.cri.nz/PDF_surveillance/NZPHSR/2004/NZPHSR2004December.pdf>

41 Korobeinikov, A. et al. 2003. "Estimation of effective vaccination rate: pertussis in New Zealand as a case study". *J Theor Biol.* September: 21; 224(2): 269–75. PMID: 12927532. "The obtained figures indicate that in New Zealand the effective vaccination rate against pertussis is lower than 50%, and perhaps even as low as 33% of the population. These figures contradict the medical statistics which claim that more than 80% . . . in New Zealand are vaccinated against pertussis (Turner et al. 2000). This contradiction is due to the mentioned unreliability of the available vaccine."

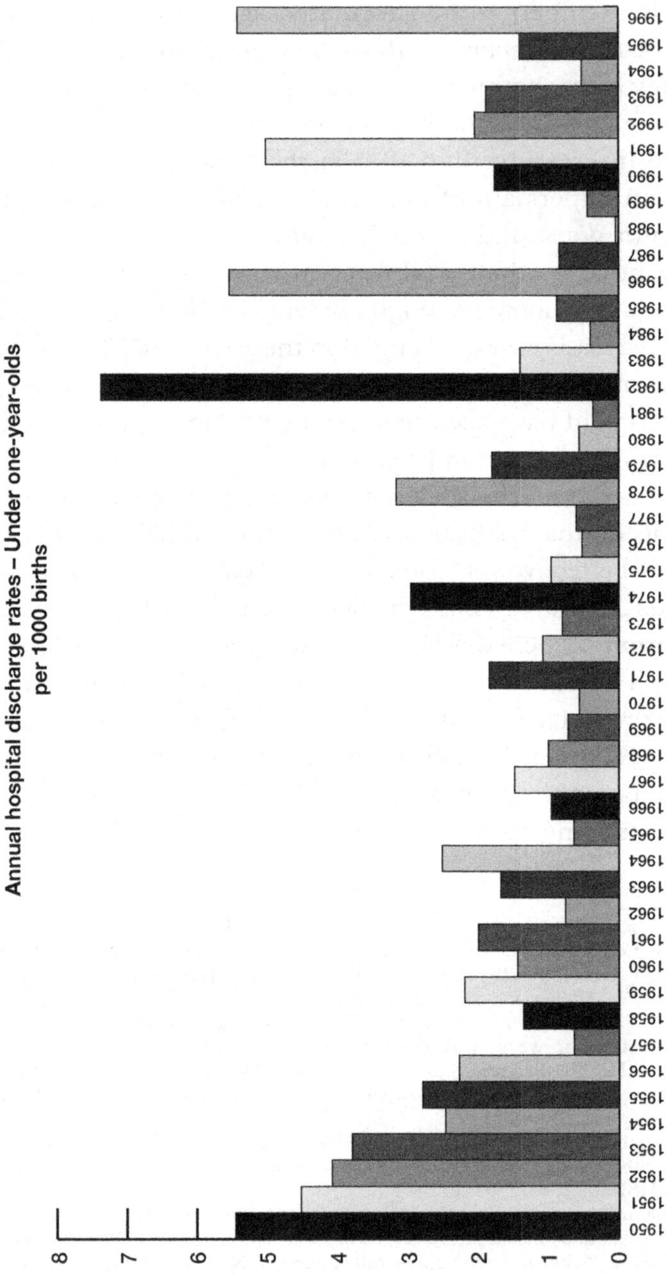

Source: *NZ Family Phys*, Vol 24: No 26; Dec 1997: p. 46

medical profession will have to admit that the pertussis vaccine never prevented community spread of whooping cough. It's a mystery to me why it was ever promoted as doing so. Doctors might also have to admit that they have made a tiny sector of the community who chose not to vaccinate, unfair convenient scapegoats in their effort to wield the big stick.

Before vaccines a person got one significant clinical attack of pertussis between the ages of 3 and 11. There may have been regular minor infections through the later years that looked like bronchitis, but long-term immunity was reinforced by regular exposure to circulating bacteria. With increasingly unpredictable gaps between natural exposure, it is now commonplace overseas for adolescents and adults to get the actual clinical disease several times, which mostly presents as a few weeks of bronchitis and coughing, a pattern that may emerge here in the future.

I believe that it won't be long before adults are told they should have regular life-long booster shots for whooping cough in order to mimic the very patterns of nature the vaccine programme has altered overseas. Doctors will say it's safer to use a needle instead of risking disease, but that's debatable.

So far, in this country, clinically severe whooping cough hasn't spread to rest-homes as it has in the USA and the Netherlands. Perhaps that's because the bacteria is still very persistent in the community, no matter how loathe the medical people have been to correctly diagnose it in vaccinated children in the past.

The increase in serious whooping cough in babies under one in New Zealand started as a trend in 1982.[42] The recent deaths have mostly been in very young babies too young for vaccination and ESR documents show that two of those deaths happened in babies with pre-existing conditions.[43] Even in England, a recent upsurge of whooping cough in children under seven weeks of age has been seen, and concerns are increasing about this new phenomenon.[44] Likewise, in the USA in 2004, 25,827 total cases were reported. Of these cases,

42 Cullen, R. et al. 1997. "Pertussis hospitalizations and mass vaccination in New Zealand 1948–1996" *NZ Family Physician* December, Vol. 24(6), Figure 2. (Not accessible on Pubmed.)

43 *PHS* "Annual Report 2004 Notifiable and other diseases in NZ" Table 30. Reported deaths from selected notifiable diseases 2000–2001, p. 55.

44 Smith, C. et al. Early infantile pertussis: increasingly prevalent and potentially fatal. Eur *J Pediatr* (2000) Vol. 159, pp. 898–900. PMID: 11131347.

2622 cases (10%) were in infants less than six months, 611 cases (2%) were in infants 6–11 months old, and 2562 cases (10%) were in children aged 1 to 4 years. Twenty-seven deaths were also reported in 2004, twenty-four of which occurred in infants less than three months old.[45]

The medical profession worldwide, continues to blame unvaccinated children for spreading whooping cough, when the real problem is the fact that the vaccine does not provide good individual or herd immunity. Dr Liz Segedin, said recently, in spite of all the evidence ***"The only way to fix it is to improve the immunization rate within the country. If everyone else isn't carrying it, they can't give it to those little babies."***[46] Again, the assumption is that if you're vaccinated, you can't carry it.

Dr Rob Everitt could tell her, if she asked, how a presumably vaccinated doctor can pass whooping cough on to his vaccinated son.[47] Dr Everitt's story as reported in the *New Zealand Herald*, was that he caught whooping cough after treating three babies who had it, then passed whooping cough to his fully vaccinated 10-month-old son. Interestingly Dr Everitt said that ***"Timothy was a very healthy baby when he caught the cough so he was coping well"***. Which is not the message that is normally passed on to parents of healthy babies. The excuse in the article as to why Timothy caught whooping cough from his father was that ***"Timothy appears to be amongst the 10% of the population for whom the vaccine doesn't work."*** A percentage which we know is far higher than that. Another question here is that if the vaccine failed to induce immunity in a healthy baby, what happens in not so healthy children? Just maybe, the vaccine isn't very good at all.

The first warning that changes had been made to the New Zealand vaccination schedule came on Thursday 9 March, when the news[48] said that at least 24 eleven-year-olds were given the higher strength whooping cough vaccine normally given to babies.

There was no publicity about this change. However, a Ministry of

45 17 November 2005, data from Dr Manisha Patel, MD., CDC Atlanta Georgia.
46 Johnson, M. Whooping cough kills baby. *New Zealand Herald* (2004, 7 July), p. A3.
47 Mold, F. "Whooping cough strikes early" *New Zealand Herald*, (2000, 23 March), front page.
48 "Children Given Wrong Dose Of Vaccine" 2006. Retrieved on 18 September, 2005 from <http://www.newswire.co.nz/main/viewstory.aspx?storyid=306268&catid=0>

Health booklet[49] sent to doctors lists the 15 month dose of whooping cough vaccine rescheduled to eleven years of age, supposedly because the primary schedule of three should last six years, and in the 2004/5 epidemic that we never heard about, there were higher numbers of cases in the 11–15 years than previously seen. Page 5 also stated that:

> *"Waning immunity and less frequent boosting of immunity from circulating pertussis mean adolescents and young adults may be at risk of pertussis disease."*

The blame for this was again low immunization coverage with *"waning immunity"*.

Given that as of March 2003:[50] *"New Zealand's pertussis vaccination programme appears relatively ineffective at controlling this disease. Epidemics are continuing to occur at 4–5 year intervals, and the rate of disease during inter-epidemic periods appears to be increasing, based on notification and hospitalization data for 2002"* why would these people think there was any decrease in circulation of whooping cough?

Here's my future prediction. Slowly, new policy will implement boosters for health workers and doctors, grandparents, and maybe teachers and pregnant mothers as well, to stop all these previously multi-punctured people giving it to newborn babies . And when that doesn't work either... there will be plenty more doses of whooping cough vaccine left over for everyone else vaccine policy makers didn't think of, to add to a never ending cycle of free cradle-to-grave on-going pricks.

Question: will any proposed new vaccines for adolescents and maybe adults be any more useful than the reported low rate of 33%–50% effective vaccination from the current baby vaccine?

Remember all this, when you think back to the days when we were told that those two little whooping cough pricks meant you wouldn't catch "it", gave immunity for life, and wiped out the deaths and cases in the past.

---

49 "National Immunization Schedule 2006" 2006. Ministry of Health. January.

50 PHS Annual Surveillance Summary 2002 (May 2003) p. 47.

13 How Parents can Whop the Whoop

In order to justify as high a figure of vaccination as the only means to protect babies against whooping cough, we are told that mothers don't pass immunity to their children. With pertussis death numbers increasing in babies under one, in a group who previously gained natural immunity from their parents, it is interesting that there are references that show mothers can, and do pass immunity through the placenta, at least, for three months.[1,2] This is one of the reasons doctors are again looking at vaccinating pregnant mothers in the last trimester of pregnancy.[3]

---

1 Goshima, T. et al. 1990. "Passive Transmission of Pertussis Antibodies". Manclark, C.R. (ed) 1990. Sixth International Symposium on Pertussis. Abstracts. Department of Health and Human Services, United States Public Health Service, Bethesda, Maryland. DHHS Publication No (FDA) 90–1162. 260 pages. "Antibodies pass easily through the placenta according to the antibody levels of the mother. Passive immunity transmission is, therefore, thought to be possible in pertussis infection." Abstract 48, p. 174.

2 Bass, J.W. and Zacher, L.L. 1989. "Do newborn infants have passive immunity to pertussis?" *Pediatr Infect Dis J*, Vol. 8: 352–3, "Therefore mothers in the pre-pertussis vaccine era, most of whom had natural pertussis as children, may have passively transferred specific antibodies, which had protected them against reinfection, to their newborn infants, providing them with protection against pertussis throughout most of the first year of life . . . in contrast it is well accepted that vaccine-induced immunity . . . is partial and transient so that most young women of childbearing years are susceptible . . . there is no reason to expect that passive immunity to pertussis should be transferred to their infants." PMID: 2748237.

3 Rosenthal, M. 1996. "Vaccinating moms to protect baby may be a practice whose time has come" *Infectious Diseases in Children*, August: p. 28. "A study of whole cell pertussis vaccine in 1945 showed that the vaccine was safe and there was transplacental passage of antibody in 57 immunized pregnant women."

The other popular misconception spread by the medical profession is that breast milk is of no use against whooping cough. While it's not a topic that garners enthusiast research money there are some older studies which show that colostrum[4] and breast milk carry specific IgG and IgA antibodies to four organisms: whooping cough, *Haemophilus* B, *Streptococcus* pneumoniae and *Neisseria* meningitidis,[5,6] all of which have corresponding baby vaccines: whooping cough or pertussis vaccine; Hib vaccine; Prevnar vaccine; and various types of meningitidis vaccines, the most recent of which was MeNZB vaccine.

Even for mothers who cannot give their babies disease specific antibodies, breast milk has other large arrays of antibacterials that should provide the baby with considerable immune support.[7]

It seems that mothers vaccinated with whooping cough as children,[8] may be facing the same situation as measles-vaccinated mothers did in the 1990s, who unlike their naturally immune mothers, were unable to pass long-lasting immunity to their baby.[9,10] This could explain why more and more very young babies are dying from whooping cough. The lucky mothers are the vaccinated girls who then got whooping cough naturally when our children did, or later on. They are more likely to be able to give their young babies reasonable levels of immunity particularly if they breastfeed as well.

The medical profession started looking at vaccinating pregnant mothers in the last three months of pregnancy way back in 1996.[11]

---

4 Helmy, M.F. et al. 1992. "Bordetella pertussis FHA antibodies in maternal/infants sera and colostrum. *J. Egypt Public Health Assoc*, 67(1–2): 195–212. PMID: 1295946.

5 Kassim, O. et al. 1989. "Class-specific antibodies to Bordetella pertussis, Haemophilus influenzae type b, Streptococcus pneumoniae and Neisseria meningitidis in human breast-milk and maternal-infant sera". *Ann Trop Paediatr* December 9(4): 226–232. PMID: 2482004.

6 Tripodi, V. et al. 1988. "Vertical transmission of immunity against B. pertussis". *Boll 1st Sieroter Milan*, Vol. 67(5–6): 357–62. PMID: 2908739.

7 Hakannson, A. et al. "Apoptosis induced by a human milk protein". *Proc Nat Acad Sci*, Vol. 92(17): 8064–8. PMID: 7644538. "Breastmilk 'furnishes a wide array of molecules that restrict microbes, such as antibodies, bactericidins, and inhibitors of bacterial adherence. Multimeric alpha-lactalbumin killed all transformed, embryonic and lymphoid cells, but spared mature epithelial elements . . . milk contributes to mucosal immunity not only by furnishing antimicrobial molecules, but also by policing the function of lymphocytes and epithelium . . .'"

8 Bass, J. et al. 1989. "Do newborn infants have passive immunity to pertussis?" *Pediatr. Infect Dis J*, 8:352–3. PMID: 2748237.

9 Darmstadt, G.L. et al. 1992. "Measles in mother-infant pairs". *Pediatr Infect Dis J*, June 11(6): 492–3. PMID: 1608688.

10 Kacica, M.A. et al. 1995. "Measels antibodies in women and infants in the vaccine era". *J. Med Virol*, Feb; 45(2): 227–9. PMID: 7775944.

11 Rosenthal, M. 1996. "Vaccinating moms to protect baby may be a practice whose time has come." *Infectious Diseases in Children* August: Newsletter. p. 28.

But to vaccinate a mother in the last trimester of pregnancy, poses considerable medical and legal hurdles.

Whooping cough hospitalization rates for illness complications, are higher for Polynesians and Maori than for Europeans,[12] a situation which applies in the case of pneumonia, measles, and meningitis, as well serious chronic ill health. It is these groups who need more constructive help than offered at present.

Without any publicity, the medical profession appears to have done a recent about-face on methods to prevent the spread of whooping cough. In 2004, the Immunization Advisory Centre admitted that vaccinated children were now coming down with whooping cough. In the past, unvaccinated children were banned from school for however long the outbreak lasted in the school. The vaccinated coughers, diagnosed as something else, stayed in class. Now vaccinated children who are diagnosed with whooping cough, are sent home, but allowed to return to school after five days on antibiotics, or three weeks after coughing starts.[13] And Dr Marguerite Dalton, from IMAC, says that the vaccine was "not one of the best we have."[14]

So what do you do if you or your children have whooping cough? You could opt for the medical approach, which is an antibiotic called Erythromycin, but in my experience a lot of children get very upset stomachs and are more upset by the antibiotics than by the coughing. Nowhere have I seen convincing scientific information in the medical literature that five days on antibiotics or a three-week period at home is a fool-proof way to prevent whooping cough spreading. For a start, other family members come and go.

Antibiotics don't make the disease better, and can sometimes make it worse. Three studies[15,16,17] have related the use of antibiotics to the prolongation of symptoms. The 2003 and 1992 studies both

---

12 Grant, C. et al. 1997. "A comparison of two pertussis epidemics in Auckland." *NZMJ*, May 23; 110(1044):182–4. PMID: 9201203.

13 Johnston, M. 2004. "Coughing kids may be banished." *New Zealand Herald*, 9 December: A3. Quoting Dr Will Paterson, Auckland Regional Public Health.

14 Johnston, M. 2004. "Coughing kids may be banished." *New Zealand Herald*, 9 December: A3. "Dr Dalton admitted the vaccine was 'not one of the best we have'."

15 Tozzi, A.E. et al. 2003. "Clinical Presentation of Pertussis in Unvaccinated and Vaccinated Children in the First Six Years of Life". *Pediatrics*, November: 112(5): 1069–75. PMID: 14595048.

16 Farizo, K.M. et al. 1992. "Epidemiological Features of Pertussis in the United States, 1980–1989". *Clinical Infectious Diseases*, Vol. 14: 708–19. PMID: 1562663.

17 Mertsola, J. et al. 1983 "Intrafamilial spread of pertussis". *J. Pediatrics*, Sep; 103(3): 359–63. PMID: 6886900.

mentioned that children treated with antibiotics have a longer duration of cough than those not given antibiotics. They reasoned that:

> ***"antibiotic treatment was found to be a marker of severe disease."***

I don't accept this reasoning, because I've seen children with mild cases of whooping cough being given antibiotics and within 24 hours the coughing will become substantially worse. I believe there is another mechanism at work here, which shows up two related problems.

Whooping cough is a *toxin-mediated* disease, which means that the symptoms you see and hear are caused partly by the toxin released from the bacteria sticking to the hairs in the bronchials. The toxin cuts off the hairs in the bronchials. Normally the mucus in the lungs and bronchials circulates around, being swept up the bronchials by those cilia that the toxin cut off, then moving down into the stomach where stomach acid deals with potentially problematic bacteria. This steady circulation of mucus out of the lungs is important to keep the lung mucus surfaces healthy and stop bacteria multiplying and causing infections.

With the hairs in the bronchials being gradually chopped off as bacteria numbers increase, the mucus from the lungs comes to the base of the bronchials, and then the problem occurs, because there are fewer cilia, and they don't cope as well with moving the mucus upwards. Mucus starts to pool at the bottom, and interferes with breathing so the child starts to cough to move it up. As more hairs are cut off, mucus pools more, and coughing it up gets harder, and takes more coughs, as the body tries to get the excess up, so that the mucus in the lungs can be replaced. The pertussis toxin also irritates the bronchials and increases and thickens mucus production.

The pertussis toxin from the bacteria can also cross through the mucus membranes and is degraded in the body in two ways. Firstly, through the kuppfer cells in the liver chomping up the endotoxin, and secondly, by antibodies in the blood.

The antibiotic used for whooping cough is erythromycin, which indiscriminately kills gut flora and other toxin producing bacteria in the body. Throughout this book, you will see mention of endotoxaemia from e-coli in the gut.[18] It is well known in medical literature that if

18 The current theory is that most e-coli are beneficial in humans, but that a few types are

you try to treat e-coli problems with antibiotics you make the problem worse, because the bacterial die-off in the gut means that the bacterial envelopes (which are the toxin) become a huge source of curlin, or endotoxin, which the liver then has to get rid of. Exercise-induced endotoxaemia doesn't come from an E-coli with an aberrant gene. It comes from a generalized release of E-coli curlin from the gut into the bloodstream.[19]

If you give antibiotics to a child who has substantial levels of gram negative bacteria in their gut flora[20] and who are also processing whooping cough endotoxin via the liver and antibodies in the blood, the antibiotics will cause massive general bacterial die-off. Not just e-coli in the gut, but also other gram negative bacteria die. These other bacteria release their toxins into the body as well, placing a huge amount of extra stress on the liver and on the antibodies in the blood. I believe it is this general die-off that causes extra stress on the body when erythromycin or zithromax is prescribed, that makes some patients with whooping cough worse.

So what are the options?

High doses of Vitamin C (sodium ascorbate[21]) have been written up in the medical literature of old by many doctors in the past, even surprisingly a Japanese doctor.[22] A pub med search showed

---

not. These types are considered to encode a protein that causes cell death in humans. However, if you look at the huge amount of early research, you will see that all types of *E-coli* were considered potentially dangerous IF there were greatly increased numbers in the proximal ileum and jejunum. Invasion of *E-coli* into these more absorptive portions of the small intestines results in absorption of increased amounts of lipopolysaccharides (LPS or endotoxin or curlin) which can then set up a cascade which can potentially lead to death. *E-Coli* is normally kept in check, in place by a good balance of other gut flora and a well functioning liver, but the body requires good levels of Vitamin C to deal with endotoxin. Other gram negative bacteria can also produce an almost identical endotoxin. Endotoxemia is a complicated subject. A pubmed search using Endotoxin and Vitamin C is a good place to start. Also see <http://www.acnem.org/journal/24-1_april_2005/endotoxin.htm and http://tomlevymd.com/vcthree.htm>

19 Ashton, T. et al. 2003. "Exercise-induced endotoxemia: the effect of ascorbic acid supplementation." *Free Radic Biol Med.* August: 35(3): 284–91. PMID:12885590.

20 Such as formula-fed babies, or children who have had their gut flora altered by several courses of antibiotics where doctors have not corrected the antibiotic damage with probiotics.

21 I use *Vitamin C* and *Sodium Ascorbate* as interchangeable terms. The biochemically neutral and preferred form of Vitamin C is always Sodium Ascorbate. Never allow yourself to be conned into buying anything else. Other forms will work in the short term, but they have affects on the body chemistry which, in the long term, are not desirable.

22 Professor Hattori, 1936. "Concerning the vitamin C therapy of whooping cough." *Klinische Wochenschrift*, December: 15(51): 1884–1885. Retrieved on 18 September, 2005 from <http://www.seanet.com/~alexs/ascorbate/193x/otani-t-klin_wchnschr-1936-v15-n51-p1884-eng.htm>

many studies[23] where Vitamin C was used successfully for treating endotoxaemia from many types of gram negative bacteria.

The medical profession's stonewalling of the use of sodium ascorbate for toxin neutralization is paralleled by ignoring, until recently, the use of Vitamin A to reduce complications and deaths in measles, and other viral conditions which increase the body's need for Vitamin A.

It also parallels the ignoring of the literature which shows selenium to be crucially important for all viral infections, especially influenza, Hepatitis B, coxsackie, Hantaan haemorrhagic fever, entero and polio viruses, HIV, and rheumatoid arthritis. It seems farmers who give selenium to their animals, know more about selenium than many in the medical profession do. A recent newspaper article[24] said that no attempt has been made to increase New Zealanders' intake of selenium, because Otago University made the astonishing claim there have been no adverse consequences for our health and that we have adapted to a low selenium intake. Funny how this country has some of the highest rates in the world of the acute and chronic diseases that you would specifically expect to see in people with a selenium deficiency.

We first came across the literature used for treating whooping cough with Vitamin C in a strange way. We had known about it vaguely, but had no guide as to dosages, so the amount I was giving to our coughing children was an uneducated guess. One morning, an American doctor rang me as I was trying to help our younger son pull on a long-sleeved T-shirt, which got stuck as I answered the phone. In the struggle to get his arm through, David started coughing and whooped. The doctor recognized the whoop, and asked what my treatment protocol was for the cough. When I told him, he told me my dose of Vitamin C for him was far too low. He sent me some medical articles on the use of Vitamin C in toxin-mediated diseases.

After I increased the doses to the correct level for each child, there was a dramatic improvement. Our younger, who has a different immune system to the older (who never whooped), required a much higher mg rate per kilo of body weight than the older one. Also, the

---

23 An internet search engine for medical articles at http://www.nebi.nlm.nih.gov/entrez/query.fcgi. Where you see a reference with a PMID number that is a pubmed ID number.

24 2002. "Selenium too important to ignore". *Christchurch Press*, 22 June: D15. Quoting Otago University.

greater the amount of the toxin level, the higher the dose you will need until the toxin is neutralized. It took 12 hours to get a marked improvement in the coughing, but 48 hours to clear toxin out from the whole body. The symptoms dramatically reduced, and the pink eye disappeared in the younger (ocular pressure from coughing). When both children got diarrhoea I was able to reduce the dose to a stable dose, which was different for each child. As the infection process ran its course, the doses reduced further, so I ran a sodium ascorbate chart stuck to the front of the fridge so that I would remember which child received what amount. David only whooped about five times.

Using references from the articles sent by my American doctor friend, I hunted out other articles on the treatment with Vitamin C of any toxin-mediated disease, and books with extensive documentation, solely from the medical literature. I was astounded that so much information existed, and even more astounded at how ferociously it has been disparaged. If the saying is, ***"where there's smoke there's fire"***, then this was a massive forest blaze. The two more recent books explain how Vitamin C works, and when and how to use it,[25,26] but best and most comprehensive from a clinical point of view, is a three-volume medical text written by Professor C. Alan B. Clemetson and published by CRC Press in 1989.[27] Like all medical books, it was priced far too high, and was never reprinted. Perhaps doctors thought they knew all there was to know about Vitamin C just from the old stories about scurvy, not realising that sodium ascorbate is far more than just a vitamin. It has so many biochemical actions on the body that this extremely powerful and versatile substance warrants far greater use in many areas of medicine.

If you do choose to use Vitamin C though, be warned. Don't expect any doctor or hospital system, to treat you as anything other than an eccentric. Be prepared for some to treat you as if you are a positive danger to your child. You might even be told that your child could get kidney stones or rebound scurvy, neither of which is true.

Perhaps stimulated by antibiotic resistance, and desperation at the

---

25 Levy, T.E. 2002. *Vitamin C, Infectious Diseases, and Toxins: Curing the Incurable*, Philadelphia, Xlibris Corporation. ISBN 1-4010-6964-9.

26 Hickey, S. and Roberts, H. 2004. *Ascorbate: The Science of Vitamin C*. Lulu Press. ISBN 1-4116-0724-4.

27 Clemetson, C.A.B. 1989. *Vitamin C*. CRC Press Inc, FL. 33431, USA. Volume 1: ISBN 0-8493-4841-2 318 pages. Volume 2: ISBN 0-8493-4842-0 236 pages. Volume 3: ISBN 0-8493-4843-9 264 pages.

idea that medics may soon be looking down a very empty therapeutic barrel in terms of antibacterial treatments, there have been a lot of interesting articles in the medical literature regarding Vitamin C and the treatment of another toxin-mediated disease: bacterial meningitis or sepsis.[28,29,30] Following these through on cross-searches reveals huge amounts of other information which details how and why sodium ascorbate is a logical treatment modality for all toxin-mediated diseases.

Had information published recently in the *NZMJ* on the subject been taken seriously,[31] perhaps some of the recently well-publicized meningitis cases would not have died, or would not have undergone amputations. What was there to lose?

In the case of whooping cough, throughout the by-choice-unvaccinating community, the information on use of Vitamin C in pertussis and other toxin-mediated diseases has spread like wildfire in the last 20 years. It is very effective, and reduces the severity of the cough in all ages, by 75%, usually within a day. Babies and children don't lose weight, don't lose condition, don't vomit nearly as much, if at all; have far less thick mucus, very few problems with breathing, they stop whooping, and seem to have no visible apnoea attacks. The coughing becomes nuisance value only.

Something else you are not told is that for six to nine months after having had whooping cough, any cold or infection in the chest will result in the same characteristic cough because until those hairs grow back again fully, to sweep away the mucus with ease, any infection will cause an increase in mucus which will pool, and the child will have to cough it up, just as with whooping cough.

No, there have never been any controlled scientific studies done on Vitamin C and whooping cough. Giving official recognition to an effective treatment for whooping cough would remove a potent emotional lever in promoting the vaccine, namely, ***"there is nothing***

28 Long, C.L. et al. 2003. "Ascorbic acid dynamics in the seriously ill and injured". *J Surg Res*, 109(2): 144–8. PMID: 12643856.

29 Galley, H.F. et al. 1996. "Ascorbyl radical formation in patients with sepsis: effect of ascorbate loading". *Free Radic Biol Med*, 20(1): 139–43. PMID: 8903690.

30 Voigt, K. et al. 2002 "Decreased plasma and cerebrospinal fluid ascorbate levels in patients with septic encephalopathy". *Free Radic Res.* 36(7): 735–9. PMID: 12180123.

31 Godfrey, M.E. 2004. "Haemorrhagic meningococcal meningitis: is it scurvy?" *New Zealand Medical Journal*, August: 117(1200) Retrieved on 18 September, 2005 from <http://www.nzma.org.nz/journal/117-1200/1029/> PMID: 15475995.

***we can do to treat whooping cough"*.**

It is to be hoped, for the sake of clinical meningitis or sepsis cases of any type to come, or babies with pertussis, that doctors won't wait another two decades to figure out that by using Vitamin C, no pneumonia[32,33,34,35] or damage need continue[36] to young or premature babies from the whooping cough toxin, or from most other toxin-mediated diseases for that matter.

32 Hemila, H. et al. 1999. "Vitamin C and acute respiratory infections". *Int J Tuberc Lung Dis*, Sep; 3(9): 756–61. PMID 10488881.

33 Hemila, H. 2004. "Vitamin C supplementation and respiratory infections: a systematic review". *Mil Med*, Nov; 169(11): 920–3. PMID: 15605943.

34 Wintergerst, E.S. et al. 2006. "Immune enhancing role of Vitamin C and zinc and effect on clinical conditions". *Ann Nutr Metab*, 50(2): 85–94. PMID: 16373990.

35 Bakaev, V.V. et al. 2004. "Ascorbic acid in blood serum of patients with pulmonary tuberculosis and pneumonia". *Int J T ubercl Lung Dis*, Feb; 8(2): 263–6. PMID: 15139458.

36 Johnson, M. 2004. "Whooping cough kills baby". *New Zealand Herald* 7 July): A3. Quoting Dr Liz Segedin, "little babies suffering from the disease were often untreatable. Antibiotics could kill the bacteria that caused it, but it was a 'toxin-mediated disease' and the damage could continue, particularly in young, prematurely-born babies. They could develop high pressure in lung blood vessels and pneumonia."

14 Pearls of Wisdom

All vaccines are first tested on animals for "safety". The flu vaccine is tested on chickens using the ***"chicken challenge assay"***. Monkeys are given an intraspinal injection of the oral polio vaccine, rats are injected with the injectable polio vaccine, and guinea pigs injected with tetanus and Hepatitis B vaccines.

A good example of some of the science behind these tests is the mice testing of the whooping cough vaccine, which looks at what whooping cough toxins will do to mice. The only test specified by regulatory authorities such as the World Health Organization is the weight gain test, but two others are also done.

Mouse weight gain test for safety

> Testing laboratory staff inject vaccine into the abdomens of mice, then weigh them regularly. If the mouse loses lots of weight, apparently the vaccine is more likely to cause brain damage in your child.[1]

1 Corbel, M.J. et al. 2004. "Toxicity and potency evaluation of pertussis vaccines". *Expert Rev. Vaccines* 3(1): 89–101. PMID: 14761246. It is stated that this test "correlates with adverse reactions" yet in the next breath they go on to say its "mechanism is unclear". (I can't work out how weight loss equals brain damage either, actually.) They also say it's not a useful procedure for acellular vaccines.

Kendrick test for effectiveness

> Staff will use several groups of mice and inject into their brains different amounts of whooping cough bacteria several times, until they establish the exact amount that will kill exactly half of the injected mice.

When the right dose is established they use two new groups of mice. Group A is injected with the vaccine. Group B get none. After a few weeks the exact amount of bacteria that killed half the mice is then injected into every mouse's brain.

Then they watch the mice. In the unvaccinated group, presumably half the mice die. In the vaccinated group, if fewer mice die than in the unvaccinated group, then they assume that vaccine is going to work in your baby.

The Kendrick test is supposed to *"correlate with protection"* or prove that the vaccine works. Which is patently a nonsense. The biggest proof of that stares you right in the face. Vaccinated babies and children catch whooping cough. Another proof is the fact that the number of injections you are told your child needs increases every few years.

The article says that the Kendrick test is inadequate.[2] So even they must see that it isn't relevant to humans.

Hist test for how much residual toxin is in the vaccine

> Vaccine is injected into the stomach of the mice. Four to five days afterwards they are injected with histamine, and the number dying within 24 hours is recorded. If too many mice die, there is too much residual toxin in the vaccine for your baby.

This one, they say[3] is so inadequate it ***"must be regarded as a priority for replacement"***.

Of course concerns about these tests have been voiced.[4] Especially

2 Corbel, M.J. et al. 2004. "Toxicity and potency evaluation of pertussis vaccines". *Expert Rev. Vaccines* 3(1): 89–101. PMID: 14761246. "A better potency assay is needed."

3 Ibid p. 94.

4 Christopher, P. et al. 1991. "Committee to review the adverse consequences of pertussis and rubella vaccines". *American Institute of Medicine*, Appendix (C): Available from <http://www.nap.edu/catalog/1815.html> "Bordetella pertussis does not naturally cause disease in animals . . . The causes of toxicity (manifested as poor weight gain) in the test are not well understood . . . Results of the test have been shown to vary with the adjuvant or absorbent used with the vaccine, mouse strain, diet, size of cage, ambient

the fact that mice do not exactly correlate to human beings anyway.

Yet despite stated misgivings, 58 years after these mouse tests were first developed, they are still the benchmark for proving that whooping cough vaccines are safe and potent.

The other interesting point is that test results depend on the age and breed of mice. Some tests have to be in *"infant or suckling mice"*.[5] But most are in adult mice. Old mice aren't susceptible to respiratory infections. Some breeds are hardier, or die in larger numbers. The best breed is "ddy" (Ref 1, p. 95) but in 1991 the preference was for a "HSFSN" mouse (Ref 4, C2).

Interestingly, only one strain of whooping cough-type bacteria (strain 18-323) works well in mice. This strain is more closely related to Bordetalla brochoseptica than b-type pertussis raising further questions regarding its applicability to natural disease in humans (Ref 4, C2).

You have to ask the question: ***"Are the human breed 'mice' supposed to keel over like the 'mice' mice?"***

There are a million mechanisms by which a foreign substance like a vaccine can cause harm. These safety tests are only designed to look at a very narrow spectrum of the blatantly obvious, and even that isn't done very well. But doctors see an official report saying that the potency is effective, the vaccine is safe, and assume that these tests prove that the whooping cough vaccine is safe in all possible aspects, for every possible reaction.

So if your child dies, or maybe gets serious brain damage, autism or behavioural disorders which the tests aren't designed to look at, doctors think that that damage can't come from the vaccine, because the Ministry of Health has a piece of paper saying that the vaccine is *"safe"*.

The reality is that mouse tests are irrelevant to human biology in many ways. Some people attempt to argue that they are only regulatory stepping stones to more relevant human trials. In human trials, though, what equates to what happened to the mice? In many ways, human trials can be worse in design concept than the mouse tests.

I have two problems with human trials. The first is the exclusion of anyone who doesn't fit the healthy criteria. The second is that

---

temperature and durations of exposure to light. These vagaries further illustrate the difficulty of generalizing to humans the results obtained from studies in animals . . . It cannot be concluded with confidence that data from animal models relate to findings in humans."

5 Corbel, M.J. et al. 2004. "Toxicity and potency evaluation of pertussis vaccines". *Expert Rev. Vaccines* 3(1): 89–101. PMID: 14761246.

the control group are now given a comparable drug, usually another similar vaccine.

If a study of drugs comparing one with the other shows that both test the same, does that mean both are safe? If one comes out better, what is that relative to? One that's equally as bad, or not quite as bad? To use one product which has its own level of harm as a base-line to try to detect potential harm from a similar product is unethical and unscientific. Particularly if what you want to know is what would happen in comparison with a person who wasn't vaccinated at all. How else can you determine what is the actual risk of a side effect occurring?

Human vaccine trials usually have at least three phases, though the MeNZB[6] vaccine had only two phases.

Phase One trials are usually conducted on healthy adults, in so far as the medical profession can see that they are healthy from medical checks and records. Each phase of vaccine has two groups: the group that gets the trial vaccine, and a control group receiving a vaccine of a similar type. If, say, the adult trial is considered to provoke antibodies and doesn't cause a side-effect thought to be from the vaccine, a similar trial will test the vaccine on a couple of hundred children and adolescents. And if they go okay, then another trial might test about 100 healthy babies over the age of six months.

All trial participants have to be healthy. You won't find babies in these trials who have ongoing health issues, family history of immunodeficiency, failure to thrive, or any ill health.

Then perhaps they will test 100 healthy babies under six months.

Fifty-five per cent of the healthy six month-old babies in the MeNZB vaccine trial tests developed antibodies, but that's better than none, they say.

Normally, a vaccine proceeds to Phase Three trials in a country where that particular disease is circulating continuously in the community. In a third-phase trial, a large number of people are vaccinated, and then the disease rates in this group are compared with the disease rates in a group that is not vaccinated. That trial is the trial which usually detects post-licensure vaccine safety issues. In the case of the MeNZB vaccine, the nationwide use of the vaccine is, in essence, the third-phase trial.

So the human trials are done, and the vaccine is then pronounced

6 A meningitis vaccine of a new strain B which originated in New Zealand.

safe. Most people don't realize that the findings from these trials always include a *no public disclosure* clause, and you are not allowed to see the data gleaned from these clinical trials.

Even the FDA or CDC in the USA gets to see only the filtered final statistics. In New Zealand, the committee approving the MenZB vaccine didn't even get to see that. They took the vaccine manufacturer's word for it,[7] based on data on a similarly manufactured vaccine in a different trial on the other side of the world.

The Immunization Awareness Society requested all information pertaining to the development, data from trials, documents relating to licensing and administration of the Meningococcal Meningitis Group B vaccine for the current meningitis vaccination programme, under the Official Information Act. Almost everything we asked for, even the protocols, were withheld under confidentiality provisions of section 9(2)(ba)(i) of the Act. We only got to see the clinical trial applications and information to volunteers.[8]

An example to consider : A study of five vaccines at birth

With so many new vaccines to add into the new schedule over the next few years, there is talk about putting several of them together into one needle, and starting the schedule earlier. The vaccine policy makers are worried about vaccine fatigue; parents who are sick of never-ending needles for one thing or the next.

You're an ordinary parent, right? Then imagine you are asked to participate in an ongoing trial[9] where they are giving DtaP, Hepatitis B, IPV in one shot to 260 babies at birth. The trial is to compare what these vaccines do to babies at birth in comparison with using the same combination vaccine in another group of babies at 2, 4 and 6 months and a DtaP vaccine booster at 15 months of age. They want to assess age-specific antibody responses following each vaccine dose and assess T- and B-cell correlates of immune responsiveness.

You are asked to read all the information and you find that your baby

7 Minutes of the Vaccine Sub-committee meeting, dated 5 April 2004, p. 5: "The committee was concerned that there was no efficacy data for the proposed vaccine."

8 Letter dated 30 July 2004 from Medsafe to Immunization Awareness Society.

9 Retrieved on 18 September, 2005 from <http://www.clinicaltrials.gov/ct/show/NCT00133445?order=5 Pentavalent> DTaP-Hep B-IPV ClinicalTrials.gov identifier NCT00133445 Study ID Numbers: 03-062 Last Updated: November 18, 2005 (Screen shot of page taken 23 November 2005). (DtaPIpv = Diphtheria, Tetanus and Pertussis, Hepatitis B, and injectable polio).

will be excluded from either group if any of the following apply.

- You, the mother, are a Hepatitis B carrier, or have AIDs or syphilis. Or have had Hepatitis B vaccine yourself.
- Your doctor gave you drugs that suppressed your immune system in the last three months of pregnancy.
- You were given blood, blood products, Hepatitis B immune globulin, or antibiotics for infection.
- You have diabetes.
- If you had a pregnancy problem such as the placenta coming away suddenly, or pre-eclampsia (which is a problem with toxaemia), something in the pregnancy that might cause known congenital defects or you are requesting cord blood to be retained for stem cell preservation.
- A member in your family has an immune system that doesn't work normally.
- You had problems before or in labour, such as prolonged rupture of membranes lasting longer than 18 hours.

Your baby will be rejected from the trial if it:

- was born before 37 weeks' gestation, and weighed less than 2500 grams at birth;
- needed resuscitation, received IV medication antibiotics for suspected infection, or might have any suspected medical, congenital, developmental, or surgical disease involving the immune system, central nervous system, congenital abnormalities, seizures or multi-organ dysfunction that they can't see, but could be a possibility;
- has any other health problem after examination by doctors that is considered sufficient for your baby to be excluded.

Each Phase trial (which takes a vaccine closer to being given to every baby on the planet) has very similar strict criteria to refuse babies where there is any whiff of a family health problem. That means that while a vaccine may end up being considered safe, it's ONLY safe in that tiny segment of people it was tested on, within larger society.

If it's not acceptable to vaccinate babies with any possible health problem in any vaccine study, why does it become acceptable after the vaccine has been licensed to vaccinate premature babies? Or to vaccinate at birth, babies from at risk mothers who have exactly these problems that excluded them from the study in the first place, or babies who have just come out of intensive care?

If these researchers stopped studying vaccines in some utopian mini-bubble that doesn't make up the whole real-life planet Earth, and trialled vaccine in all the babies these vaccines will eventually be given to, might they find out that there were safety issues they had not seen before?

We don't know, because the first time that happens is when the vaccine is let loose on the general public.

That's why the data which say vaccines are safe, looks so good. Researchers don't take the risk that a vaccine might somehow tip sick babies over the edge, making them worse. They don't include sick babies in the trial, because the not-quite-normal babies and children might suddenly die in larger numbers, and make the study look bad.

Think about this for a minute. Think about those animal safety tests as well.

If the animal and human trial safety and efficacy data would help sell the vaccine in any way, the vaccine manufacturer would not just release the results, they would purchase millions of dollars' worth of advertising space to make sure that everyone saw it. Patent monopolies outlaw competition, so there is no logical reason for the safety and efficacy data to be withheld from the public, except that the information contained in them could motivate parents to avoid the vaccine.

We, the public, and ordinary doctors, are left to assume that the test results are comprehensive, cover all possibilities, and would address every concern. Why should I consider injecting any vaccine into my baby when the company selling it, and the doctors trialing it, won't release all of the safety and efficacy data?

BUT parents believe the health authorities when they say:

"By the way, the vaccine is also safe for all the sick (especially for the sick, because they need it the most), the premature, babies with congenital defects and, if the vaccine is not live, immunodeficient children also need it."

Does that make sense when none of these categories of babies were included in the trials at any point, because they were too unhealthy?

So parents are reassured that if they turn up at the surgery with their apathetic child who has a little bitty fever, to be vaccinated, that's fine. So long as they are not too sick.

Exactly what is this mild sickness? The beginning of meningitis maybe, but you don't know that yet? Developing flu maybe, but not quite there yet? Perhaps your child's mild sickness is the beginning of something much bigger, and you don't know it right then?

Perhaps you ask that question. "Don't worry about it," you'll be reassured. If you ask if the vaccine could make that sickness worse, you'll be told that that's impossible. And if they do get really sick afterwards, it will be the pre-existing condition, not the vaccine that will be blamed because the vaccine is always perfectly safe. Even if that pre-existing condition could be one which would have excluded your child from any vaccine trial.

Even a visit to A&E with two broken legs is now a vaccinating opportunity. I know an adolescent admonished with: "What? You're not up-to-date on your tetanus, Hepatitis B, dT and Polio? Well, we'll do them all now, to save you time." Never mind that his body had better things to do, like heal some broken legs.

And if something unusual happens to your child after the vaccine, it must be something else because they didn't see that in the trials.

Somehow, the following recommendations for giving the measles vaccine to sick children in hospitals, from the World Health Organization,[10] didn't come as a surprise. My emphasis is added to the text:

> *"Since there are virtually no contraindications to measles vaccination, measles vaccine should be administered regardless of the patient's health status. Measles vaccination is particularly important for malnourished children and for those with chronic illnesses, as they are at increased risk of complications due to measles. An exception to this recommendation are children who on admission are so ill that they are at serious risk of dying. Although administration of measles vaccine is not dangerous in such cases, parents may incorrectly attribute a death to the vaccination."*

10 Biellik. R.J. et al. Strategies for minimizing nosocomial measles transmission. *Bulletin of the World Health Organisation* (1997), Vol. 75(4), p. 371. PMID: 9342896.

To me, the statement that the vaccine should not be given to people at serious risk of dying, because parents might mistakenly consider the death to be from the vaccine, proves that the author's priority is the reputation of the vaccine and NOT the health of the person it might have been given to.

15 A Vaccine-Free Interlude

House and houses.
Mouse and mouses. Right? Wrong!

Goose and geese.
Mouse and meece. Right? Wrong!

House and mice.
Mouse and hice. Right? Wrong.

Louse and mouse.
Lice and mice, right? Right at last!

English has some interesting inconsistencies and they can provide teachers (which includes parents of course) with a lot of laughs.

Howlers, I think they're called.

It's not just singulars and plurals, or collective nouns that can confuse children, but also the shades of meaning that have to be grappled with.

Vocabulary can produce howlers too.

This little story isn't exactly a howler, and it could be classified as *irrelevant to the book's main theme. It could be criticized for confusing the thought flow of the dedicated reader. It is included to provide a unique segment identified by the title. It's a lighthearted reminiscence to go with a yawn and a stretch before settling down for another read.*

Perhaps the children could read it.

It's an anecdote with a kink in the tale – or should it be tail?

Hilary walked into our living room the other day carefully carrying a small cardboard carton.

"I've got a new mouse," she said as she opened the lid. In amongst the "bedding" a long tail could be seen. For some unknown reason the words of the nursery rhyme flashed into my mind: "And she cut off their tails with a carving knife . . ."

I hoped this wasn't a blind mouse, and that blind or not, it would not meet the same fate.

It didn't, although an old one was sent away to be recycled.

This new mouse was a replacement computer mouse. The other had worn out through research-related over-use.

These days I think computer mouses are better known than ordinary meece.

There are many different kinds though!

Many years ago, I kept some mice in my school classroom. Apart from being a bit (?) smelly they did what mouses do well, and as their numbers increased there were plenty of willing human helpers to attend to their needs.

The joy of learning was written on the children's faces for many weeks as they observed mouse antics and life cycles.

Then came the school holidays.

Well, the old saying that meece have about cats, was rewritten.

"When the teacher's away the mice do play."

Did they ever!!!

After a couple of days I popped in to do a few housekeeping duties for the mouses.

Alas.

The display case was empty.

Hanging nearby were the blackout curtains, ruined now.

They were full of holes where the mice had wreaked havoc.

No doubt, somewhere in the wall cavities, or under the floor, another litter was being provided with nice soft bedding.

I thought I had started with the ordinary grey "house" mouses. But I have since learned about the **"ddy"** *strain. Hilary discovered in her research that the* **"ddy"** *breed of mice were the best to use for testing the whooping cough v—. Whoops! This was supposed to be a vaccine free story!!*

I think I must have had some of those meeces. Their IQs would put them in the ranks of the gifted. Being able to escape from laboratories would be a far greater incentive than my classroom breeding ground!

16 1986 – A Whole New World

After the *New Zealand Herald* article on vaccination was published in 1986, anonymity was no longer possible. Privately and publicly, many people who had reservations about vaccination contacted me. The media became half-heartedly interested, but only half-heartedly. At the *Herald* itself, there was much hostility against the reporter who had taken me seriously and annoyance that somebody had challenged medical orthodoxy.

Whereas most other social issues could be intelligently discussed across all types of media, when it came to vaccines there was a barely disguised contempt for questioning. For the first time, I realized that the topic of vaccination was more untouchable and hallowed than any other facet of medicine. If you didn't vaccinate, you might as well be breeding rats, carrying black plague, and all other pestilential diseases, judging by the reactions from the medical profession and some parents who vaccinated their children.

At playcentres, parents of vaccinated children would whisk their children away if they heard there were unvaccinated children among them. This is ironic, since the same people presumably believe in the complete protective powers of vaccines.

Dr Mendelsohn spent a lot of time talking to me about the media after this introduction to irrationality. In America, editors and journalists would report his doubts about vaccines because he was a board-certified paediatrician, and had a CV that the most conservative doctor would envy. I, on the other hand, had no formal medical qualifications, and it was easy for some journalists to dismiss me as a crank.

Anyone with the capacity to learn and think, armed with medical dictionaries and a few decent textbooks can easily understand medical literature. And Health Department decline graphs from 1872 aren't that hard to understand. The Health Department told journalists I wasn't qualified to comment. So I'd hand them graphs from the Health Department reports in the Appendices of Parliamentary journals, and new ones with subsequent data from the Morbidity and Mortality reports cross-referenced with the *Official Year Book* figures and ask, "What is so hard to understand about these graphs? Are you telling me that this doesn't say something to you?" The issue was simple really. Even the old official prevaccine deaths graphs from 1872 showed the huge decline of many of the historic immunable diseases, and speak for themselves. A 12-year-old could have a reasonably accurate analytical guess.

The medical people were forced to admit the graphs were easily understood, so changed tack by telling journalists that everything I said was misinterpreted. So I'd get a journalist to read a relevant paper, and tell me what they thought. Often their conclusions were the same as mine. Which led to the next obvious question as to whether the journalist was stupid as well.

1987 was a personal watershed year for several reasons. In March, Dr Mendelsohn came to Auckland to give a talk in his usual entertaining style, except for one not very funny comment right at the end when he announced that he and I would be writing a book together, to which I responded that that was the first I'd heard of it. He looked straight at me, and said, "Well, I want it to happen. Now."

We started protracted and complicated negotiations between Contemporary USA and Hodder and Stoughton New Zealand, but in the meantime, both of us had our hands full. Dr Mendelsohn had his busy schedules, and Auckland was in the middle of the media hysteria required to make parents scared enough to give their children a Menomune A (meningitis) vaccination. Ultimately the plan for a book came to nothing, as Dr Mendelsohn died at the beginning of 1988. In those days such a book was nothing without the selling name behind it.

The disappointment of his death was a major factor in the setting up of the Immunization Awareness Society the following year. Many people stepped in to help, wanting there to be a group of people who could provide help to each other, encouragement to mothers, and create a sense of community and they wanted to do something too. I was starting to find the speaking circuit very tiring, and without being able to publish a book, a newsletter sounded like a reasonable alternative.

17 The Truth Isn't Always the Truth

Years ago, Dr Robert A. Good,[1] who was a world-renowned teacher, researcher and paediatrician, and who would become very famous in immunology, was at a conference talking about when he was a medical student. He told how he had sat in the front row each class, writing down everything the professor said into morocco bound notebooks with all extra information he could find from textbooks and medical journals. He said:

> ***The scheme seemed to work, because it gave me very high grades in school, top scores in state and national board examinations and my choice of training spots and fellowships. I closed my notebooks however, for 10 years. When I opened them again, and studied them 10 years after so carefully completing them, I was astonished to find that they were almost entirely filled with lies. Except for a few descriptions such as well-established anatomy, everything that seemed so orderly and beautiful with the rather comprehensive treatment I had given it for one moment in history, had changed, grown, and been reordered by the scholarship of the intervening ten years. That is why it is***

1 Good, R.A. 1974. "The Immunoglobulin A system". *Adv. Exp. Med. Biol*, 45: 513–531. Impressions, summary and questions raised by the IgA Symposium. International Symposium on the Immunoglobulin A System, Birmingham, Alabama, 1973.

so important so frequently to take stock . . . and to consider what has been happening in the research laboratories and in our thinking on so many subjects.

Parents generally have little concept that what is thought to be true today, won't be tomorrow. Few know any medical history, to put into context a world where drugs and vaccines are expanding in numbers, and are big business in a way which has never been seen before.

Few know, as was so eloquently revealed in the UK paper, *Independent*[2] by Glaxo's drug expert, Dr Roses, that ***"our drugs do not work on most patients."*** Not that such knowledge gets in the way of aggressive drug promotion.

Pharmaceutical companies are now upping the stakes, by actively becoming involved by funding nurses in the state system. Fortunately some in the British system do see it for what it is.[3]

"Alan Maynard, a professor of health economics at the University of York, expressed concern. "This gives the drug companies a way in, the chance of more direct contact with patients. Ultimately they think that it will prove commercially advantageous or they wouldn't be doing it."

Should we be happy with a future system that might allow our health to be held hostage by the aims or objectives of companies which see returns from sickness primarily in terms of long-term corporate financial gain?

Actually that system already exists, in some doctors' surgeries. Stand up anyone who doesn't think a doctor's practice is a commercial business. The last thing we parents need is more control exerted by anyone who may already be under the control of vested interests, and who perhaps don't recognize that. Doctors are paid by pharmaceutical

2 Connor, S. 2003 "Glaxo chief: our drugs do not work on most patients." "It is an open secret within the drugs industry that most of its products are ineffective in most patients but this is the first time that such a senior drugs boss has gone public. His comments come days after it emerged that the NHS drugs bill has soared by nearly 50 per cent in three years, rising by £2.3bn a year to an annual cost to the taxpayer of £7.2bn. GSK announced last week that it had 20 or more new drugs under development that could each earn the company up to $1bn (£600m) a year." Retrieved on 18 September, 2005 from <http://www.ghchealth.com/glaxo-chief-our-drugs-do-not-work-on-most-patients.html>

3 Day, M. 2004. "Drug manufacturers' role in NHS raises fears over ethics". *The Sunday Telgraph*, 29 September. Available from <http://www.telegraph.co.uk/health/main.jhtml?xml=/health/2004/09/29/ndrugs26.xml> last accessed 26 February 2006.

companies to attend seminars or conferences which are financed by the companies whose products are mostly used. Some UK doctors seem quite happy to let pharmaceutical drug reps[4] examine files to see who might be a risk of certain diseases. How common will this become? Interestingly, the medical profession has a history of NOT seeing their involvement with drug companies as a conflict of interest. Particularly when it comes to matters of dissent from others.

So when the Immunization Awareness Society put on an International Vaccination Symposium in 1992, funding was, of course, an issue. Weleda, a company that makes homeopathics, gave IAS $500.00 to print the programme. The rest of the money was put up, up front, by IAS which hoped to make ends meet, and pay the bills from what people paid to attend the Symposium. We invited as many in the medical profession as we could. We wanted them to hear medical information and see the human face of what they were doing.

One of those invited was John Newman, then the Director of Child Health Services in the new children's hospital, called *Starship*. John Newman was also well known for his pithy and blunt columns in the newspapers, and articles about immunization. To him vaccination was not a dilemma, but pretty much a black-and-white choice. You chose to do it.

Those who stepped outside the paradigm of the moment, and tried to write independent research, were suddenly not independent. I already knew all the pro-vaccine stuff, but I had questions, so wrote under the banner of IRONI, which stood for Independent Research On Non-Immunization. There was no funding from the Government, pharmaceuticals, or clearing-house organizations for pharmaceutical money. I considered myself independent from compromising or vested interests.

That's not how the medical profession saw it. The minute you questioned their paradigm you are not independent, you are now biased against them.

Vaccine-promoting doctors whose whole basis of employment is to raise the vaccine uptake to saturation level, don't consider that they are biased, or compromised because they are pro-vaccine, even though

4 Templeton, S.K. et al. 2006. "GPs open up patient files to drug firms" *The Sunday Times*, 5 Feb. Retrieved on 18 September, 2005 from <http://www.timesonline.co.uk/article/0,,2087-2025628,00.html> "It emerged last week that 'nurse advisers' funded by drugs firms are also given routine access to confidential patient files."

similar areas of conflicts of interest have recently been well aired in the *British Medical Journal*[5] and other journals as well.

John Newman had said verbally that he would come to the conference called *Vaccination Dilemma*, if we would go and see his ward full of children with whooping cough. We agreed, but there were no children to see. Shortly before the conference, I was handed a copy of letter on Auckland Area Health Board letterhead:

19 March, 1992

Judy Gilbert

The Immunization Awareness Society . . .

Dear Judy,

Thank you for the information on your seminar. I have consulted with my family and will not be attending your conference. That is a pity as there will be a lot going on there that I am sure I would like to hear.

I have read your handout and am concerned that

1. It is financed by a multinational with financial interests in the field.
2. The bias of speakers is evident.
3. There are assumptions which are unwarranted and are presented as established facts.
4. There are judgements and pejoratives which betray a political bias.

With kind regards,
Yours sincerely,

John Newman, F.R.A.C.P. Director Child Health Services.

As this letter was passed around the committee, everyone read it in silence. Faces were a picture. First incredulity, then wry smiles. How droll.

5 Ferner, R.E. 2005. "The influence of big pharma". *British Medical Journal*, April 16: 330(7496): 885–856. PMID: 15831847.

18 Meningitis, then . . .

In 1987 the media woke up to the fact that not all was well in vaccine-machine land. The Auckland Menomune A meningitis vaccination campaign had become a public relations disaster. Some children were in a bad way after the vaccine. The Health Department was forced to admit that it had lost the plot by claiming it was all *"hysteria"*, so for once, the media had half the other ear open as well.

Strange things happen when a person writes in the newspaper that nutrition, housing and other social factors have everything to do with increasing the risk of catching infectious diseases, especially meningitis. And that the face of vaccine campaigns shouldn't be posters, brochures and consent forms, covered with lotteries, prizes and draws, paid for and sponsored by Homestead Chicken.

The telephone rang and at the other end was a mother so angry that even though the onslaught hadn't started, you could feel the sparks before the illogic.

> *"It's the likes of you people who won't vaccinate your kids, that make all the rest sick. Your snotty-nosed little brats are the ones who carry these bugs and put all the rest at risk."*

Even worse, at one talk in Auckland a doctor stood up and berated me, saying that the unvaccinated kids were a hazard to the vaccinated kids.

I held up for all to see, the then current Health Department wallposter. It read: *"Immunization MEANS THEY WON'T CATCH IT"*. "It doesn't always work . . ." he blustered. I asked him if he ever told his patients that. Silence. I also asked him if he could explain to our children how they got measles from vaccinated children who became sick, not unvaccinated children. More silence.

I explained to him that those of us who chose not to vaccinate our children are not telling those who want vaccines, NOT to vaccinate. All we want is to make our own choices based on all the information. Not a select few sound-bites. We want to know WHY certain people, or groups get sick and whether our child fits in that group. If they do, and we still don't want to vaccinate, what can we do to make our children healthier and safer? If they don't, then we will still want to make our children healthier and safer. We want to have enough facts to make our own decisions, about what all the risks are. It's called INFORMED CONSENT.

Yet, here we were in 1987 (and again, in 2004–2005), at the mercy of medical spin meisters.

The advent of vaccines has so far paralysed most "pavement epidemiology"[1] and gagged research into the really important risk factors of meningitis, and most other infectious diseases as well. What is the point in knowing what the risk factors are if the only thing that will be pointed at the problem is a needle and the assumption is that that will fix everything? The reason meningitis is important in terms of shoe-leather epidemiology, is that various experts predicted long ago that in spite of vaccines, meningitis would become epidemic in the future.[2]

When the 1987 promotional campaign was launched, it focused on how terrible this disease was for children, with documentaries on how this killer disease causes death, brain damage, gangrenous legs and arms, deafness and a whole host of permanent nasties enough to scare any mother watching. In 2004–2005, the tactics were similar, maybe even worse, depending on whether the children were shown "that" video.

1 "Pavement epidemiology" is where epidemiologists would walk into communities and homes to look at everything and analyse what social factors were contributing to the seriousness of various diseases.

2 Lambert, H. *Radio Pacific New Zealand* broadcast, 7 January 1988, at 7 a.m. "The trouble with this germ is that it's sort of like an iceberg. A lot of people carry the germ in their throat, and then every now and again it hits someone who's susceptible and bingo: they get the disease."

Auckland city's one million people had it drummed into them that unless 250,000 children between the ages of 3 months and 12 years were vaccinated with Menomune A, they could all drop dead. It was monotonously repeated that in two years, 141 people had caught it, and 14 had died.

During those two years before the campaign was launched, one million relaxed people didn't worry their grey matter over it, then suddenly, three weeks before the vaccine campaign, everyone went hysterical. The fact that ***"meningitis bacteria hardly ever cause disease"*** was lost in the hype, as was the really important information from the statistics.

The tactic employed by the Health Department of using lots of prizes, was to catch the attention of people who aren't usually interested in jabs, but were interested in something for nothing. Homestead Chicken supplied $25,000 worth of prizes: 2000 packs of chicken, hundreds of iceblocks, 50 Barbie dolls, 50 Masters of the Universe, 20 Postbank accounts of $100.00 each for winning children; and for the parents, 2 video recorders, 3 stereo ghetto-blasters, and a microwave oven.

All these could be yours with three chances each, but only for children who were vaccinated. Most of the space on the consent form was taken up by competition pictures and details, which were, after all, the really important information. Not only were these forms handed out at schools, but there were letter-box drops as well.

Parents who didn't want to be part of this campaign faced considerable pressure, not just from children who felt they were missing out on a chance to win if they got a jab, but also because teachers and nurses were telling the non-vaccinated children they could now turn blotchy and die. Even school principals got into the act.

Initially I thought the kids were getting the wrong end of the stick, but then teachers started to ring me because they felt they were being required to socially engineer compliance. Then a few doctors rang to say that their children had come home with the same stories.

One teacher was so upset with the Education Department education units that she supplied me with copies. Then I understood the concerns.

The important information that parents needed in order to discuss the issues were: ***"What is the risk to my child of catching this disease?", "What age are the children who are most likely to***

catch this disease?" and "Who are the groups most likely to catch this disease?" To figure that out, data was needed. After some reluctance, the following data was handed over by the Health Department, and it showed that for every 1 European meningitis case, there were 10 Maori cases and 14 Polynesian cases.

Ethnicity	No of cases	Proportion of population.	Strike rate per year
European	58	83%	20 per 100,000 per year
Maori	73	11%	200 per 100,000 per year
Polynesian	80	6%	300 per 100,000 per year

The distribution of Type A cases were:

Takapuna = 13
Auckland = 47
South Auckland = 79

Most of the North Shore cases were not Type A.

When I eventually published this data, the Health Department contacted me, and the media,[3] to say that I was being a racist. I thought I was being a realist.

Amongst survivors, there were four profoundly deaf children and six partially deaf children. There were no gangrenous, amputated limbs and no brain-damaged children. However, I was interested to see that the antibiotic used to treat those children had ***"deafness"*** written as a common side effect. So was the deafness caused by the meningitis or by the treatment?

The youngest case was 3 weeks old, the oldest 85 years, and the mean average 13.7 years of age. The majority of the 1986 cases had been older than the proposed vaccine target group, and the 1987 cases had followed that pattern even more closely.

Some people did simple division and decided 1 million people divided by 72 cases each year meant that they or their children were less likely to get meningitis than they were to get smashed up in a car crash on the road. But regardless of logical thinking, parents were never told information from the medical literature on meningococcal disease which

3 1988. "Anti-jab lobby effectively racist-doctor". *The Evening Post*, May 18.

said that only one in every 5000 carriers might get a clinical infection and only one in every 1000 clinical infections would get the actual disease.[4]

Parents were not told that meningococcal bacteria of many types are ***"commensal"*** bacteria that sit there doing nothing other than create immunity in at least 400,000 Auckland throats at any one time; that there are many meningitis varieties; that they circulate in the community all the time, and that during outbreaks, the bacteria can be found more commonly than the common cold.

It's not rocket science. But even the media didn't do simple maths and ask why it was that, if this bacterium is so common, it does nothing to most people, most of the time, and then suddenly descends like a relatively predictable axe on a few specific individuals?

Yet at the time the *Manukau Courier* screamed out, ***"About half a million South Aucklanders live in poverty, a Mangere budget adviser estimates."***[5] South Auckland would have been the first place anyone would expect to find an increased rate of infection. Not just of meningococcal disease, but of most diseases.

The Health Department line was simple. A flyswat vaccine will fix it all up now.

I tried to point out, through the media, that overcrowding, poor housing, smoking, poor general health, acute respiratory diseases, anaemia, and immune deficiencies were very important risk factors.[6] Much of the medical literature on risk factors in meningitis in 1987 was observational, whereas the very comprehensively detailed information now is more from the immunological perspective.

N. meningitidis is a bacteria carried in the nose and throat on 10 per cent of adults but[7] ***"the organism rarely colonized the proximal airways of healthy young children."*** Healthy children. How do you define healthy?

The New Zealand experts[8] said in their own publications that ***"Susceptibility is generally very low and a large proportion of***

---

4 Peltola, H. 1983. "Meningococcal Disease: Still with Us". *Reviews of Infectious Diseases*, Jan–Feb; 5(1): 71–91; 82. PMID: 6338571.

5 Ashton, A. 1987. "Hundreds in real poverty". *Manukau Courier*, June: 13(48).

6 De Voe, I.W. 1982. "The Meningococcus and Mechanisms of Pathogenicity" *Microbiological Reviews*; June: 46(2): 162–190. PMID: 6126800.

7 Pollard, A.J. et al. 2001. "Development of natural immunity to Neisseria meningitidis". *Vaccine*. 19; 1327–46. PMID: 11163654.

8 Baker, M. et al. 1992. "Epidemiology and Control of Meningococcal Disease in New Zealand in 1992". *Communicable Disease New Zealand*, July: 92(7): 57–61; p. 60. ISSN 01133-1974.

the population is colonized without ill effects." But the Health Department's 1987 response to my comments about housing, overcrowding, poverty and diet, was to say that fixing those things is too hard, and takes too long. Then they would dismiss all that by saying, ***"anyway, it hits the rich too, you know"***.

As if the rich might not also have immune system problems? Yes, it can hit the rich. But the statistics from 1985 to now show that it hits the poor far more frequently than it hits the rich.

Dr Jane O'Hallahan still tells us in 2005, that ***"meningococcal disease knows no social and economic boundaries".***[9] Another doctor[10] tells us of ***". . . unequal incidence of meningococcal disease (with rates of 28.9, 20.5, 12.1, and 6.8 per 10^5 population respectively in Pacific, Maori, European and 'other' ethnic groups) . . ."*** Dr Nikki Turner[11] told the country that, had housing and other problems been solved earlier, maybe New Zealand wouldn't have the epidemic we see today.

What can be said, is that meningococcal bacteria take advantage of IMMUNOLOGICAL WEAKNESSES, which have many causes; risk factors which are most often operative in lower socio-economic communities, but which can also occur anywhere people live under stress; or where people ignore basic aspects of health care, nutrition and environmental risk taking.

If meningococcal meningitis was an indiscriminate killer that knew no boundaries, we would all have been dead of it, long before vaccines were invented.

Even the worst type of meningitis, which is the C-type, has a reasonably low strike rate. In the UK which introduced a vaccine against the most serious C-type (one which has a hypervirulent strain ET-37) doctors said that when there isn't an epidemic, 3–9% of meningococcal bacteria found in the throats of symptom-free people was the hypervirulent strain.[12] UK had 1500 cases every year, but they also stated that as many as 500,000 people in the UK could

9 2005. *Sunday Star Times* 10 April: p. A3.

10 Thomas, M. 2004. "Prevention of group B meningococcal disease by vaccination: a difficult task". *New Zealand Medical Journal,* August: 117(1200). Retrieved on 18 September, 2005 from <http://www.nzma.org.nz/journal/117-1200/1016> PMID: 15475986.

11 Television Broadcast on *60 Minutes* on 11 April 2005.

12 Maiden, M.C.J. 1999. "Meningococcal conjugate vaccine: new opportunities and new challenges". *The Lancet,* August: 354: 615–616. PMID: 10466659.

carry it at any time, all the time, which means that as the bacteria shift around, and another 500,000 people have it, and pass it on to the next 500,000 people, eventually the whole population of the UK will have been exposed. That is, after all, how the majority of us already have acquired natural immunity.

I have listened to parents say that their children are perfectly healthy, when their children's blood tests have just returned showing clinically significant anaemia. To some parents, so long as their child isn't in bed all the time, *"they are perfectly healthy"*.

I've also heard parents who are chain smokers and who also smoke marijuana and drink alcohol, whose children are fed junk food, whose teeth would make most dentists cringe, whose children live in dirty houses, run around bare-foot, unkempt with running noses, say with a straight face that their children are perfectly healthy and well fed.

Like most of us, their children will have carried other meningococcal bacterial strains many times before, or maybe even that strain before, but that child or person may be at risk of contracting meningitis at that time, because of immune system issues, life-style factors, nutritional factors, or family dynamic stress, but to suggest the illness was just one of those things, would be ridiculous. During an epidemic, and particularly when a vaccine is being promoted, the medical profession and politicians deny that real social risk factors are relevant. Our culture prefers to blame some outside monster so that parents feel they can't control the problem and feel helpless and afraid.

Dr Mark MacDonald, the Medical Officer of Health from Hamilton, was the speaker at a May 1987 meeting in Onewhero, organized by a local doctor to promote the upcoming Menomune A vaccination campaign. He commented that on the basis of statistics that year, up until the meeting, there had been far fewer meningitis A cases than the previous two years, and that they believed that the epidemic was running out of steam. Then he said:

> *"But we can't really tell, because now is the time when we have increases in meningitis case numbers."*

I asked him, "If you are right and the epidemic is running out of steam and we do this vaccine campaign, what will get the credit? The vaccine or the natural epidemiological trend?" He didn't know how to answer that question.

The Menomune A vaccine got the credit for wiping out the epidemic[13] not just on radio, but in all subsequent articles.

After the Menomune A vaccination campaign started, there were rumblings of trouble, but nothing that gave me much concern. Reports filtered out from the media about a group of children in school vomiting, fainting, being unable to walk, feeling nauseous, looking pale and wobbly. The Health Department investigated and said it was adolescent hysteria because of an hour's delay which got the children upset. But the children didn't know there was a delay, because they weren't told. They just stayed in class until lined up for their dose.

Some of these kids got a lot sicker, and the parents weren't very happy with the *"hysteria"* tag. Worse was to come when they tried to talk to doctors in the Health Department. Some parents rang me to say that it had been inferred by the medical profession that they were being *"neurotic"*.

Then it was revealed that similar reactions had happened in other schools, too. I filled an exercise book with names and addresses of people whose children had been affected. Soon the issue was so large that hotlines had to be set up by the Health Department. The problem was, the hot line didn't work half the time, and many parents whose children did have side effects, didn't know about the hotline. Some who rang it, either couldn't get through, or got the brush-off.

About this time, Television New Zealand contacted the American office of the vaccine manufacturers, who confirmed to TVNZ that this specific vaccine had only previously been trialled in Burkina Faso, for which there were no results, and in some US Army recruits.

The news presenter, Lindsey Perigo was brave enough to confront the Health Department representative, on TV. On the same programme, I also tried to drive home the point that this vaccine was actually an experimental vaccine being used on our children. This comment brought forth howls from the Health Department who quoted studies to prove that it wasn't. When it was pointed out that the studies hadn't used the vaccine we were using here, their retort was that it was *"so similar, it made no difference"*.

By the next morning, radio reported that the vaccine manufacturers

13 Dr Dell Hood, *National News Radio* broadcast on 26 June 1987.

weren't talking to anyone. The Health Department's further "proof" that the vaccine had been trialled overseas showed that, in many studies, the vaccines used were multi-strain vaccines, not Menomune A. In the end, the Department resorted to saying that the vaccine had "passed all standard tests".

Parents started telling me about symptoms which I considered serious, and I was becoming very concerned. The medical profession brushed them all off. One of the worst cases was a young boy of 11, who was vaccinated on Friday, 5 June 1987. All Saturday he felt unwell; for three days he lay around lethargically, vomiting consistently. A ripper of a headache continued for days. Then, one morning, two weeks later, he woke up, and his arms were so sore he couldn't move them. He had stomach pains, and was as white as a sheet. By the following week his feet and legs were sore, his back was aching, and his mother, Anne, described his walk as being like that of a spastic. "He crawled into his room, sobbing . . . a total blithering mess . . . so we lifted him into his bed, but he complained that when we touched him, it hurt. He was so sore, we couldn't touch him at all. The doctors just scratched their heads." All the doctors would say was, "It can't be the vaccine." Well, what else was it then?

For months this child was lethargic, with constant headaches, sore legs and nausea, often in cycles of three weeks. The family eventually went to America in search of treatment for their son.

Out of all the cases parents related to me, only one was blood-tested correctly. This little 8-year-old girl was vaccinated on 21 June 1987. After a week of severe and painful symptoms, she was blood-tested. The liver tests were grossly abnormal, the rheumatoid test was very high, and some of the other results were also very abnormal, but in view of the fact that she was no longer in pain when the doctor finally rang to tell the parents the results a week after the tests were done, no diagnosis was offered. In fact, nothing more was said, and the doctor never reported any ***"reaction"***. The mother rang the hotline but said that no one there was interested in looking at any of the blood test results done on her daughter either.

Others reported that the examining neurologist set up to investigate reactions reported to the hotline, was pleasant enough, but wouldn't listen to parents' concerns.

At this point, Finlay Macdonald from the *Listener* wrote the first thoughtful article on poverty and overcrowding risk factors for meningitis, the side-effects of the vaccine, and presented one of the children who reacted to the vaccine.[14] He tried to pose the questions as to why so many of our children were at risk from these diseases and the socio-economic factors involved to Dr Salmond, who in my view, ducked the issue by saying that it had just crept up on them, so they had to do what they could now, and maybe later, *"We have to go back and look at the implications for other infectious diseases."*

They didn't. Then when the meningococcal B crept up on them, the medical profession did a study which confirmed their previously stated link between meningococcal disease, poor housing, overcrowded living conditions, and passive smoking. Annette King posted it on the Government website as a press release, saying that the Labour Party had said all that for years, but National had denied it and done nothing to fix it.[15] ***"The NZHS identified 'the unacceptable reality that some New Zealanders live in unhealthy housing, have poor nutrition and, in rural areas, have limited access to clean water and sewerage systems' . . ."***.

Finlay MacDonald's 1987 article brought a swift response from the Health Department who then placed the blame for unwarranted media exposure on *"anti-vaccine propaganda"*.

Looking back, the Health Department's strategy had been fascinating. First, it tried to prevent publication of unfavourable articles by delay tactics and constant denial. By July 5, the Department admitted in *Sunday Star Times* that it hadn't published material on the reactions, in order not to *"threaten"* the campaign.[16] Then, as more parents reported trouble a few Health Department people spoke out contradicting each other, so by the time the *Listener* article was published all responses to journalists were handled by one medical spokesperson and mainly consisted of comments about how well the vaccine campaign had gone.

Public disquiet was so persistent by the end of the first vaccination shots that the Health Department had to postpone the booster programme until the Adverse Effects Committee had considered the

14 Macdonald, F. 1987. "Meningitis A campaign goes astray". *New Zealand Listener*, 29 August: 17.

15 King, A. 2000. 10 January. "Findings of Meningococcal Disease study". Retrieved on 18 September, 2005 from <http://www.beehive.govt.nz/ViewDocument.cfm?DocumentID=8176>

16 Roberts, J. 1987. "Health Dept admits cover-up". *Sunday Star*, July 5: pp 1 and 3.

vaccine reactions. The committee decided on the basis of an Auckland neurologist's report that because there was *"no pattern"* to the side-effects, they were probably not caused by the vaccine, therefore it was most likely safe and effective. This was a situation that journalists found somewhat ironic, since their lists of cases showed the same distinct patterns as mine. But to be cautious, the Committee also advised that any child who had had any reaction didn't need a second dose.

Less than a third of those parents whose babies were supposed to have the second dose, allowed their babies to have it.

The Adverse Reactions Committee report studied 546 children whose parents requested full investigation. Of these, 217 were excluded for reasons of insufficient information, or were judged to be due to *"other causes"*. Of the remainder, 92 had peripheral nerve involvement, 80 of which involved weakness and heaviness in limbs, 57 had sensory disturbance with paraesthesia, dyasthesia or pain in a limb separate to injection site. Some had both sensory and motor disturbances.[17]

Guillain Barre (which used to be called *"ascending paralysis"*) was never considered to have been a side-effect, yet several children had the exact symptoms you would have expected, starting off with heavy legs, pins and needles in the extremities, and loss of balance which can then progress to breathing difficulty. Ninety-nine out of 100 cases of Guillain Barre don't result in loss of ability to breathe or swallow, but if the condition gets to the lungs, it can kill the patient if there is not appropriate medical support. It's a condition which can have long term sequelae. Anyone who experiences Guillain Barre after one vaccine should not have another one.

The Committee's conclusion was that ***"a final causality cannot be attributed according to the current data"***.[18] All the fainting, nausea, dizziness and slurred speech etc., at the time was attributed to psychological reasons. Needless to say, there were many very unhappy parents out there, who felt they were being dismissed, and seen as a vocal minority.[19] Although one consultant leapt to their defence in a medical journal,[20] no one leapt to their defence in public.

17 Hood, D. et al. 1989. "Meningococcal vaccine – do some children experience side-effects?" *New Zealand Medical Journal*, Feb 22; 102(862): 65–7. PMID: 2919016.

18 Conclusion in report (received from Minister of Health David Caygill on 13 July 1988, by Centre for Adverse Reactions Monitoring, Dr Ralph Edwards.

19 Ellis-Peglar, R.B. 1987. "Meningitis vaccination in Auckland". *New Zealand Medical Journal*, Aug 12; 100(82a): 501. PMID: 3455519.

20 Newman, J. 1987. "Meningitis vaccination in Auckland". *New Zealand Medical Journal*.

The other reason stated for considering this vaccine safe, was that such reactions had not occurred in Finland, and their vaccine was classified as safe.

I was told later, by the then Medical Assessor for Adverse Reactions, that he had been to an overseas meeting where the vaccination campaign was discussed. He said he tried to table the report, as a potential side-effects signal, but it was rejected on the basis that no other country had seen those side-effects.

Side-effects, obviously have to be seen somewhere for the first time. Why is it then, when it comes to vaccines, that no one wants to know, if your country happens to be the first?

So the reputation of the Menomune A vaccine will remain squeaky clean, by virtue of the fact that no other country, before ours, saw side-effects. The side-effects seen with Menomune A looked remarkably like the ongoing problems seen now with Menactra (A, C, Y, W135) vaccine in America.[21,22] I wonder if they too will be finally listed as coincidental.

A Department of Health national working party for the implementation of Hepatitis B in New Zealand,[23] compared the rates of doctors who reported Menomune A reactions to the Centre for Adverse Reactions Monitoring (CARM) with the numbers of parents who had heard about reporting on the hotline, and reported their children's reaction. The working party stated that:

> *". . . the 1987 meningitis campaign reporting rate was only 0.8%".*

What does that tell you about how seriously doctors viewed parental concerns? What might the real figure have been if all parents had been heard?

Oct 14; 100(833): 636. PMID: 3132658. "Unfortunately so long as we see dissatisfied customers as 'a vocal minority' we will continue to alienate groups of our clientele. Perhaps the message is starting to get through that a more literate population, a more discerning population and a more skeptical population does not look to the medical profession for magic but looks to us rather for advice, for technical expertise and above all for accountability for our actions."

21 FDA News. 2005. "FDA and CDC issue alert on Menactra meningococcal vaccine and Guillain Barre syndrome". 30 September. Available from <http://www.fda.gov/bbs/topics/news/2005/new01238.html>

22 Medscape Medical News. 2006. April 7. Available from <http://www.medscape.com/viewarticle/529405_print>

23 Minutes of 6th meeting, "Department of Health National Working Party for the Implementation of Hepatitis B in New Zealand" dated 20 January 1988, p. 3.

19 And Meningitis Now . . .

In 1990, not long after Meningitis A was pronounced "vanquished", Meningitis B case numbers started to creep up. In 1992, we were told that there was a new, different meningitis crisis caused by Haemophilus B. In 1994, the Hib vaccine was inserted into the schedule. This is a vaccine which, wherever it has been used, has drastically reduced meningitis cases caused by capsular haemophilus B. It also appears to remove the capsular strain from circulating in the community. Other Hib strains continue to circulate.

One year after the introduction of Tetramune (1995), doctors were worried that the proportion of very young children admitted to hospital was getting higher,[1] and mentioned illnesses such as pneumonia, asthma, meningococcal disease, fevers and bronchiolitis. The reasons for this increase in hospital admissions weren't clear, but it seemed lack of money to pay doctors' bills was a factor. What else might keel over as a result of lack of money? Nutrition, by any chance?

I had read an American article which stated, ***"We have great concern for the increasing prevalence of relatively or absolutely penicillin-resistant pneumococci coupled with the increased relative frequency of pneumococcal disease as a result of universal***

1 Barber, F. 1995. "Children sicker and lots more attending Starship hospital". *New Zealand Herald*, 26 December: Section 1, p. 3.

***Haemophilus vaccination.*"**[2] I fired off a letter to Bill Birch,[3] then the Minister for Health asking him whether or not, in shooting off the grey wolves (Meningitis A) then the white wolves (Haemophilus B), we were simply clearing space so that other, different meningitis strains could walk in and take their places? He wrote back politely suggesting that was a ridiculous thing to say.

The trouble is, there is some reason to believe that this is exactly what happens. The concern is not so much that it can happen, because out of the 13 meningococcal serogroups, only 5 commonly cause disease[4] . . . the concern is that:

> ***"the vacancy created by the elimination of serogroup C organisms may be occupied by meningococci of other serogroups . . . of particular concern is the possibility that serogroup B, W-135, or Y variants of the ETE-37 complex might exploit this opportunity."***

In Finland[5], Belgium[6] and Sweden[7] after the use of the Hib vaccine, haemophilus declined, and the rates of invasive pneumococcal infections increased. The increase in numbers of pneumococcus was real and serious, and it's harder to treat than haemophilus.

But this wasn't exactly what was happening in New Zealand. It seems to me that after the decline of first Meningitis A and then Haemophilus out of the bacterial mix in the community, as would also happen in any epidemic cycles or swings, the bacteria that developed and took over the vacuum was a unique-to-New Zealand home-grown type of Meningococcal B.

By 1996, Meningitis B had filled the hole well. 2001 was the peak year for Meningitis B cases and deaths. Since that year, we have seen substantial decreases in both the numbers of cases and deaths caused by Meningitis B. Looking at the graph which shows a decline of 50% in

---

2 Nelson, J.D. 1992. "The perilous pneumococcus". *The Pediatric Infections Disease Journal Newsletter*, June; 18(6): 12.

3 Letter from H. Butler to B. Birch, dated 1 May 1993.

4 Maiden, M.C.J. 1999. "Meningococcal conjugate vaccine: new opportunities and new challenges". *The Lancet*, August: 354: 615–616. PMID: 10466659.

5 Baer, M., Vuento, R., and Vesikari, T. 1995. "Increase in bacteraemic pneumococcal infections in children". *The Lancet*, March: 345(8950): 661. PMID: 7898220.

6 Van Hoeck, K.J. et al. 1997. "A retrospective epidemiological study of bacterial meningitis in an urban area in Belgium". *Eur J Pediatr*, 156: 288–291. PMID: 9128813.

7 Schonheyder, H.C. et al. 1997. "Increase in pneumococcal bacteraemia in Sweden". *The Lancet*, 1997 March: 349(9053): 699–700. PMID: 9167485.

cases since 2001 and 75% in deaths, it would also be logical to suggest, just as Dr Mark MacDonald did, back in 1987 in Onewhero, that the historical natural cycle of Meningitis B, like other meningitis types before it, was well on the downturn before the vaccine was even used.

Why do epidemic cycles happen? Most people will carry different bacterial meningitis types many times, and simply acquire immunity. However, immune people repeatedly carry and continue to spread most of the bacterial types circulating, but fewer cases will occur of that strain, because there are fewer people at risk of the disease, who haven't been exposed to it. Once there are no infections to keep the carriage rates higher, cases from other strains which exploit the same risk factors rise in numbers, just as happened with all the other meningitis epidemics in the past.

What will happen next? We are told that Meningitis C vaccine is the next vaccine the medical profession wants to give to children, along with a pneumococcus vaccine called Prevnar.

In the UK, research was done[8] on carriage of the hypervirulent C strain after the Meningitis C vaccination campaign, testing 15,010 vaccinated individuals and finding 19 carriers. They tested 1170 unvaccinated people and found 4 carriers. Statistically, there were 63% fewer carriers in the vaccinated than the unvaccinated group. So the MenC UK vaccine may reduce carriage. I use the word may because bacteria tend to sit around in isolated corners and play musical chairs, which people who take throat swabs can't see. Those tests, repeated in other places over time, could have found higher or lower rates of carriage.

Studies are also being done to see if the ET-37 hypervirulent strain will be replaced by ***"vaccine escape variants or virulent non-serogroup C strains".*** Just as bacteria become resistant to antibiotics, they can and do become resistant to vaccines.

Prevnar knocks out carriage of the vaccine types, but other pneumococcus types step in.[9] The overseas studies show that while Hib vaccine seems to knock out carriage to the type in the vaccine, and that in the USA between 1995 and 2003, there was a decline in

8 Maiden, M.C.J. 2002. "Carriage of serogroup C meningococci 1 year after meningococcal C conjugate polysaccharide vaccination". *The Lancet,* May: 359(9320): 1829–31. PMID: 12044380.

9 Lipsitch, M. 2000. "Bacterial Vaccines and Serotype Replacement: Lessons from Haemophilus Influenzae and Prospects for Streptococcus pneumoniae". *Emerging Infectious Diseases,* May–June: 5(3): 336–45. PMID: 10341170.

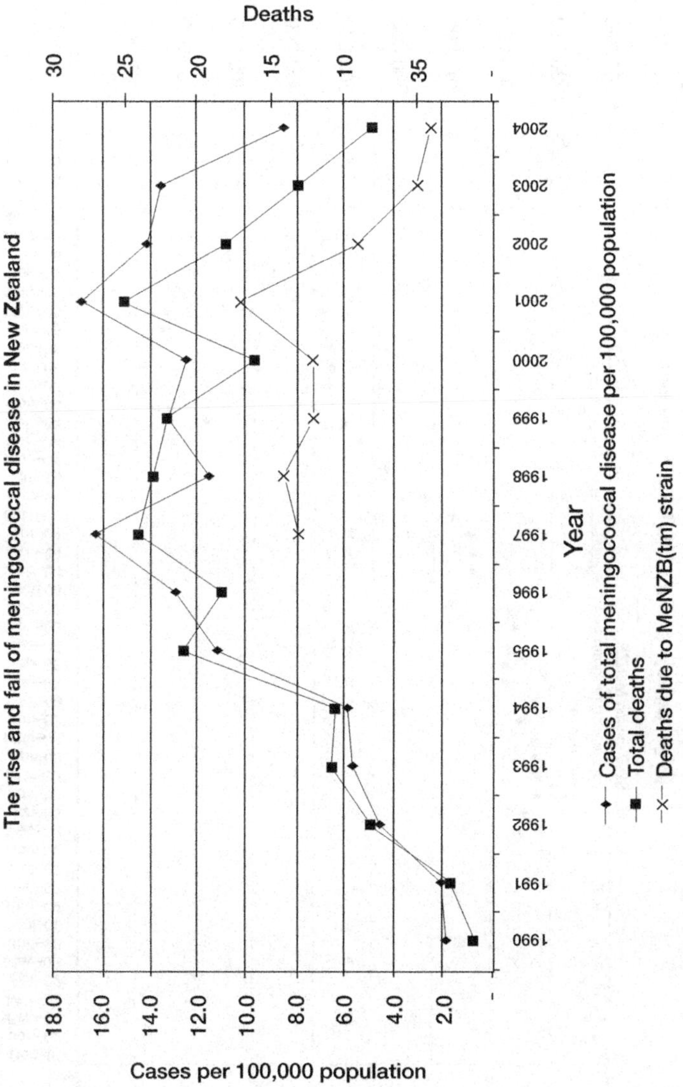

Source: Ministry of Health, ESR, NZ Stats

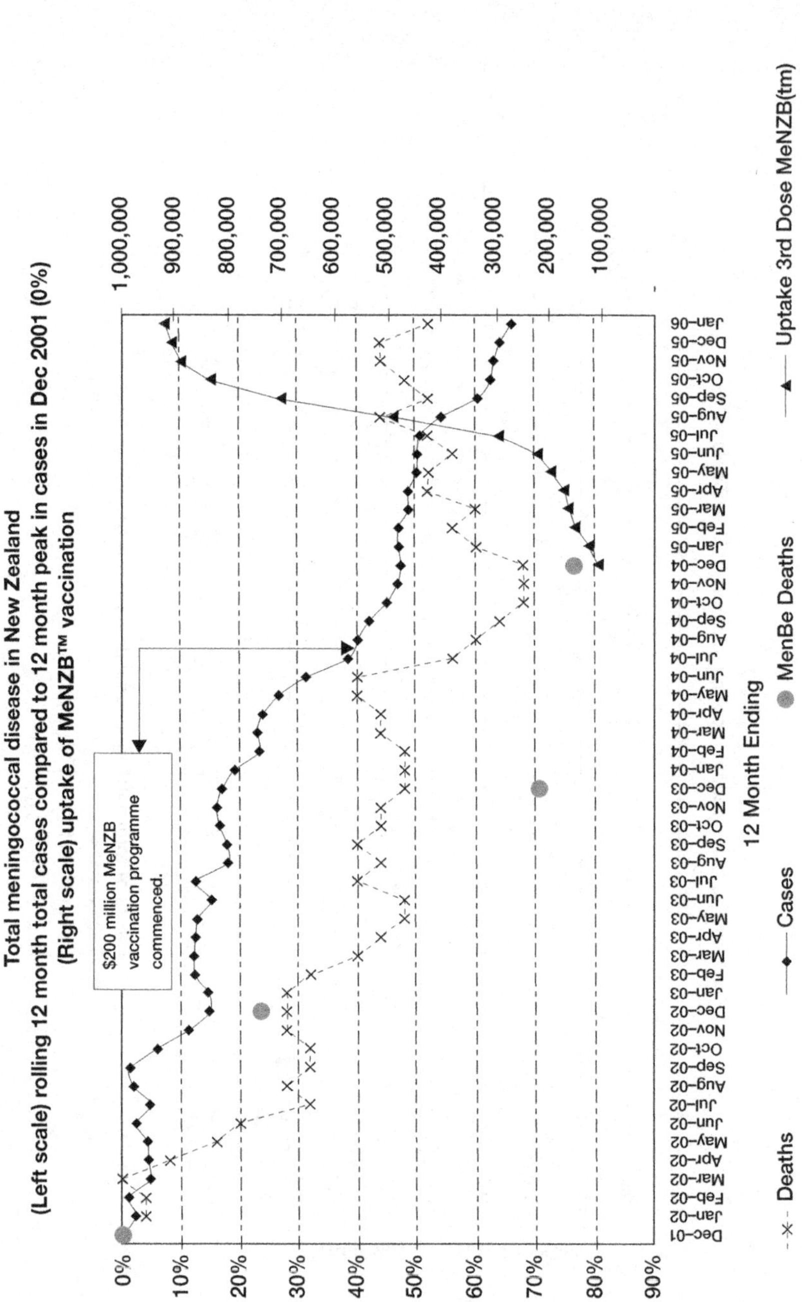

Change Deaths & Cases Compared to
12 Month Total at Dec 2001

Source: Ministry of Health/ESR

pneumococcus ear infections, there was an increase in haemophilus ear infections.[10] Not all children were immunized with Prevnar though. The reasons for the changes are stated as unknown.

Pneumococcus has 90 known strains and since the introduction of the 7–strain Prevnar in the USA, there has been a slow and definite rise in infections not covered by the three doses of the vaccine. One article[11] said,

> ***"Recent studies have found that strains of pneumococci not covered by Prevnar multiply in the noses and throats of children after they are given the vaccine. Although Prevnar reduces the amount of the seven strains it covers, other strains completely fill in the gap – so the total amount of pneumococcus found in children's noses and throats is not reduced by vaccination."***

The article also stated that Wyeth and GlaxoSmithKline now have vaccines in development to tackle the next *pneumococcus* epidemic. So what will happen here?

In New Zealand we have come full circle with another vaccine campaign started in mid-2004 and having been completed in 2005. What will be given the credit for the decline in Meningitis B cases since 2001? The vaccine used in 2004 and 2005?

The history of medicine is very clear in terms of all infectious diseases. Nature abhors a vacuum. Epidemics come in cycles. The use of vaccines won't prevent the next vacuum opportunist, or get rid of the individual risk factors.

Many families, including ours, have lived through decades when we have been told that we are at risk from Meningitis A, Haemophilus B, Meningitis B, and now Meningitis C, Pneumococcus and whatever else is floating around. We've been told that in order to survive, our children needed all the vaccines available. We, and they have not had any of those vaccines, and none of us have had meningitis.

Yes, you can say that some people have had meningitis, and that is a fact. If that's all you are going to say, then you've missed the point.

---

10 Casey, J.R. et al. 2004. "Changes in Frequency and Pathogens Causing Acute Otitis Media in 1995–2003". *Pediatric Infect Dis J*, 23(9): 824–828. PMID: 15361720.

11 Hochman, M.E. 2005. "Childhood vaccine saves lives, but may lead to other infections". *The Boston Globe* 21 June. Retrieved on 9 March, 2006 from <http://www.boston.com/news/globe/health_science/articles/2005/06/21/childhood_vaccine_saves_lives_but_may_lead_to_other_infections/>

The point is that if people want vaccines, they are welcome to have them. But if people don't want them, they should not be hounded to have them. And if parents get upset and talk about the fact that official information is unfactual and biased because it omits critical information, they shouldn't be pilloried for doing so. After all, if the pamphlets were accurate, there would be nothing for anyone to criticize. People should be given all the information instead of snippets in emotionally loaded pamphlets, and be allowed to make their choices based on all balancing facts.

As was stated in the *Boston Globe*, the medical profession has recognized that in order to attempt to eliminate all types of meningitis, there will have to be lots of new vaccines to inject into people.

And perhaps we should get rid of another myth. New Zealanders appear to really believe that state funded vaccines are free. But vaccine manufacturers don't donate vaccines out of the goodness of their hearts. The actual cost of the vaccines comes out of the back pocket of every tax payer, whether they want their tax to go towards vaccines or not. Given that the Health Department has just put a wide variety of meningitis vaccines on the *"free"* list for *"at risk"* people, let's get facts straight. These vaccines are taxpayer funded. How many billions might that be in the future?

There is another way of looking at the actual meningitis risk issue and it's this.

New Zealand's population is approximately 4,250,000.

NO meningitis VACCINES for 60 years and let us assume we used the epidemic figures for the last 15 years carried on for the next 45 years:

	Cases	*Deaths*
Department of Health statistics for last 15 years	5000	200
Estimates for next 45 years	15,000	600
Total over 60 years, 1990–2050 =		
With *no* meningitis vaccines:	20,000	800

Using these figures in 60 years without vaccines 4,230,000 out of 4,250,000 New Zealanders would never have had any type of meningitis illness at all.

In ***60 years without vaccines***, 4,249,200 people out of 4,250,000 would never have died either.

So for all those four million people plus any alleged vaccine benefit from all types of meningitis vaccines is NIL and the huge costs will be totally wasted, even more so if rapid decline in antibodies means repeat doses will be advised every year or two.[12]

That is the statistical history of meningitis.

However, the *reality history* for those 20,000 cases and 800 deaths over 60 years is that the reasons the people got meningitis in the first place will not have been remedied, while the huge cost to this country of lots of vaccines to people who would never have got the disease anyway, would have long since gone over the multi-billion dollar mark.

In 1925, a doctor had this to say:

> ***"It is fortunate for the world that pre-immunization against the typhoid group was not discovered in the days of laissez-faire; had it been, many more thousands would have died of typhoid than actually did. Eighty years ago it would have been hard to persuade the possessing classes to spend money on safeguarding water supplies if so cheap an alternative method of protection could have been provided."***[13]

This is what upsets me most about this whole issue. Vaccines are a cheaper option than real preventive medicine. ***"Jabs rushed in to save a gazillion children,"*** would sound much more heroic than ***"Manukau poor now have warm, dry housing and good food".*** Using vaccines does nothing to get rid of bad nutrition, anaemia, obesity, overcrowding, bad housing, stress, despair, dislocation, social discord, drug abuse, smoking, and alcoholism. Deal with these risk factors, and you will get rid of most serious cases of TB, and other infections of most types; viral and bacterial meningitis; you will drastically reduce diabetes, rheumatoid arthritis, and a whole range of other chronic complaints which will become an impossible financial burden in the future.

A fence at the top of the cliff is better than an ambulance at the bottom.

Nikki Turner was right about one of those factors on TV.[14] If the

12 Thomas, M. 2004. "Prevention of group B meningococcal disease by vaccination: a difficult task." *New Zealand Medical Journal*, August: 117(1200): PMID: 15475986. Available from: <http://www.nzma.org.nz/journal/117-1200/1016/> Accessed 11 November 2005.

13 Greenwood (Major). 1925. *Epidemic and Crowd Diseases, An Introduction to the Study of Epidemiology*. London: Williams & Norgate. Page 75.

14 Television broadcast on *60 Minutes*, 11 April 2005.

reality issues in South Auckland (and everywhere else), had been dealt with all those years ago, we might not have had to worry about any wolves: white, grey, black or green, in the future. Or any more meningo-vaccines, for that matter.

In 1987 in both print media and on radio, I said that I saw little hope that either politicians or the medical profession would ever commit to real educational, or social reforms, which could radically slash rates of both infectious and chronic disease in this country. Nearly twenty years on I see nothing on the horizon to change that view, either here or overseas.

All over the world vaccines are now used as a cheap substitute for basic necessities, which the WHO has admitted in the past, is the best immune caretaker of all: warm dry housing with sanitation, clean water, adequate nutrition and basic medical care. The *New York Times*[15] recently inflicted upon readers misleading statements like this: ***"Vaccinating children against measles is the greatest return on investment for child health that we have," said Dr. Mark Grabowsky, who for five years was the adviser to the Red Cross for the Centers for Disease Control and Prevention. "It's the low-hanging fruit."***

Best of all in this world that looks for feel good media sound bites, the measles vaccine only costs 15 cents per child, and no-one notices the factors that cause severe measles or any other diseases in Nepalese children. Has one "fruit" been picked off, only for those children to fall to another for the same reasons? What might be the greatest future return on investment for overall health in Nepal or India, if the medical profession really cared? The Vitamin A programme studied by Professors Sommer and Keith West from John Hopkins University,[16,17] and forcibly pushed by 49,000 Nepalese grannies.[18] This programme, not any vaccine, has resulted in substantial reductions in disease and death in Nepalese mothers and children. Next on the list for Nepal should be overall diet, clean water and sanitation.

---

15 Dugger, C.W. 2006. "Mothers of Nepal Vanquish a Killer of Children." *New York Times*, April 30 from http://www.nytimes.com/2006/04/30/world/asia/30measles.html

16 Sommer, A. 2006. "Global Health Champions" April from http://www.pbs.org/wgbh/rxforsurvival/series/champions/alfred_sommer.html

17 West, K.P. Prof. "Vitamin A for Health, Vision and Survival" (no date) from http://www.healthnet.org.np/sachetana/ss.html

18 PBS TV special 2006 "Rx for Survival – The Heroes" April from http://www.pbs.org/wgbh/rxforsurvival/series/about/special.html

20 Does the Talk Match the Walk?

Let me return to what I have called "our unique lifestyle".

It is so important to recognize what may appear at times to be an uncompromising position that is being mentioned.

"Living Beyond Conformity" cannot be reproduced here for obvious reasons, but very simply, conformity is produced by mindsets.

We all have them. Many are inherited from customs and traditions. Many are passed on to us by our parents.

Because most of us resist change (for a wide range of reasons), mindsets tend to stick around for a long time.

When we live **beyond** *conformity, transformations to lifestyle will be taking place. Each transformation needs to be a metamorphosis. From the chrysalis will emerge the butterfly. There will be no resemblance to the old mindset.*

Questions have been asked.

Answers have been evaluated from many different points of view.

Convictions based on solid foundations provide a sure path to follow.

The dangers of following along like a lost sheep can be recognized and steps taken to rectify the situation.

Falling into the clutches of "blind leaders of the blind" can be minimized by giving high priority to the learning of clearly defined life skills.

The **cost of being different** will be seen as part of living beyond conformity.

But this is not the complete picture.

The missing ingredient is a **consistency** that will eliminate double standards, hypocrisy and the shifting sands of situational ethics.

The lifestyle we chose as a family was an attempt to move away from the common practice of putting daily living into separate compartments or boxes, such as nutrition, exercise, education, leisure, wellness and sickness, morality – you name it. For example, the fact that what we eat may produce wellness **or** sickness will probably mean that the standards acceptable in one area are **not consistent** with those used in another.

Our unique lifestyle-related curriculum meant that every area of living would be integrated as far as is possible. It involved the teaching of skills to achieve this as well as involving self-control and self-discipline, respecting other people's views and beliefs (which might be different to our own), and to differentiate between the **"action"** that may result, and its consequences, and the **person** who is entitled to consideration and acceptance as a fellow human being.

Now I'm sure you can see that the work Hilary does relating to immunization and other health issues associated with this, has frequently brought us face to face with the "person" and the "system". This can often mean a clash between love and hate, war and peace!

One of my roles has been to try to keep the peace as far as I am able to do this.

It is my desire that as you read on and consider these things as they affect our involvement and your own, in days to come, we shall understand more clearly that we are not fighting against people made of flesh and blood, but against systems, structures, policies, deceptions and the manipulation of truth, political agendas, vested interests and so on.

These things affect **every** area of life and what weapons and strategies we use are crucial to the outcome.

21 Tuberculosis – a Foundation of Shifting Sands

Do you remember the day when you were lined up at school in the school corridor, for the TB Manteaux test?

That morning the teacher reminded us in subdued tones, what a scourge TB had been. We pretty much knew that, as the way history was slanted you couldn't help but know. Our parents had been brought up on Greta Garbo's 1936 rendition of Alexander Dumas' *Camille*. Stories reinforced history lessons about how TB in the 1800s was the women's "in" social disease, which made you look pale and exquisite. Unfortunately its consequences were anything but elegant.

I went to a school where history and literature were important. Mental images of TB's place in history, which made us shudder, had been well hammered into most of us because who would want to have TB? We were told that the BCG vaccine had overcome this terrible scourge, and had changed the course of history for the better.

We all believed this little prick was worth it. The funny thing was, no one told us when the BCG had been introduced, and neither did they show us the death decline statistics that went before. But then, we never thought to ask.

The first nurse went along the line swabbing the inner part of everyone's right forearm. The next nurse came along with a somewhat formidable looking thing which went bang and left some little pricks in a round circle. The old school had no air conditioning, but the doors at the end of the corridor leading outside were open, because it was so stifling. No one fainted, and everyone felt like honoured soldiers, very proud and dutiful to the cause.

A few days later, another corridor inspection. Forearms were inspected and like sheep in a sorting pen, most of us were herded one way, a few another way. Those of us in one corridor had our sleeves rolled up on the left side, and we were NOT allowed to watch. This time, we weren't told it was a little prick. I don't know what did it to me, but it was not comfortable. A sticky plaster was applied and we all went back to class.

When the others who hadn't been whacked in the left arm came back to class, all eyes were on them. What had happened, eager minds wanted to know? In a school where talking in the classroom was a cardinal sin, such intelligence was gathered through whispering as the opportunity presented itself, or the sly passing of notes with breath held, avoiding the eye of the teacher so as not to end up for an hour in detention after school on Wednesday.

By the end of the day we found out that the others had to go see their doctors for "X-rays, or something."

That day vanished from my memory until after our older child was born, and the Cavalry arrived to say that I wasn't doing my national duty because I was refusing the BCG. With a supposedly very sick baby, all sorts of questions went through my mind. I stood my ground, and refused.

Not long after that, New Zealand abandoned the BCG. There was no public announcement or explanation of the vaccine's withdrawal . . . it just vanished . . . silently.

I wondered why. Much later, when I was studying the Mortality and Morbidity books in the Philson Medical library, and reading all the historical medical literature, it came as a huge shock to find that way back in school I'd been told a load of lies.

Medical literature made it plain that the BCG vaccine could never provide protection against the spread of the disease at all, just as the disease itself could not. Why did they use it then? After looking at the graphs of TB death and disease decline in New Zealand and in other countries, which showed that the dramatic decline in deaths and cases happened long before the vaccine was introduced, I looked at disease decline in the USA, and parts of Europe where the TB vaccine had never been used at all. The trend was exactly the same.

So how was it that TB had declined in Europe and the USA without a vaccine, at the same rate as it did everywhere else? One of the trials USA did to look at effectiveness of the vaccine stuck out like a beacon. Not the trial itself, which showed a minus four per cent effectiveness, but the concluding comment:

> ***". . . it is particularly tragic that the use of scarce resources to administer BCG must still be based on blind faith."*** [1]

Even worse was an offshoot of this study which showed:

> ***". . . Although no statistically significant protective effect of BCG could be demonstrated, the vaccinated group had a slight deficiency of leukemia cases, and an excess of lymphosarcoma and Hodgkins disease."*** [2]

As time passed I followed two huge World Health Organisation studies quietly undertaken to try to resolve some previous disappointing studies of the BCG which also found that the vaccine was useless. The first was mentioned in an editorial in the *Lancet*[3] which pointed out that the gloomy result of a zero protective effect was not without precedent. The whole point of this trial was to iron out what the WHO considered were study flaws in previous trials. The complete study[4] was even more interesting to me, as it was a vaccine trial with a real placebo – dextran, which is a carbohydrate polymer – in other words, it was actually an honest trial, which really compared vaccinated with unvaccinated. The results were a major disappointment to WHO. It was followed by a further study,[5] which again, showed ***"There was no statistically significant protection by BCG against tuberculosis in this population. These findings add to the evidence that BCG vaccines afford greater protection against leprosy than against tuberculosis."***

These studies never appeared in newspapers either. Myriads of other medical articles on BCG were added to my collection as time

---

1 Comstock, G.W. et al. 1974. "Evaluation of BCG vaccination among Puerto Rican children". *American Journal of Public Health*, 64(3): 283–91. PMID: 4811772.

2 Snider, D.E. et al. 1978. "Efficacy of BCG in prevention of cancer: an update". *J. Natl Cancer Inst*, April: 60(4): 785–8. PMID: 344899.

3 1980. "BCG: bad news from India". Jan 12; 1(8159): 73–4. PMID: 610419.

4 Bailey, G.V.J. et al. 1980 "Tuberculosis Prevention Trial, Madras". *Indian Journal of Medical Research*, Vol. 72 (suppl): 1–74. PMID: 7005086.

5 (No authors) 1999. "Fifteen year follow-up of trial of BCG vaccines in South India" . . . Tuberculosis Research Centre (ICMR). *Indian J. of Medical Research*, Aug: 110: 56–69. PMID: 10573656.

New Zealand deaths from Tuberculosis
Death rates per million 1872–1960

Source: Director General Yearly Reports in Apendices to Parliamentary Journals

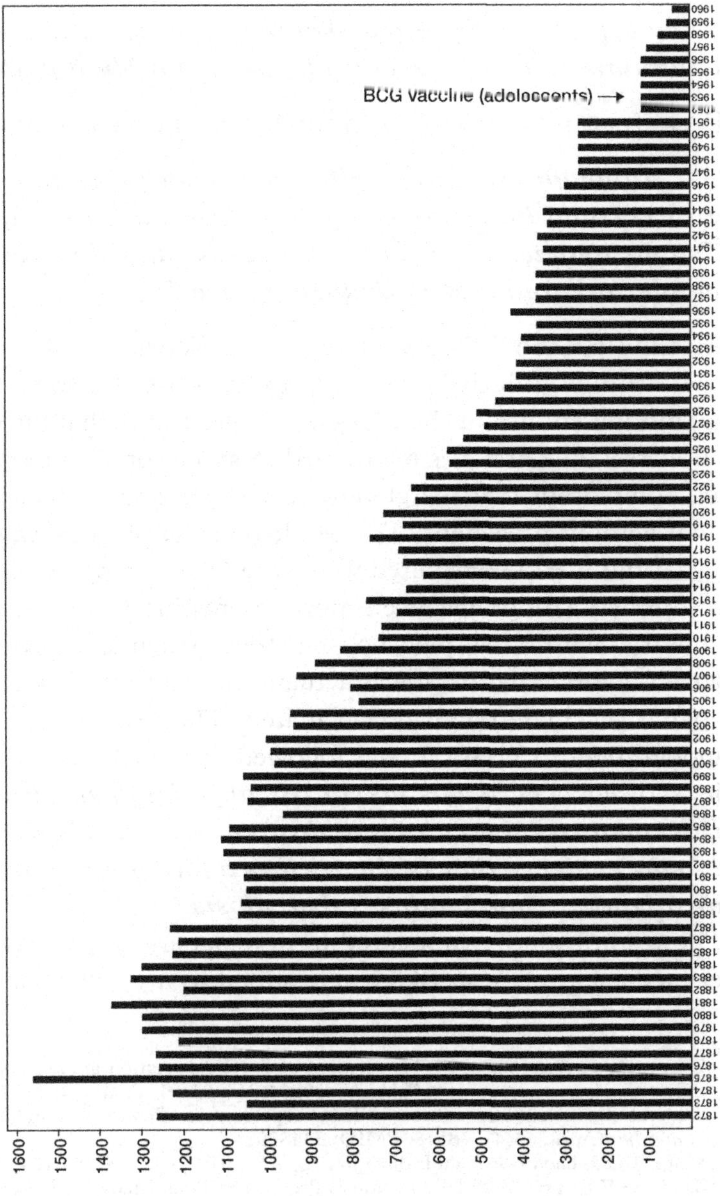

passed. What possible benefit could there be from this vaccine? Apart from leprosy protection, which is about 50%.[6] This Malawi study also showed no protection against TB from the BCG vaccine.

These piles of medical literature raise a few issues:

1) What else I might find to show me that my past knowledge was conditioned compliance, based on factual inaccuracies?

2) Why had the medical profession so stoutly defended such a shonky vaccine?

Some meta-analyses consider the BCG to be protective against meningitis and miliary TB in childhood,[7,8] but I have my doubts. To me, these two studies seem like a last-ditch stand to retrieve something out of the mess of misinformation we have been subjected to for years.[9,10] Particularly when push comes to shove, and recent events like those in Leicester, UK reveal that the majority of students found with active disease had been immunized.[11] Yet at a time in history when TB is increasing, the UK has just abandoned the use of the school BCG vaccine[12] in favour of targeted vaccination of babies and older adults from the very countries where TB is endemic and where the BCG didn't work in WHO trials. Where is the logic in that? Perhaps the real logic lies in the fact that since 1989 the factory that produced the BCG had released batches that failed quality control checks and never informed anyone that children might not have been

6 Ponnighaus, J.M. et al. 1992. Efficacy of BCG vaccine against leprosy and tuberculosis in northern Malawi. *The Lancet* 14 March, Vol. 339, pp. 636–9. PMID 1347338.

7 Rodrigues, L.C. et al. 1993. BCG against tuberculous meningitis and miliary tuberculosis: a meta-analysis. *Int J Epidemiol*, Vol. 22(6) (December). pp. 1154–8. PMID: 8144299.

8 Colditz, G.A. et al. 1994 Efficacy of BCG vaccine in the prevention of tuberculosis. Meta-analysis of the published literature. *JAMA*, Vol. 271, pp. 698–702. PMID: 8309034.

9 Rodrigues, L.C. 1993. "Protective effect of BCG against tuberculosis meningitis and miliary tuberculosis: a meta-analysis". *Int. J Epidemiol*, December: 22(6): 1154–6. And *JAMA* 1994. March: 271(9): 698–702. PMID: 8144299.

10 Colditz, G.A. et al. 1994. "Efficacy of BCG vaccine in the prevention of tuberculosis. Meta-analysis of the published literature". *JAMA*, Mar 2; 271(9): 698–702. PMID: 8309034.

11 Watson, J.M. et al. 2001. "TB in Leicester: out of control, or just one of those things?" *British Medical Journal*, 322: 1133–4. PMID: 11348891.

12 Meikle, J. 2005. "TB immunization to be targeted at high-risk groups". *The Guardian*, 7 July. Retrieved on 18 September, 2005 from <http://www.guardian.co.uk/medicine/story/0,11381,1522820,00.html?gusrc=rss>

protected.[13,14] Nobody thought to ask the real question as to whether any alleged protection was even worth having.

Natural resistance to TB, and what prevents it getting out of control is a concept for which pharmaceutical companies looking for profits have no use. Even before a TB vaccine was invented, some doctors understood this:

> *". . . Let the public understand that since the discovery of the bacillus tuberculosus the disease has been added to the list of diseases that are preventable by attainable means. Let the public school-master understand that he may render his healthy boys and girls immune by gymnastics and calisthenics which increase their vital resistance, for while the object of hygienic regulations is the prevention of the propagation and spread of the tubercle bacilli, yet we know that the healthy tissue cell has a demonstrable power of resistance, so by increasing vital force we may build up a nearly impenetrable barrier against bacillary invasion."*[15]

In 1997 various papers reported this:

> *"Wellington researchers believe they have made a major breakthrough in the fight against tuberculosis . . . In their search for an effective vaccine, they have discovered that by boosting a small section of the immune system it will fight back and control the disease . . . it was a stunning discovery for the researchers who believed that the immune system was incapable of effectively fighting the disease."*

> *"We are looking forward to the future, to convincing people that we have found another way to make a vaccine . . . for tuberculosis." (Profession Le Gros)*[16]

---

13 Weston, A. 2005. "Drugs firm stayed silent over its faulty vaccines". *Liverpool Daily Post*, 21 November.

14 "Lord linked to TB vaccine concern". 2005. Retrieved on 18 September, 2005 from <http://news.bbc.co.uk/1/hi/uk/4453676.stm> "Official documents show that from 1989 some of the TB vaccines manufactured at the factory were faulty . . . It was only when health inspectors staged a crash inspection in July 2002 that Whitehall – not the public – was informed."

15 Hamilton, J.R. 1887. "The Prevention of Tuberculosis". *JAMA*, Jun 12; 28: 1110–1114.

16 1997. "Researchers believe they have Tb discovery". *Westport News*, 20 August.

Note the underlined words. This was the first tacit admission I had ever read that the vaccine we use now in newborn babies of so-called at-risk groups isn't effective. Yet no reporters thought to follow up the logical next question, which was: ***"Oh, you mean the BCG used now isn't effective in preventing the spread of TB? How is it we weren't told that?"*** Why is it still used in the very selected South Auckland communities from countries where the effectiveness trials were unsuccessful?

Why do these doctors believe that the immune system doesn't have the ability to effectively fight TB? Had they not studied all the New Zealand prisoners of war from World War II, who came back from camps at half their normal body weight and riddled with TB?[17] Yet even in 1946 doctors knew that prisoners of war, receiving supplementary food with 30 g protein daily had a TB rate of only 1.2% compared with a rate of 15–19% in other prisoners.[18] It's crystal clear that susceptibility to TB has a lot to do with poverty and malnutrition.[19,20,21,22]

In 1988, the *Sunday Star*[23] featured two of New Zealand's Stalag VIIIB prisoner-of-war heroes, Ray Lomas and Charles Croall, who returned emaciated and riddled with TB. Lomas later lost a lung to TB, but in 1947 walked out of Waikato Hospital having been told he had three months to live:

> ***". . . I said, 'To hell with that. I'll take no notice of what the doctors say'." He took 12 months' leave of absence from his work at the Post Office and set off for Britain with his English-born wife for "a working holiday".***

The 1988 article even went on to say that up until recently he smoked 120 cigarettes a day and had changed to a pipe. At the

17 Macdonald, J. 1988. "Death camp Terezin nightmare for New Zealand POWs". *Sunday Star* 24 April: A12.
18 Leyton, G.B. 1946. *The Lancet*, 2: 73.
19 Ramsden, S.S. 1988. "Tuberculosis among the central London single homeless". *J R Coll Physicians Lond*, January: 22(1): 16–7. PMID: 3339569.
20 Tekkel, M. et al. 2002. "Risk factor for pulmonary tuberculosis in Estonia". *Int J. Tuberc Lung Dis*, October: 6(10): 887–94. PMID: 12365575.
21 Ruck, N. 1997 "Human factors in the TB epidemic". *Afr Health*, November: 20(1): 23–4. PMID: 12348377.
22 Hawker, J.I. et al. 1999. "Ecological analysis of ethnic differences in relation between tuberulosis and poverty". *British Medical Journal*, October: 319: 1031–4. PMID: 10521193.
23 Macdonald, J. 1988. "Death Camp". *Sunday Star*, 24 April: A12.

interview he was cursing his recent loss of mobility having punctured his remaining lung after falling off his motorbike at the age of 70.

If doctors had spent more time understanding how it was that so many of our war-time heroes overcame TB by eating well, working the land, and generally increasing the functioning of their immune system, they would understand how it is that the immune system has had the ability, given the right conditions and food, not only to effectively fight TB, but also to live in symbiosis with TB, contain the bacteria, and provide a defence against the worst excesses of TB.

Certainly there are problems with the concept of any TB vaccine. And here's one reason why it's unlikely that an effective vaccine will be found any day soon:

Dr Annelies van Rie of the University of Stellenbosch in Tygerberg found that people who recovered from one TB infection, could acquire a new one, because strains in any country appear to change quite quickly.[24]

It's just a shame researchers didn't look at host factors instead of just blasting the TB bacteria with potent drugs which have very serious side-effects, and leaving the very risk factors there, that resulted in the person coming down with TB in the first place. Paul Fine, a TB guru, says in the editorial in the same medical journal:

> ***"If natural infection does not confer protective immunity . . . the development of improved vaccines against tuberculosis will be especially challenging."***[25]

Further he says in a different article:

> ***"natural immunity to tuberculosis is generally associated with persistent, rather than self-limited infection . . .***
>
> ***. . . There has been little discussion of herd immunity with reference to tuberculosis. A major reason for this silence is the rudimentary level of our understanding of the nature and implications of either natural or vaccine derived immunity to this disease . . . there is no convincing evidence that the use of BCG vaccines has reduced the risk of infection with***

24 van Rie, A. et al. 1999. "Exogenous reinfection as a cause of recurrent tuberculosis after curative treatment". *N Engl J Med* October: 341: 1174–1179. PMID: 10519895.

25 Fine, P.E. et al. 1999. "Exogenous reinfection in tuberculosis". *N Engl J Med* October: 341: 1226–7. PMID: 10519901.

the tubercle bacillus in any population. In the absence of greater basic understanding of the nature and implications of the immune response to tuberculosis, it is of questionable utility to ponder its theoretical herd implications."[26]

So why were we all told that the BCG, given to all adolescents from 1953 onwards had saved New Zealand and the world, from white death, when TB had already decreased in this country from an incidence of 1560 per million, to 110 per million before BCG even hit the market?

And why is the medical profession's understanding of TB still so rudimentary even today?

We know how and why TB deaths and its incidence declined, and how to keep it under control. The justifications used to continue the flyswat use of a vaccine that doesn't work, and should never have been used in the first place, are baffling.

Is it easier to offer a vaccine that doesn't work but let people think it does, and let them listen to the sound-good media stories, than to deal with the real risk factors that lie behind TB in the first place?

---

26 Fine, P.E. 1993. "Herd immunity: history, theory, practice". *Epidemiologic Reviews*, 15(2): 294. PMID: 8174658.

22 1987: the Issue Gains Traction

Following on from the Homestead chook shot campaign, in September 1987 the *New Zealand Woman's Weekly* joined the article queue and interviewed Suzy O'Brien, the Wellington mother of Sophie, who was one of an early group of seriously vaccine-damaged children to be accepted for compensation by the Accident Compensation Corporation (ACC). *Woman's Weekly* also touched on some of the meningitis issues. The article was valuable primarily because it started to show some of the true stripes of the tiger.

The article detailed an infectious disease doctor talking about America, presumably on the assumption that people here wouldn't know what the facts were. E.g. the fact that there was wide acceptance of vaccination and disease prevention in USA, and ***"you simply aren't allowed to enter school without a vaccination certificate"***.

Far from being totally uncontroversial in the USA, vaccination was the big buzz word there, and had been for several years. Vaccination rates were plummeting in the wake of television programmes showing the other side to vaccines. There had been huge numbers of USA civilian legal cases for vaccine damage; so many, in fact that the manufacturers felt that they needed government indemnity from prosecution of any kind, and had just pushed through legislation securing that. Furthermore, all American states had legal provisions allowing vaccine exemptions on religious, medical and even philosophical grounds.

In 1987 media portrayal of vaccination was generally what Dr Mendelsohn called **articles of faith**.

The question line of most journalists who interviewed me was usually the same. A series of philosophical probes, to see if I was of the *flower power* generation . . . maybe I did dope? Surreptitious looks would scan titles of books on my shelves. Pretty soon, I arranged the house so that journalists could have the guided tour first, suss out my character and philosophy over a cup of coffee, while sitting down to interview me next to some of the bookcases.

At the point where they realized that I wasn't some fruitcake from bat land, I'd take them to where the medical literature was kept. That was usually where things became interesting, because most journalists didn't expect there to be anything from the medical literature to back up what I was saying. In answer to each question, evidentiary heaps would be constructed from the relevant medical literature.

At the end, I'd always ask, "When you spoke to X doctors, did you ask them to give you the proof from the medical literature to justify their statements?"

The answer was always "no", so a subsidiary question would be, "Why not?" The answer was usually that . . . well . . . you didn't do that with doctors, because they'd been to medical school, and they just . . . "know". Did they think that fair?

More often than not, the last question remained unanswered. Usually by this time, any truly thinking journalist could see that their nice little pre-planned 1000 easy words, had just become a nightmare.

23 Reaction, Side-Effect, or Direct Action?

The term *side-effects* has a very subtle effect on the brain. You hear the word and it sounds almost as if whatever has happened is irrelevant and *to one side*.

A vaccine will create within a baby, direct effects. Some are wanted, and others unwanted.

The wanted direct effects of a vaccine are, according to the medical profession, the development of antibodies presumed to give immunity. The unwanted but equally direct effects of vaccines can be toxic effects or immunological responses which the medical people don't want to see, or to recognize.

Perhaps that's why they (and many unwanted direct effects of any drugs) have been called *side-effects* so as to emotionally brush them off in a slightly dismissive way. The newer term, *"adverse effects"* is slightly more accurate, but still so impersonal as to have no real form.

During 1987, I started to get some answers to a long-standing problem of my own, which had started way back in 1973. I had been working in the physically demanding job of herd-testing, and was told to have shots against rubella and measles, which were given to me in the second week of the third month of testing.

After the shot, I was okay to begin with, then started to feel tired beyond belief, and my elbows and joints started to hurt. The doctor diagnosed what they called *"carpal tunnel syndrome"* which is now called OOS.[1]

By the end of the month I was ready to throw in the towel, and talked to my boss. The doctor had queried whether the problem was sample flasks which you had to twist off every milk meter on each milk machine line. That action, he thought, might cause OOS. So head office changed my flasks to new flick-off ones to lessen the strain on the wrists.

The next month wasn't much better with what now felt like creaked up joints which even axle grease wouldn't loosen. The doctor, on reviewing my history, saw that before I'd been a crock in bed three years previously, I'd also been dumb enough to have done competitive gymnastics. His diagnosis of the joint pain was, "Any idiot who thinks vaulting, floor work and crazy contortionism doesn't have a price to pay, is dreaming."

So, the verdict was that my health problems were arthritis from gymnastics, and OOS from my job.

The OOS got worse, and I landed up in hospital having both wrists operated on. After time off, I went back to work, with not much OOS but still plenty of joint ache. In 1974 I tossed herd-testing in. It was just too hard on the body.

I went back herd-testing in 1978. That year wasn't so bad. The aching joints had settled into a pattern where from December through to February there wasn't much pain, as the heat of summer seemed to ease everything up.

In 1980, Peter and I got married. In 1981, I was pregnant. Amazingly, the pain switched off totally during pregnancy. Over the years I'd forgotten what painlessness was like, until I had none for a longer period of time.

The year after our first child was born, the pain returned with a vengeance. In 1983 I was pregnant again, which meant more pain-free bliss.

By March 1984, I was in serious need of a major grease, lube and frontal lobotomy.

Some would say it was my fault, because I won't use pain relief. When pain relief crashes your blood pressure and causes you to become horizontal, what's the point? With two babies, you have to be able to do more than issue orders to no one from the bed.

I'd done a comprehensive Medline search in 1982 on various

1 Occupational overuse syndrome.

vaccinations including rubella, but hadn't paid any attention to the rubella section. Why should I? Rubella wasn't in the children's schedule then. And my problems were due to gymnastics and my job.

What I couldn't understand, was why pregnancy had switched off the pain.

In 1987 I went back to the Rubella part of the Medline search, and page after page was full of OOS, arthralgia and arthritis. I pulled lots of articles from the med library and found it hard to escape the conclusion that the problems I had were far more likely to be vaccine-induced, than caused by overwork or gymnastics.

I quizzed the local doctor about previous diagnoses and he just shrugged, though he provided one brief moment of light relief, by suggesting that the solution was in my own hands; "Why don't you just get pregnant every two years?"

He couldn't see how any vaccines could possibly cause arthritis because the Health Department said they didn't.

After checking the Medline search for potential authors who might have some answers, I wrote overseas. Replies indicated that specific tests might reveal certain things. I had the doctor do those tests in December, when I was in my annual pain remission time. But even so they came back with some strange findings. I had positive tests for arthritis, but they weren't the 'normal' abnormal tests. Furthermore, the immunoglobin tests came back with some really strange results.

After some investigation from my doctor, and talking to immunologists, and consulting texts, it was concluded that I had an immunodeficiency called dysgammaglobulinaemia.

The immunodeficiency provided even more grist to the argument that ***"no, the problems were nothing to do with the vaccine"***, even though the OOS and arthritis started developing days after the shots and got progressively worse thereafter. Serial denial was the medical order of the day, because it was the immunodeficiency, not the vaccine that allegedly caused the problems. I copied all my files and test results and sent them overseas to some of the researchers, telling all of them who else I had sent them to.

One of them replied. The letter was very interesting. Parts of it read:

> ***"My colleagues . . . and I have received many letters since . . . from women such as yourself . . . In all cases their GPs have strongly denied any vaccine association***

> *(particularly the American doctors who fear litigation) . . . your symptoms fit exactly with our findings . . . it is more than likely that your personal diagnosis is correct.* (Emphasis in original letter.)
>
> *. . . Many of the patients we have seen, or corresponded with, have complained less of the symptoms themselves than of the attitude of the medical profession in denying the problem exists and offering neither sympathy nor understanding. There is unfortunately no cure, but it is our experience that the recurrences of symptoms tend to become less and less prevalent with time. This is not a progressive destructive disease, but a recurrent acute one, much like a cold sore."*

The doctor discussed the fact that there was no good test for who might be susceptible to rubella arthritis after the vaccine. A paper[2] which she had authored, and had included with the letter, said:

> *"Patients who develop arthritis have probably been infected by rubella virus previously and have responded to this previous infection with an abnormal immune response. This aberrant response may lead to the development of arthritis on subsequent contact with the virus, or possibly through the reactivation of virus from a latent carrier state."*

I took all this to New Zealand doctors to see what they would say.

They all dismissed the theory. An immunologist told me that the vaccine simply showed up the pre-existing weakness in my system. He also said that in his opinion, people who got arthritis after wild rubella virus probably already had a strange immune system as well.

He talked a lot about people who got certain other diseases because they had aberrant immune responses.

Over the coming years, I was to discover an awful lot of people with aberrant responses to the rubella vaccine, who were very interested in what the medical literature had to say, even if their doctors weren't. Most of them, though, didn't have immunodeficiencies, or strange

2 I have kept the paper which has a reference number, but no publication details on it.

blood test results like I did, but did have the same symptoms as I had had. I showed some of this material to some of the women journalists. A couple were stunned, as they had been diagnosed with OOS shortly after rubella shots. None of them had immunodeficiencies either.

Written media journalists were about to take a back seat because 1987 also marked another watershed point for me, in the form of Leighton Smith. It was he who introduced me to the world of us and them.

24 1987 – "Us" and "Them"

In March 1987, I challenged Leighton Smith about a singularly obnoxious pro-vaccination broadcast aired on Radio 1ZB. In response, Leighton invited me to do a talkback session. I was very nervous about appearing on live radio, and irritated that at the last minute, instead of being on my own, I was going to appear with Dr Michael Soljak of the Health Department, supposedly to provide the right balance to what I was saying. You never got this sort of balance in reverse when ***"you must vaccinate"*** programmes were being presented.

The broadcast went very well, despite a moment in the middle where all sound cut out of my headphones while everyone else sailed on without me. My husband, who had been listening at home, thought I'd got stage fright. I just didn't know what was going on.

I was to discover later what a reasonable and open-minded person Dr Soljak proved to be. Most unexpectedly, he came and visited us at home, prepared to discuss issues openly, to be honest, and to admit when he did not have answers to a lot of my questions. He did ask me about my personal motives and whether I was being influenced unduly by my negative birth experience and reaction to the rubella vaccine. And he shared some of my concerns about informed consent and about the need to question accepted wisdom. He later involved me in trying to write fair and genuinely balanced brochures on immunization, but the project wasn't a success.

Dr Soljak's brainchild was an immunization register system which he had set up in Northland, and wanted to extend countrywide. We discussed various forms this might take, and the need to collect a far more comprehensive base of information such as vaccine reactions any child had and enough family and medical history to assess why a child had reactions. He understood the rationale behind the detail, and indicated willingness to do that, but there was none from the top. It seemed that people at the top considered the only relevant data to be names and addresses, in particular if possible, those of people who were not vaccinated.

When I publicly expressed concerns about certain aspects of the Hepatitis B programme, various study protocols were sent to me for comment, and I returned possible contributions to the thinking processes. But as time went past, though Dr Soljak said little, I felt he was striking opposition from within the Health Department about his dealings with me, although I didn't know for sure.

By 1989, I started to feel as if I was taking part in an invisible game of chess, losing myself and becoming too single focused, so I returned to a hobby I've always buried myself in when the head seems to spin: embroidery.

25 Choosing the Right Frame

A wheat ear. I liked that.

Seahorses. They were great too, especially in the right light.

Then things changed.

Fans and cords. Goldfish. Pansies. No beads in this lot. More colour though. Shiny too. Like silk.

And the cranes. Now they are exquisite. I say hello to them each day as they look haughtily at me from their position on our sitting room wall. I admire their sheen. Silver, gold and white on the black. Beautiful.

Lots more pieces too. All works of art displayed in frames which bring out the very best in them.

The frame makes all the difference.

Hours of patient, careful, intricate, stitching of silk threads on silk fabric.

The transition from beaded needlework to Japanese embroidery had taken place.

The ***artist*** *– the creator of these beautiful and valuable art forms is Hilary.*

Yes, my wife has many skills at her fingertips.

And I have a feeling that, at times, her fingertips itch for more skills.

Like building a clay oven!

Or making soap!

I'm very proud of her though. Really I am.

But I get frustrated too.

Like when she decided to become a cricket scorer!

So many of these skills are very time consuming. So excluding of other people. Sometimes it's very difficult to find a suitable stopping place, or a time to ***interrupt****!*

What do you do when your priorities and interests are different?

It's a bit like the owl and the rooster in different disguises! (You'll read about this later!)

The daily composition of our unique lifestyle gives us plenty of variety. There's no doubt about that. Sometimes it ticks along quietly, but at other times it can become too overloaded. That's when it's not always easy to determine the order of priorities.

So into the mix of the vaccination and immunization issues, plus all the other health matters which are directly or indirectly related, have to be added:

- *"normal" routines and chores of family living, which includes the needs of* ***all*** *members of the family unit*
- *leisure-time activities determined by how much leisure time there is and who will be involved in it*
- *inflexible segments such as appointments, employment, meetings, sports fixtures and the like*
- *hobbies and interests.*

The total mix could be viewed as a delicate juggling act as well as walking through an uncharted minefield. You never quite know when you'll make the wrong move and what the consequences will be.

Perhaps that's why living selfishly is the easier way to go for lots of people.

Choosing the right frame should direct the focus onto what lies within the limits of its boundaries. We can all be works of art that others, especially those closest to us, can appreciate, value and enjoy.

26 Hepatitis B Publicity, a Runaway Train

Hepatitis B is a nasty disease. I know, having had it, not once, but twice. The question is how do you assess how nasty it can be and what ongoing consequences it might have? Health Department information in 1984[1] said: ***"Most people expect a patient with hepatitis to go yellow or 'jaundiced'. However, a lot of people with hepatitis B never go yellow. This means that they may never realize they've had it."***

Later, the booklet prepared for the New Zealand Department of Health[2] said, ***"The majority of those infected (at least 60%) do not have clinically recognized hepatitis."***

So the only hepatitis statistics we have are from the minority of people who get enough symptoms to feel sick enough to go to the doctor and have a blood test. So how likely was it that these people would become carriers, or die?

In 1983[3], doctors were reassured by the people who did the original

---

1 Clements, C.J. 1984. "Hepatitis B", *Health*, Autumn: 36(1): 6.

2 "Hepatitis B infection, A guide for Health Professionals in New Zealand". Hepatitis Research Unit, Whakatane Hospital, New Zealand.

3 Milne, A. 1983. "Hepatitis B vaccine: priority for use". *New Zealand Medical Journal* Oct 26; 96(742): 810–11. PMID: 6578456. ". . . the main objective must be to reduce the reservoir of HBV carriers, particularly childhood supercarriers . . . a suggested priority for vaccination is 1) newborn of supercarriers 2) All Polynesian newborn regardless of HBsAg status of the mother. This would involve about 6500 Maori

research into Hepatitis B that:

> ***"Doctors might like to assure their patients that in New Zealand, clearance of HBV following the acute illness appears to be the rule, whether the patient is an adult or a child."***

The laboratory concerned had followed 300 cases of clinical acute Hepatitis B over seven years, and ***"not even one became a carrier."***

What was the concern then? Babies. The concern was pregnant women who were carriers, who were having babies who were becoming carriers. (And Hepatitis B carriers might get liver cirrhosis, cancer and die.) The researchers mentioning this concern advised quite limited vaccination.

The reason for the extended hours I spent in the medical library from 1987 onwards, was that it was becoming plain that the next vaccine to be put into the New Zealand baby schedule would be the one for Hepatitis B. This had been heralded by articles with titles like *Undercover Epidemic*[4] which described Hepatitis B as a threat to the health of all New Zealanders, not just babies.

Talk was that this vaccine had been very useful in Alaskan Inuit and so should be used in New Zealand.

The information I was seeing did not give parents an objective assessment of the disease or its risks, but consisted solely of emotive points doctors wanted people to know, in order that all parents of all races, would agree to their babies and children being vaccinated. This feeling was echoed by a dissatisfied Whakatane resident describing the public meetings held by doctors as being ***"like revivalist gatherings; light on fact, heavy on emotions,"***[5] though Mr Milne did admit that during the eight years of his research in the area, nobody had died from Hepatitis B-related causes.

Parents were told that Hepatitis B was linked to children in bare feet:[6]

---

and 3500 other Polynesians per year; 3) Selected European newborn in areas with known high rates of HBV infections. 4) Preschool susceptible Polynesians and selected Europeans, then older children if finance allows up to the age of about 12 years after which infection appears to result in elimination of the virus; 5) Health workers at high risk, homosexuals, sex partners of known acute cases or 'supercarriers' and other groups where appropriate."

4 Guerin, L. 1985. "Undercover epidemic". *New Zealand Listener*, 16–18.

5 Letter by K.L. Hawkes. 1985. "Hepatitis B". *New Zealand Listener*, 28 September.

6 Stockdill, R. 1986. "Hepatitis B linked to children in bare feet". *Sunday Star*, 7 December.

"'The virus is apparently transmitted at schools,' says Rotorua medical officer of health Alister Millar . . . (who) said, 'Children playing at school spread the virus through playing without wearing footwear.'"

Dr Millar though refused to discuss *"high-risk"* groups considering it a *"New Zealand"* problem. Which is very strange given that Dr Moyes[7] stated that:

"vertical transmission from carrier mothers (to babies) remains a problem mainly in Polynesian and Maori groups."

Parents who are trying to figure out what the problem is, and how it might affect them, or their children, ask questions like:

Can our children get it from other children? (horizontally)

Can they get it from us? (horizontally)

If I am pregnant and I have hepatitis surface antigen only, can baby get it from me? (vertically) (*That's unlikely.*)

If I am pregnant and have the infectious core infective antigen, can baby get it from me? (vertically) (*Most likely. This parent needs to be told about immunoglobin, and the vaccine, but should also be told that the vaccine and immunoglobin may not protect*[8] *their babies.*)

What is in the vaccine? What does the manufacturer's information say about side-effects?

These were the basic things parents should have been told.

The other thing that parents should be told is that selenium deficiency vastly increases the likelihood of Hepatitis B infection and liver cancer. When selenium was added to the diet of people in a Chinese province known to be selenium deficient in the soil, the results[9] showed a significant protective effect against viral hepatitis and liver cancer. Another Chinese study[10] pointed out that:

7 Moyes, C.D. 1988. "Hepatitis B – how does New Zealand compare?" *Update,* 20 May: 10.

8 Farmer, K. 1987. "A combination of hepatitis B vaccine and immunoglobulin does not protect all infants born to hepatitis B e antigen mothers". *New Zealand Medical Journal,* July 8; 100(827): 412–4. PMID: 2967932.

9 Yu, S.Y. et al. 1997. "Protective role of selenium against hepatitis B Virus and primary liver cancer in Qidong". *Biol Trace Elem Res.* January: 56(1): 17–124. PMID: 9152515.

10 Yu, S.Y. et al. 1989. "Chemoprevention trial of human hepatitis with selenium supplementation in China". *Biol Trace Elem Res.* Apr–May: 20(1–2):15–22. PMID: 2484394.

> ***"Epidemiological studies have demonstrated that a low grain Se content is associated with a high regional incidence of hepatitis B virus infections."***

Given that New Zealand soil is selenium deficient, and these trials began long before New Zealand opted for a Hepatitis B vaccine, you wonder why selenium hasn't been tried here.

The only medical research I could find on bare-foot playground spread of Hepatitis B was much later, when Australian research[11] reported that a study of 3000 Sydney school children in 50 schools found no evidence for transmission of Hepatitis B between schoolchildren. But then, perhaps inner-city Sydney children don't play barefoot, or the sorts of rough and tumble rugby and other contact games that New Zealand children did in the mid-1980s.

Australia, however, had no problem identifying high-risk children infected horizontally and vertically who had come from countries such as Vietnam, Thailand, Cambodia or South America, with more than 20% of those children positive to Hepatitis B markers, and a third of them chronic carriers.

A very useful suggestion made by Mr Milne in the 13 February 1985 *New Zealand Medical Journal* was this:

> ***"To those who still doubt, or are unaware of, the extent of this problem in the North Island of New Zealand, we would suggest that they perform similar simple studies in this valuable indicator group (fourth formers) in their own districts."***

Mr Milne then conducted a study in Tauranga area to ***"help parents make considered judgements before getting their children vaccinated"***. He tested children in Matua, Bethlehem and Maunganui who surprisingly (to him) showed only a 4% infection rate among European children and 6% in Maori and Pacific Island children. He concluded that children in low-risk areas need not be vaccinated against Hepatitis B[12,13] though they could, if they wished.

This was the first suggestion that perhaps things were not equal throughout New Zealand, and that perhaps Hepatitis B wasn't a country-wide problem.

---

11 Overy, S. 1992. "Kids don't spread hepatitis B". *Australia Dr Weekly*, November.
12 NZPA. 1989. "Hepatitis survey surprises expert". *Dominion Times*, 14 May: 5.
13 1989. "Tauranga has low hepatitis rates". *Bay of Plenty Times* 13 May.

Various schools in Auckland, including Dilworth, did their own surveys, and found that either carriage didn't exist, or that it was at much lower levels than in the eastern Bay of Plenty, or in Northland.

In Marlborough, in the South Island, Drs Dave Durham and John Welch and Wairau Hospital's principal technologist, Gerard Verkaaik, tested 400 fourth-formers and found no carriers, and no difference between Maori and non-Maori in the small numbers who did have immunity.[14] But because the vaccine was considered "so safe" and because of the mobile nature of New Zealand's population, they thought it made sense to use it anyway.

Likewise in Te Anau in the South Island, local school children about to receive immunization were tested and there too, no carriers[15] were found.

While Mr Milne was clear that vaccination of children was best in high-risk areas, and only of babies in low-risk areas, the problem I saw coming was that it wouldn't stay that way for long. To vaccinate selected at-risk groups is too hard to explain, and words cost time and money. It also could create racial disharmony. By March 1988 it was obvious that in order to make the vaccine campaign nice, simple and sanitary, the KISS[16] principle of just-jab-everyone, no matter the age, was being introduced. That way, no one feels picked on, blamed or targeted. If it can be done, why not just do everyone? But if I were a carrier, I'd rather know.

Vaccines weren't always administered in this blind fashion. In the 1930s when the diphtheria vaccine first came on the market, the medical profession started testing everyone after finding high rates of serious reactions in those with pre-existing immunity. The rates of natural immunity were quite high, and the first testing done in Auckland found that 72.8% of children were immune. This is what was said about testing first:[17]

"By using [the] Schick test . . . over 3000 injections have

14 1989. "Low incidence of hepatitis B here". *Marlborough Express*, 13 March. "Testing in the area showed no carriers, and very low numbers with immunity . . . The low incidence raised the question of whether Marlborough children should be immunized . . ." but apparently because the vaccine was "so safe" it made sense to reduce the risk throughout the country not just the North Island. (quoting Dr Dave Durham).

15 Walker, T. et al. 1986. "Hepatitis B survey at Te Anau". *New Zealand Medical Journal*, May 28; 99(802): 380. PMID: 3464883.

16 KISS = Keep It Simple, Stupid.

17 *Appendices to Parliamentary Journals* H-31, page 96, 1938.

been avoided. This means a large saving financially while there is the personal satisfaction of knowing that unnecessary injections are avoided and one's time is being economized . . . it is frequently stated that [the] Schick test may be dispensed with . . . those who hold those views give themselves more work in the long run and also give to a considerable portion of naturally immune children quite unnecessary injections of potent material."

However, many districts did just jab, and as a result the diphtheria vaccine got a very bad name amongst the public, with huge fall-offs in numbers because of children reacting badly to the first or second doses.

The message to all mothers nationwide about the Hepatitis B vaccine, was similar to the one given to the 60 European non-carrier mothers in South Auckland who refused the vaccine and were publicly berated for it by the South Auckland Medical Officer of Health:[18]

"unprotected babies who catch the disease can develop liver failure and die."

They can't, if their mothers aren't carriers of any sort. No one was told there were two sorts of carrier. Surface antigen carriers who were not infectious, and core DNA carriers who were potentially infectious. Wouldn't it have been a good idea to have told those non-carrier mothers that in their case, the chances of Hepatitis B causing liver cancer in European cancer patients, was zero?[19]

Or how about telling parents, based on the literature of the time, that the majority of chronic carriers don't develop cirrhosis, and the majority of those with cirrhosis don't develop primary liver cancer?[20]

---

18 Roberts, J. 1987. "Mothers refuse jabs for babies". *Sunday Star* 19 April. Dr Allan Cowan.

19 Simmons, G.C. et al. 1983. "The association of Hepatitis B infection and hepatocellular cancer in New Zealand". *New Zealand Medical Journal,* Sep14; 96(739): 669–71. PMID: 6310459. "The total population incidence rate of hepatocellular carcinoma in Auckland of 1.1/100,000 is comparable to that found in Europe and America. The incidence rates for Pacific Islanders and Maori are much higher than this and coincided with a higher HbsAg carrier incidence in their subpopulation. In general (non-tumourous) populations, the hepatitis B surface antigen carrier rate was 7% for the Pacific Islander and Maori and 0.5% for the Europeans. In the tumour patients where HBsAg were tested, 66% of Pacific Islanders, 100% of Maori and 0% of Europeans had positive antigenaemia."

20 Blumberg, B.S. and London, W.T. 1980. In Essex, M. et al. (eds). "Viruses in naturally occurring cancer, Book A, Cold Spring Harbour Conferences on Cell Proliferation." p. 403. "Some of the chronic carriers develop chronic active hepatitis, but the majority do not; some proportion of the individuals which chronic active hepatitis develop

Suddenly it was being intimated that we could eliminate all cancer developing from chronic hepatitis with this vaccine, which isn't true. No one mentioned that:

> ***"In Auckland, 30–40% of all chronic hepatitis is due to HBV infection."***[21]

Well, what causes the other 60–70% of chronic hepatitis?

Why did no one mention at the time that a significant number of liver cancers aren't caused by Hepatitis B?[22] Why had none of the European liver cancer patients in Auckland had Hepatitis B? What was causing non-Hepatitis B liver cancer here and in the USA?

> ***"In the United States, alcoholic cirrhosis more commonly leads to primary hepatic cancer than does chronic Hepatitis B infection."***

Nor was there any discussion with New Zealanders about the fact that:

> ***"It has been clearly shown that symptomatic Hepatitis B carriers are much more likely to develop hepatocellular abnormalities when they drink alcohol . . . it is thought that hepatotoxic substances exert a synergistic effect on the liver and that liver cell injury is more likely to occur in the chronic carrier state."***[23]

---

cirrhosis, but most do not: and finally, some of the individuals with cirrhosis develop PHC (liver cancer) but again most (~75% from the Japanese study) do not. Therefore it is important to investigate which factors lead to progression from one stage to another and which lead to arrest of the process or even reversal."

21 Lane, M.R. et al. 1985. "Hepatitis B viral infections: clinical, pathological, serological features and treatment". *New Zealand Medical Journal*, Feb 13; 98(772): 57–61. PMID: 2983271. p. 58.

22 Blumberg, B.S. and London, W.T. 1980. In Essex, M. et al. (eds). "Viruses in naturally occurring cancer, Book A, Cold Spring Harbour Conferences on Cell Proliferation." p. 426. "More interesting are (liver cancer) patients apparently not actively infected with HBV . . . tumors from most such patients studied appear to be free of detectable viral antigens and viral DNAs. The failure to find viral DNA base sequences in these tumours suggests they are not viral in origin . . . No evidence of HBV DNA base sequences or any other viral markers was found in numerous HCC from American and African patients, in particular those without HbsAg in the blood . . . If in fact, the viral genome is not present in these tumours an etiological (causal) relationship of HBV with the tumors would seem unlikely. In that case, a significant fraction of HCCs in man (particularly those in populations, such as the United States, with low incidence of HBV infection), must be caused by factors other than HBV."

23 Murray, B.J. 1986. "The Hepatitis B carrier state". *Am Fam Physician*, Apr; 33(4): 127–33. PMID: 2938461.

The 14th edition of *Harrison's*[24] had a long list of toxins and prescription drugs that could also cause liver cancer, including oral contraceptives. Another book described an immune system defect, which stopped some people clearing the virus from their bodies and increased the chances of liver cancer. A vaccine trial suggested a similar defect in vaccine non-responders.[25]

Does that mean people who don't get antibodies from the Hepatitis B vaccine have an immune system defect? Are they the ones at greater risk of liver cancer, from multiple other sources? What might those factors be?

Ironically, at about this time the *Star*[26] carried an article saying:

"A single nutrient deficiency can result in total impairment of the immune processes" and it quoted a study showing that 88% of American hospital patients had at least one nutrient deficiency and 59% two or more.

As mentioned before, New Zealand's soil is chronically selenium deficient. Farmers know that. How many people do? Selenium deficiency is known to be linked to immune-system dysfunction, as well as prostate cancer amongst other problems, so might it also be linked to liver cancer? According to Chinese studies, yes.

Given that 70% of people who contract Hepatitis B never have any symptoms, but simply develop immunity, might not the serious Hepatitis B that I had, (and liver cancer of all types), actually be a nutritional issue?

Add to that a *Herald* article[27] which stated ***"Nicotine in tobacco may act as a tour guide for cancer cells, helping the disease spread through the body"*** and some questions need to be asked, because it was the norm at that time (and probably even now), for the high-risk carrier and liver cancer groups to have a high use of

24 McGraw-Hill, T. 1998. in Fauci S. et al (eds). *Harrison's Principles of Internal Medicine*, pp. 1798–9.

25 Ryder, R.W. et al. 1985. "Response of Children of Patients with Primary Hepatocellular Carcinoma to Hepatitis B virus vaccine". *J. Infect Dis.* January: 151(1): 187–91. "The non-responders closely resemble many patients with PHC (primary hepatic cancer) who produce high titers of antibody to hepatitis B core antigen and to hepatitis B E antigen, but who do not develop anti-HBs. Inability to produce anti-HBs despite high levels of circulating hepatitis B surface antigen suggests the presence of a specific immune defect. These non-responders, unprotected by the HBV vaccine, might be that portion of the population at greatest risk of developing PHC. Failure to consider this possibility could seriously compromise any mass attempt to prevent PHC through widespread administration of HBV vaccine." PMID: 2981276.

26 1987. *The Star*, 20 January.

27 1988. *New Zealand Herald* 23 April: p. 3.

alcohol, cigarettes and prescription medicine, many of which further compromise liver function.

None of these variables in carriage rates or known data concerning diet, alcohol, smoking, drugs, their relationship with immunity, liver function and cancer were being discussed at all.

There was no sensible discussion about real risks of the disease or the vaccine being offered to anyone, except Mr Milne's perspective, which didn't fit the KISS principle.

When I expressed concern about lack of information on the risks of the vaccine, and dismissing of potentially serious side-effects, and pointed out the list in the international physicians' circular, those concerns were thrust away by Mr Milne:

> ***"You take 10,000 children and give them each a lolly, and see how many are sick tomorrow. The difficulty is establishing how much higher the rate of complaints is than it would have been in the same group if they were given no vaccine."***[28]

Which is an old-fashioned view, because these days there is never a vaccine trial written up in which one group have the vaccine, and the other group get nothing.

To dismiss potential side-effects in that way (epidemiologically) is very unscientific. The whole principle of a drug reaction is that if the individual is given something and it causes a reaction, the individual stops using it. It's called ***"challenge/dechallenge/rechallenge"*** and is also acknowledged with regard to vaccines in a 1994 book[29] which some doctors considered the gold standard of vaccine safety:

> ***"Dechallenge: did the adverse event diminish as would be expected if the vaccine caused the event . . . Rechallenge: Was the vaccine readministered? If so, did the adverse even recur?"***

If I eat tamarillos, they turn around and come right back up again. I know this, because it has happened repeatedly. I don't need a 10,000-

---

28 Calder, P. 1988. "Campaign aims to cut hepatitis risk". *New Zealand Herald*, 12 March: B12.

29 Vaccine Safety Committee, IOM. 1994. In Stratton, K. R., Howe, C. J., Johnston, R. B. (eds). *Adverse Events Associated with Childhood Vaccines, Evidence Bearing on Causality*. Washington DC: National Academy Press. (ISBN 0-309-04895-8).

person trial to tell me that penicillin could well kill me next time, or that another rubella vaccine might yet again, give me arthritis. So when is a reaction a reaction? Only when it suits?

Over the ditch in Australia where a similar campaign was being run, medical colleagues (and parents) were being given information considerably more to the point.[30]

"of all people who contract Hepatitis B nearly:

75% will only develop mild symptoms,

20% will develop "moderate" symptoms,

5% will develop severe illness,

fewer than 1% will die from the disease or associated symptoms such as liver cancer. That is, of the 1766 people who contracted Hepatitis B in 1986, about 1315 had "mild" symptoms, about 345 had "moderate symptoms", about 90 were "severely ill", and about 15 died from it.

From this we can ascertain that, all things being equal, you and your children run approximately a 105 in 16 million chance of contracting Hepatitis B and getting very ill or possibly even dying. That is, less than a one in 150,000 chance. All things being equal, you run about HALF the risk of dying from Hepatitis B as you do of contracting leprosy (there were 27 cases of leprosy reported in 1986).

The good doc then points out that *"contrary to Smith Kline and French hysteria"* Hepatitis B is largely confined to high risk groups: homosexuals, prostitutes, and IV drug users, and that medical and hospital workers are only slightly higher risk than average, but nowhere near "high-risk" groups.

He then says:

"Put into perspective, the chances of a 'normal' person contracting and dying from Hepatitis are just slightly higher than getting kicked to death by a horse."

Interesting, that a medical bulletin would use the word *"hysteria"*.

---

30 1989. "Hepatitis 'B' and aids: should you be worried?" *Inside News* September/October: pp. 12–13.

It would be fair to say that in 1988, people like me, even some medical people who questioned, were very much under the gun by the Health Department. But then something happened to make it a lot worse. A headline rang out:

"Terrorism" By Anti-vaccine Groups Alleged[31]

No-one was mentioned, but rumour spread throughout the country that it was *"anti-vaccine campaigners"* who were spreading *"gross slander"*:[32] rumours that there was an AIDS link with the vaccine, because the blood-based vaccine was made from the blood of homosexuals. The director general of health, Dr George Salmond chimed in saying[33] that the allegations were *"totally irresponsible and almost criminal"*.

Mr Milne intoned:

> *"'Let us get these people out front and ask them to explain themselves,' Mr Milne said. 'They will find themselves in court so fast that they will not know what has hit them.'"*[34]

Dr Nigel Ashworth[35] joined the fray, saying, *"It is just like terrorism – it is criminal to tell young mothers whose babies have already had the first shot that the vaccine could be contaminated with the AIDS virus."*

Over three days I was repeatedly asked by journalists why *I* had been so irresponsible as to say such a thing. The journalists just assumed that. So in order to protect myself, I had to find out what the real story was.

It turned out that Smith Kline and French (SKF) had sent a company brochure to doctors which stated that their yeast-based vaccine did not share the same theoretical risk of AIDS infection that was associated with plasma-derived vaccine, and this had been debated on radio. Two Wellington doctors then put a public notice in

31 Longdill, S. (Whangarei Staff). 1988. "Anti-immunization campaigners were using a form of terrorism, a world authority on the Hepatitis B vaccine said last night." *New Zealand Herald* 20 April: Section 1: 4.

32 1988. "Aids link to vaccine 'not true'". *Waikato Times* 18 April.

33 NZPA. 1988. "Aids Allegations 'Irresponsible'". *New Zealand Herald,* 21 April: Section 1: 14.

34 Longdill, S. (Whangarei Staff). 1988. "Anti-immunization campaigners were using a form of terrorism, a world authority on the Hepatitis B vaccine said last night." *New Zealand Herald* 20 April: Section 1: 4.

35 Jarvis, L. 1988. "Spreading AIDS link rumours 'terrorism'". *Auckland Star,* 20 April.

the *Dominion* to the effect that they couldn't guarantee their patients would not get AIDS from the vaccine.

I wrote it all up, but only one paper out of the many sent the information would publish it,[36] and even then, they wouldn't do it without also publishing written confirmation from the Ministry of Health – such is the power of silent innuendo.

What I wanted to know then, and still would like to know now, is why the Health Department didn't state right from the start who had started the rumour? I can't imagine the Department didn't know exactly where the accusatory phone calls would land up.

An anonymous advertisement appeared in the February 1989 issue of the *Listener*[37] targeting adults, which was designed to look as if it came from the Health Department. This caused Mr Milne to comment, because he considered it to be misleading and scaremongering. The advertisement said that some adults who contract Hepatitis B would die from liver cancer or cirrhosis of the liver. Mr Milne replied:[38]

> ***"The risk of a person dying of liver cancer if they contract Hepatitis B as an adult is about the same as the chances of being kicked to death by a duck."***

That's a change from a horse.

The same article was useful in that Dr Rod Ellis Pegler defined those at most risk of Hepatitis B as being Polynesians; intravenous drug users; people with multiple sexual partners; recipients of multiple blood transfusions; health care workers, and babies born to carrier mothers. Dr Ellis-Pegler also mentioned a seemingly unlikely method of transmission . . . that of an Hepatitis B-carrying orienteer running through cutty grass, who got cut on the legs, and the following orienteers cutting themselves with the same grass and contracting the disease . . .

It appeared that Smith Kline and French, the company that placed the advertisement in the *Listener* then decided to progress their cause further[39] and go public and into schools in an advance effort to

36 Butler, H. 1988. "AIDS 'rumour' came from doctors". *Franklin County News*, 26 April.
37 ADVERTISEMENT. 1989. *New Zealand Listener*, 10 February: two page, full colour.
38 Chisholm, D. 1989. "Drug company's hepatitis claims misleading, says top researcher". *Sunday Star*, 12 February: A4.
39 Calder. P. 1989. "Immunity for those who can pay". *New Zealand Herald*, 11 March: Section 2:1.

get a contract to vaccinate 650,000 school-aged children, which would provide a theoretical income of $25 million assuming a 100% compliance rate. While Fraser MacKenzie said[40] that his company:

> ***"Had spent hundreds of thousands of dollars planning the campaign and educating the public about Hepatitis B."***

Schools and the Health Department saw it very differently. The information and video supplied by the company were considered to be promotional and to provide no information upon which to allow informed consent and the Health Department requested it be withdrawn. Having heard from principals and parents about the high-pressure sales pitch and the allegedly scaremongering presentations given to pupils, it's not surprising that the contract went elsewhere. What is surprising is that in 2005, the Health Department used exactly the same tactics in the Meningitis campaign.

Mr Milne[41] said:

> ***"the plan was 'bad medicine' because it will not identify children who are already carriers of the Hepatitis B virus . . . the important thing is to identify carriers because they are at great personal risk and 'are spreading the disease'",***

And that he opposed the universal programme[42] saying it was ***"alarmist, exaggerated and grossly misleading"*** and that the company misused his data to give an exaggerated impression of the Tauranga Hepatitis B incidence, when in fact there was no factual data available for Tauranga.

The other interesting point brought out in the article was that:

> ***"Late last year Smith Kline and French had offered to vaccinate Auckland City Council workers. But the council followed Mr Milne's advice to have blood tests first and these showed about half the workers were already immune."***

Were parents getting any of these messages directly from the health

---

40 Chisholm. 1989. "Child Jab push, drug firm takes virus fight to New Zealand schools". *Sunday Star*, 19 February.

41 Chishold, D. 1989. "Hold off on jabs, asks researcher". *Sunday Star*, 26 February): A2.

42 1989. "Milne says hepatitis scheme alarmist". *Bay of Plenty Times*, 21 April: 1.

profession though? Do most parents read every paper they can get their hands on? No. Were parents told that having their adolescent children or young adults tested before vaccination might be worthwhile? No.

The Health Department's view was that blood testing was expensive and not worthwhile because the vaccine the Government was buying was so cheap. In other words, they had little interest in finding carriers.

What were other parents in really low-risk areas being told? An article and accompanying advertisement[43] in the *Saturday Express*[44] where a testing programme showed no carriers, was fairly typical. Over half the advertisement, giving the vaccination venue four days later, said:

> *"IF YOU LOVE 'EM, [Picture] PROVE IT! . . . Immunize your child against Hepatitis B."*

In the accompanying article, Dr Maree Leonard taking up two out of three columns said how bad carriage was, and how terrible the disease could be, ***"The virus will stay with you for the rest of your life . . ."*** Never mind that they had no carriers in the area, and the literature of the day stated:

> ***"Each year 1 to 2 per cent of HbsAg carriers seroconvert to an immune state. It is not unusual for hepatitis B antigenemia[45] to resolve after 20 to 30 years. In addition, the titer of HbsAG in the carrier decreases with the length of the carrier state."***[46]

There were statements maintaining that vaccinated people couldn't catch Hepatitis B after being given the vaccine which have been proven wrong in many medical articles. It was also said that the vaccine immunity mimicked natural immunity, which directly contradicted the Health Department booklet, *A Guide for Health Professionals*, which on page 13 states that ***"Following vaccination antibody levels decay rapidly, something that doesn't normally happen with natural immunity."***

When you look at the information accompanying the advertisement

43 1989. "If you love em, prove it!" *Saturday Express*, 4 March.
44 1989. "Parents strongly urged to get children immunized". *Saturday Express*, 4 March.
45 antigenaemia = hepatitis virus constantly in the blood.
46 Murray, B. 1986. "The Hepatitis B carrier state". *Am Fam Physician*, April: 33(4): 127–33. PMID: 2938461.

you can see why such tactics were used. Rather than tell people facts, it is easier to get compliance by creating guilt. Engrave on parents' brains the message that every day at school, their children could be infected by bare-foot children with scratches and cuts, every day was another day their child might get sick, and if they didn't have them vaccinated, they didn't love them.

Some parents weren't even told that, but were just being bullied. When asked about it, the authorities admitted it:

> ***"We bully the parents a bit, but it's really important for their children to have these injections"***[47]

A very upset mother was allowed space in the *Hauraki Herald* to challenge remarks by the local Medical Officer of Health.[48] Her two children had had serious reactions and her outrage was palpable when she said:

> ***"He also says that 'only a couple of children had not completed the course of injections because of health' but this again is not true, as both of my children reacted to the vaccine and neither have finished their courses."***

Another letter from an angry parent in the same paper, objecting to Dr Nicholl's statement that ***"there was only <u>one chance in several million</u> for a child to have an immediate response to the vaccines such as severe collapse", and "is one reaction too much to ask for the wipe-out of Hepatitis B?"*** said:

> ***"Parents are continually bombarded with 'fear tactic' information with the Hepatitis B promotion. Every time you switch on a radio or TV or pick up the paper you are warned of this terrible plague about to kill off all unvaccinated children . . . I spoke to Professor Ralph Edwards, the medical assessor for medicine last week because my nephew had had a severe reaction . . . Prof Edwards told me of a letter he sent to the Health Department and which was now being circulated regarding severe allergic reaction responses to the vaccine. After speaking***

---

47 1988. "Parents jabbed into action". The *Auckland Sun*, 28 June: 5. Quoting vaccination co-ordinator Atarangi Muru.

48 "Very concerned mother". 1988. "Reaction to vaccine". *Hauraki Herald* 25 June: 31.

to him, I rang the Health Department and was told this letter was not for public scrutiny as 'they were afraid of it getting into the paper'".

After that, publicity pretty much stopped, since most babies were now jabbed, the pre-school catch-up programme was complete, so there wasn't much else for the media to say.

To this day, some people who thought they were immune because they had had three shots are finding that they are carriers. Mr Milne was right. Everyone should have been tested. In my opinion, the Health Department was wrong.

Many people who decided to be tested after being vaccinated also found they had no immunity from the vaccine at all, even after six vaccinations in total. What they had never been told was that the one and only small study done in this country at that time showed that if you were over thirty years of age you were unlikely to get any antibodies to the vaccine. And how long they would last was anyone's guess.[49]

As to side-effects, what side-effects? The semantic dissembling on that was exemplified by Dr Ashworth's reply[50] to my criticism that while he was sending out memos to health professionals warning about anaphylactoid reactions, he wasn't telling parents. His response was that I'd mistaken the word "anaphylactoid" for "anaphylaxis" and that Anaphylactoid wasn't a "true" condition. "We are not talking about adverse reactions . . . we're talking about adverse effects."

And exactly what does that mean? One is a reaction and the other isn't?

---

49 Goldwater, P.N. 1984. "Successful short course for intradermal Hepatitis B vaccine". *New Zealand Medical Journal*, Dec 26; 97(770): 905–6. "We have shown that a short course of three injections one month apart is highly immunogenic in younger vaccinees but is less than satisfactory in older recipients." PMID: 6595584.

50 Parker, L. 1988. "Vaccination campaign flawed". The *Dominion*, 18 July: [PAGE?].

27 Keeping Focused

Freedoms.

Rights.

We all want them.

With them however, must go Responsibility, so that we can use those freedoms and rights properly.

The problem is: who will be the judge of that responsibility?

We talk about making informed choices that will lead to right decisions.

But what is an informed choice?

Is your "informed choice" on vaccination, for example, going to be the same as my "informed" choice?

Surely an informed choice will be based on the information you and I have available to us and are prepared to read?

We have laws that are designed to protect us from all sorts of discrimination.

There is talk of Hate Speech legislation.

What would be the implications of that?

How would **hate speech** be defined and adjudged?

For years now those who have opposed vaccination and refused to immunize their children have been subjected to considerable abuse from those who consider them irresponsible and enemies of society.

Surely such tactics seem to be denying those people their freedoms and rights? They are suffering a form of discrimination. How would such verbal abuse stand up against hate speech? The list of words can be quite disgusting, but I feel sad and sorry for those who resort to these measures.

Behind so many issues of life there are power games being played out. Huge vested interests and political agendas go to great lengths to protect themselves. Whether they will acknowledge it or not, they are wanting to play God by assuming roles that are not theirs to have. In every town of Orlsrite there will be a Dick Tait in charge of the Ministry of Conformity, Compliance and Control. (See Chapter 77.)

The systems of this world will not change. They will never become better. Legislation will be passed as it is required, and freedoms and rights will be sacrificed on the altar of expediency, for such things are expendable. All for our own good and well-being, don't you know!

Those who question vaccination threaten the profits and power of drug manufacturing companies. The more vaccines that can be invented, the greater will be the returns from a captive market – from childbirth to the grave.

Not only is it a matter of survival for the industry, but it is also a matter of survival for the large numbers of ordinary people who are dependent on the drug companies for their employment, as well as their **health**!

Within this web of inter-dependence, you and I can become the flies for the spiders.

We become pawns on a chessboard – if we allow ourselves to be.

All that I have mentioned is abuse in one form or another, but the verbal abuse employed by so many people from all walks of life can be extremely irritating and intimidating as well as identifying double standards.

I have always maintained the truth of the old saying "Mud thrown is ground lost." It represents energy that could be put to much better use. I certainly do not want to lower myself to return any missiles. Any *splatters, which may land on me, will be shed like water off a duck's back.*

The mudslingers are frequently those who, in a subtle way, are encouraged by the string-pullers' propaganda, slogans and perks freely made available to them.

Rocket launching often seems to be automatic – a response triggered by a perceived threat appearing on a radar screen. Is it friend or foe? Shoot it down and identify it later, whatever the tragic consequences! Is that good enough?

Those with their hands clean, comfortable in their plush offices may be guilty of failing to see the truth; or denying facts which cannot be ignored, on the assumption that anything coming from the "other side" must be wrong.

I have chosen a lifestyle that is based on strong convictions. Those convictions will not be compromised.

I will make responsible decisions according to my beliefs. There will be times when I may agree to disagree, but I don't have to stoop to tactics which can be so hypocritical.

I shall remain watchful, while the systems and powerful interests have their fling. There is a limit to how long it can last.

I shall try to speak the truth in love, as genuine and constructive opportunities arise.

That's not weakness.

That's strength.

28 1988 – Sinbinned

During this time, the Dean of Auckland Medical School invited me to talk to students about my views. They wanted a debate, with me talking first for an hour, them rebutting for an hour, and questions for another hour which was unacceptable because I did not want to be constantly interrupted during my speaking time, as had happened on a previous occasion. And since medical students study for four years, the students have plenty of time to hear the views of the medical school. If the students wanted to hear mine, they were welcome. If they wanted to question me, they were welcome, but the medical school was not welcome to turn it into a debate.

The Medical School changed the invitation and I went there on 29 June 1988 for two hours to speak to a full house. As always, my radar switched on early to assess the body language of people, and work out who was who. From about half way, I became aware of someone at the back, who was able to sit still and concentrate efficiently. Usually, if medical audiences disagree with what you say they stop listening and fidget because they are uncomfortable, so it's rare to see either neutral or positive body language. This person was different.

Half-way through question time, I challenged the silent listener by the door and asked who he was. Without hesitation, he said that he was an immunologist. So I asked him whether he could pick up anything said that was stupid or illogical, and he replied that he could not, and that on issues of scientific accuracy, he couldn't challenge anything I had said.

I didn't know what to do. Here was a second person in the system, who was a thinker. Perhaps the medical world wasn't as narrow as I had previously thought. Perhaps there was hope.

There had been a number of children who had had side-effects from the Menomune A vaccine in 1987, who were still unwell, and being stonewalled by doctors. There was now also the issue of large numbers of children unwell after the nationwide pre-school Hepatitis B vaccination campaign. Perhaps this person might be able to answer the question, "What is it that we are seeing here?"

This man's speciality was looking at immunology in a much broader context than just T-cells or B-cells. His interest was how the day-to-day circumstances which direct T-cells and B-cells affect the immune system overall. He talked to some of the parents involved.

Later he invited me to talk to the Immunology Department, and asked me to speak on smallpox. It was also a full house and I felt as though I was walking into a barely restrained lion's den, but I was determined to try to do it well, so definitely over-prepared. I chose to sit, primarily so they wouldn't see my knees knocking under the table. It's tough trying to say what you need to in an atmosphere that comes across as civilised, but is pregnant with aggression. I'm sure none of them realized the body language messages they sent out.

Ten minutes before the end of my presentation, someone stood up and interrupted saying that he wasn't interested in smallpox and wanted to know why my children weren't vaccinated against rubella. I calmly told him that I didn't set the topic for the day, and I would address his issues after the end of my presentation. I expected questions on the actual presentation, but got none.

Total, dead, silence.

I believed I had put together an extensive and conclusive presentation which showed that the statement that smallpox vaccine eradicated smallpox was not correct. Even worse, because of the way the vaccine was made and administered it had serious contamination issues, caused person-to-person transmission diseases and extremely serious side-effects, including cancer. All my references were from literature, and all papers used were there in person, so to speak.

And then they started. Polio, Tetanus, Rubella. Everything, but not smallpox.

I watched as two immunologists debated with each other whether Polio was a more important vaccine to give than Tetanus. They couldn't agree, and when things got heated between them, I said that it was ironic that two immunologists couldn't agree amongst themselves, yet considered it insulting when a parent exercised informed choice and chose not to vaccinate. Was there room for dissent only amongst themselves?

We adjourned for a while, and then had another meeting, chaired by Dr Lloyd Cairns, then the country's only paediatric immunologist. He wanted to know how we could progress these issues, since he didn't want to be around the same table in five years time, arguing the same points. He wanted to know why it was that I didn't accept the assurances of previous studies of vaccine effectiveness and safety.

One of many examples I gave him was the whooping cough vaccine used at that time, which had been trialled in 18-month-old children, YEARS before, in another country. That data was extrapolated without study to the 3-month age group, and then, having used it in that age group, that fact was used to justify vaccinating 6-week-old babies. There were other confounding features of the studies used, which he could not argue with.

I also presented information which showed that you can't test several vaccines separately, and then put them together, and expect them to work the same way, or guarantee that multiple vaccines at one time were safe.

I asked him several other questions like, "Exactly how much do you know about the immune system of a baby?" The answer was, "Not very much".

That was followed up with, "How much do you know about what vaccines do inside a baby's body?" That question was important because not long before, I had received written confirmation that the Hepatitis B vaccine had never been studied with regard to either the immune system of the baby, or liver enzyme function. The manufacturer of the vaccine had been asked by a doctor, who was very concerned at abnormal liver tests being returned from vaccinated newborns with jaundice lasting, in some cases, for over two months.

The more questions I put to him, which he couldn't answer, the more annoyed he seemed to get. He finally asked, "What do you want?" I answered that I wanted experts to stop pretending they knew everything about something they knew very little about, and instead to find out more. Instead of comparing vaccinated children with children given different vaccines, I believed it was time to do a long-term study which specifically compared totally unvaccinated children with vaccinated children.

If both groups were serologically tested from birth onwards, looking at the immune system parameters that the medical profession did understand, and comparing group differences in overall health as time went on, they might gain a decent understanding of the long-term health outcomes for both groups. Given that there had been a longitudinal study going on in Dunedin of a few thousand babies from birth for quite a few years, I felt that cohort might be useful, but we could provide them with another if they wished.

He asked me what such a study might prove, and I replied that, firstly, it would immediately resolve a lot of outstanding issues like the role of vaccines in endotoxic shock, which I believe was often misdiagnosed as SIDS, and whether vaccines changed the immune system and led to more allergies, asthma, chronic glue ear and other complaints. I described a study that the Immunization Awareness Society had done using parents who had immunized their first child, or two children, then had chosen not to vaccinate their subsequent children.

The study found dramatic differences between the two groups. The unvaccinated children had far fewer chronic complaints and a much better ability to cope with acute infections than vaccinated children. Vaccinated children had much higher rates of complaints like glue ear, asthma and chronic disorders. Such a study done officially would be of value in answering his opening questions, and parents' concerns.

I went out on a limb and said that, given time, IAS could provide to any study authors an unvaccinated cohort of whatever size they needed.

Much to my surprise, this was immediately discounted by a woman paediatrician who said that parents who chose not to immunize their children were more educated, and would also provide much better nutrition, and would care for their children better.

I was shocked and retorted, "Are you telling me, that you could not find a control group, in parents who chose to vaccinate, whose family situations in all other respects are equal, to match those of parents who chose not to immunize? And that you believe that parents who chose not to vaccinate are better parents?" I said that given the knowledge and resources, all parents wanted to be the best parents they could be.

I then suggested that if they wanted we could provide them with the "same family, fully vaccinated controls" to use, as an option. What better group could eliminate a lot of the possibly confounding variables between vaccinated and unvaccinated within a case and control study?

Children from these families had the same family genetics, food, house, income, schools, doctor, parents, infection exposure, with the only outward variable affecting the immune system that we could see being immunization. To have both groups within the same families in the same study would be handing them ideal research material on a plate.

She replied that only a double-blind randomly assigned trial from birth in a maternity hospital could possibly mimic reality in society. For that, you wouldn't want to allow for any confounding factors.

I didn't understand. Wasn't the whole point to eliminate confounding factors and study a situation where all social operatives are equal to see whether it was just the vaccines adversely affecting similar immune systems?

Today, I would reply that vaccine trials should be done the same way to see what happens out in the real world with no confounding factors, but back then, I didn't know that vaccine trials were done by excluding all the sick, weak, and genetically or immunologically flawed children, after which the same vaccine is given to everyone, regardless of their health.

Even worse, those who spoke around the table believed that to do any such study was highly unethical. They couldn't deprive children of all these life-saving vaccines.

Given that these children we were offering weren't going to be vaccinated anyway regardless of what they thought, such a comment seemed ludicrous.

Here was an ideal opportunity for these paediatricians to see whether or not unvaccinated children were actually healthier and what the impact of the parents' decisions upon their children was. If they believed the unvaccinated children would be much sicker as a result, such a study would surely prove their point. And if they wanted to make it a benefit-versus-risk equation, they could also compare the cost of medical care to vaccinated versus unvaccinated children over that period of time.

A woman paediatrician stunned me further by saying that such a study wouldn't find anything, because parents who didn't vaccinate would skew the study by making sure their children were better fed, and better looked after just to prove a point.

Did they not think that maybe vaccinating parents would be equally as competitive in proving their point just as earnestly?

I had never before experienced the medical brick wall that threw up every barrier they could think of as to why something wouldn't work, and therefore why something couldn't be done, and had a growing feeling that the reasons for refusal, weren't one of couldn't, but wouldn't.

The comment that they wouldn't study a group of children who were never going to be vaccinated, because it violated what they believed was the unethical withholding of life-saving treatment from children, was completely illogical to me, and told me that parents who chose not to vaccinate themselves or their children, were unlikely ever to be either respected or accepted or even listened to by the majority. Just listening to them, I felt I was already being judged as some sort of criminal.

I later took the issue up with Dr Ossi Mansoor who was then at the Public Health Commission. He raised exactly the same objections as the paediatricians at the meeting, and said,[1] ***"Of course, comparing the health of immunized versus non-immunized children is epidemiologically unsound because of selection bias."***

Then in the next letter, when I objected to his statement, he wanted to know if we could supply enough children whose parents would be prepared for them to be put in a randomized double-blind trial! But then he added:

> ***"If only we could change parental attitudes, habits and diets, not to mention poverty as easily as we could immunize, then I would agree with you. I think that should be our long-term goal, but for the moment, the practicalities and costs suggest to me that the benefits from immunization outweigh its hazards."***[2]

To this day no such study has been done. I'd still like to know what it would find.

---

1 Letter Dr Ossi Mansoor to Hilary Butler, 24.4.93.
2 Letter Dr Ossi Mansoor to Hilary Butler, 28.4.93.

29 Other Sinbinned Voices in the Wilderness

At about this time, an article came out by some scientists similarly frustrated.[1] Interestingly, one of the authors is a New Zealander. The authors wanted to discuss which specific measures had the most impact on the reduction in death rates in the United States in the 1900s.

> ***"Clearly, the medical measures considered for tuberculosis, typhoid, measles and scarlet fever were introduced at the point when the death rate for each of these diseases was already negligible. Any changes in the rates of decline that occurred subsequent to the interventions could only be minute. Of the remaining five diseases (excluding smallpox with its negligible contribution), poliomyelitis is the only disease for which the medical measures produced any noticeable change in the trends. The other four diseases – pneumonia, influenza, whooping cough, and diphtheria – exhibit relatively smooth mortality trends that are unaffected by the medical measures, even though these measures were introduced when the death rates were still notable.***

1 McKinlay, J.B., McKinlay, S.M., and Beaglehole, R. 1989. "A Review of the Evidence Concerning the Impact of Medical Measures on Recent Mortality and Morbidity in the United States". *International Journal of Health Services*, Vol. 19(2): 181–208. PMID: 2654039.

They went on to say if the poliomyelitis death rate decline was attributed to the vaccine only, then the success of medical interventions for all other diseases considered could only account for 1% of mortality decline. He said:

> "*"Rather, if we were also to attribute, more conservatively, some of the subsequent fall in the death rates for pneumonia, influenza, whooping cough, and diphtheria to medical measures . . . 3.5 per cent probably represents a reasonable upper-limit estimate of the total contribution of medical measures to the decline in infectious disease mortality in the United States since 1900.*" (Emphasis in the original.)

Medical intervention includes all forms of prophylactic and remedial protocols available to the medical profession at that time. Later on in the article, the authors state:

> ". . . *it is now generally conceded that medical interventions (as opposed to public health measures) contributed little to the decline in infectious disease mortality* . . .",

How many medical people attribute the death decline in infectious diseases to public health measures? The authors then go on to discuss aggressive management for heart conditions, strokes and cancer, and come to the conclusion that the claim to fame for all of the above is also unjustified, and ask the question:

> "*If medical measures and services were not primarily responsible for the decline, then how is it to be explained?. . . there are however, influential students of public health who continue to attribute far more to medical measures than available facts warrant (emphasis mine). Others continue to pay lip service to the importance of public health measures, while contradictorily supporting the perpetual expansion of more, but largely ineffective medical services*".

One of their major concerns was that public health continued to be "denounced" as "heretical, iconoclastic or just wrong" and that policy experts were attempting to cover up any contribution of public health in order to justify and increase the use of current medical practice and that medical students were not taught that public health had far greater contributions to offer than specific medical measures.

The authors argued that if the current view that vaccines,etc were steadily eliminating each disease, there would be no commitment to public health, but if it could be conclusively proved that specific measures actually lead to a deterioration in overall population health, then maybe there could be a priority shift and commitment to social change.

Which is basically everything Major Greenwood said in his 1925 book on Epidemic Diseases, and what I'm saying about the ever-increasing use of vaccines against all these different diseases, when real societal change could better the health of everyone, at a fraction of the cost.

In an age of corporatization, people like the McKinlays are usually consigned to the dustbin of useless ideas.

30 There's a Price to Pay

Yes, there has been, and still is a "cost" associated with Hilary's work.

The writing of this book has meant that the events it describes have had to be re-lived for both of us. Obviously this has affected us in different ways.

For me, there are many things from the past twenty years that I would prefer to forget. They bring back painful memories. However, I have been persuaded to mention a few of the "expensive" items, although I do so somewhat reluctantly.

I have already referred to the way in which many people have regarded Hilary, consciously or unconsciously, as "public" property. The worst offenders of course were those from the news media. They have deadlines to meet as well as wanting to get the most traction they can from a "hot" news item. However, organizers of meetings, seminars, workshops and conferences are also guilty, as too are those who want information.

Many have been the occasions when other people have known far more about what my wife is doing and thinking than I have. Very often I have found out about what has already been arranged by overhearing part of a telephone conversation.

It would not be an exaggeration to say that on occasions, Hilary and I might have been fortunate to get ten to fifteen minutes of meaningful conversation between us in a whole day.

Because of the need to be available to the children during the day, and to be in the house while they slept, I have been the only one who could fulfil this role. When night-time meetings have been arranged, and very often they can be held quite a distance away, sometimes involving several hours of travelling, I have had to entrust her to the care of someone else who will provide the transport. This has often meant her return in the early hours of the morning.

Because of a range and combination of circumstances and situations I have never been able to hear my sought-after wife speak at a public meeting or conference. I recently watched some videos of Hilary's past talks, and realized how rapidly the years have passed by. I looked at her animated and passionate delivery. I watched her cute pony tail (when she had one) and tried to remember her as she was then, and became quite choked up with emotion. I can't bring back those days when in a sense I had to be spectator at a distance.

Although our children no longer have to be "minded" the years have caught up with me, and night driving and late nights are far too stressful; so again, I have to make do with photographic or video'd coverage of my beautiful wife's presentations.

The emotional and physical strains of dealing with "cases", the media and the "opposition" have often resulted in Hilary's health suffering in some way, and on such occasions my role is to help pick up the pieces and get things back on an even keel again.

Over the years one of the hardest things I have had to cope with have been the times of acute loneliness, even though there may have been plenty of "action" for Hilary. Long telephone conversations, of several hours' duration; and these days, hours of time on the computer, can often reduce natural spontaneous conversation to a bare minimum, and doing things together can often be thwarted by an unexpected telephone call, or email.

There is still the "language" barrier! I have referred to this elsewhere, but I am still only a simple-minded lay person who struggles with the vocabulary and jargon that the years of research have given to Hilary. She understands the subjects so well, and can respond to the issues fuelled by the medical systems, drug companies, etc. It has become her life. She can talk the talk with so many people throughout the world who are involved in similar work. They speak the same "language" as they communicate by phone or e-mails. This is, no doubt, stimulating and necessary ***for those concerned****.*

Not many people have ever acknowledged to me, or the boys, how much they appreciate the "use" of Hilary by expressing a thank you for it.

Maybe a half dozen have. I well remember someone ringing up especially to thank me personally, for the "sacrifices" and inconveniences the family had to make.

That person's thoughtfulness, and the thoughtfulness of others like her, have done a lot to keep us going.

What of the future?

Is Hilary's work going to continue to snowball?

Is it unreasonable to look forward to being able to share my "retirement" years with Hilary? To be able to do things that relate to the health issues ***together****, as well as the other priorities which are so important too?*

If we meet you sometime in the future, let's keep things simple, shall we! I'd enjoy that after all these years.

31 Fighting Hogwash – Dr J. Anthony Morris

In 1988 and 1989 I was contacted by a small group of underground medical people, who were honestly concerned by what they were seeing in their practices. Some felt helpless in the face of what looked to them like a ticking timebomb. Somewhere, they felt, there had to be someone, brave enough to speak out, without having their head chopped off.

But . . . where?

Years before, Robert Mendelsohn had directed me to his friend, the courageous Dr Anthony J. Morris. But I was a bit scared to write to Dr Morris. I also knew Dr Glen Dettman, another person recommended by Dr Mendelsohn. He sent me medical articles which told some of Dr Morris's story. Digging around in Auckland Library archives, I gleaned more.

Most medical people have no idea of Dr John Anthony Morris's place in vaccine history and he is modest enough not to wish to dwell on his achievements. In the early days, what others had told me, and what little else I had found, was all I knew. Dr Morris brushed aside any suggestion that his story should be written up, but if everyone in the world knew, perhaps they would understand a little of what lies behind some of the current silence in the vaccination debate.

His story sets up the WHOLE of the submerged history on withheld information about modern vaccines.

Just before World War II, Dr Morris began his studies at Walter

Reed Hospital in Washington DC where he trained as a microbiologist with a special interest in viral diseases, and started working for the government in 1940. In the 1940s and 1950s he had a distinguished career researching viral and respiratory diseases. In the mid-50s the National Institute of Health set him to work investigating vaccines and the risk factors in their use. At the same time Tony was also a key figure in setting up the NIH research program on kuru and scrapie, as well as making important discoveries in responses to influenza vaccines.

In 1959, Dr Morris was recruited to the DBS[1] by Dr Joseph Smadel who drew up long-term influenza research plans for Dr Morris's laboratory. Behind the scenes, a heated controversy had been boiling in medical circles, because though the first flu vaccine was licensed in 1945, it had never taken off. People in the upper echelons argued that mass vaccination against the flu and the common cold was vital to combat the most debilitating respiratory diseases, and to forward this aim, they needed someone of Dr Morris's knowledge and calibre to do the work to prove it was possible.

Dr Morris quickly became alarmed at what he found. Regardless of the potency stated on a bottle's label, it was impossible to measure the actual strength of the vaccine.

By 1963, the studies he had done on elderly people and the flu vaccine, showed that if there was any benefit to be derived, it was so small it could not be reliably measured.

In association with Dr Galdichec (who subsequently won the Nobel prize for his investigation on croup), Dr Morris's studies on the Caroline Islands showed that, irrespective of the slight difference between the circulating virus and the vaccine, the flu vaccine was about 20% effective. Sometimes it was 40% effective, other times 0%.

To try to find out why good protection wasn't possible, other experiments showed that though the vaccine produced IgG antibodies in the blood, it didn't produce IgA in the lungs and mucus membranes where an infection might start. His studies on side-effects were also starting to concern him. In December 1966 his completed studies showed that flu vaccines were of minimal benefit, and that studies should be done to find out why.

When he communicated his concerns to his superiors, he very quickly ran into fierce opposition. He said, "*There is a close tie*

1 Division of Biologics Standards, now FDA (Federal Drug Agency).

between government scientists and manufacturing scientists. And my results were hurting the market for flu vaccines." DBS informed him he should hand over all records and materials and he would be relieved of his job. In order to prevent total destruction of his work, one of his technicians took various virus pools ***"to other places"***. But Dr Morris had no option but to destroy thousands of research animals as ordered.

His laboratory staff were reassigned elsewhere, and publication of his articles was blocked by superiors. All his research materials were crated, and taken away, the locks changed on his laboratory, he was placed in a small room with no telephone, and people wishing to see him had to get permission from the chief of the laboratory.

By 1970, over 20 million doses of influenza vaccine were being sold in the USA, making it one of the largest selling vaccines produced in the USA. At the beginning of that year, Dr Morris had just decided to leave the DBS and look for work elsewhere, when one day he was ordered to leave the DBS. He instituted a wrongful dismissal case. All charges against him were overturned, and the grievance committee unanimously found that Morris had been harassed by his superiors over an extended period of time, from 1963 to 1970, that the allegations of releasing bad vaccine was false, but made the amazing statement that Dr Morris's ***"reputation as a scientist would probably not suffer by these internal allegations"***.

It soon became obvious that his reputation had suffered, and Tony felt that his name should be cleared publicly by showing the legislators and the public that the long-term publicity that flu vaccines were being sold on was incorrect.

With a lawyer called James Turner, he drew up a detailed memorandum, showing irregularities in the handling and testing of vaccines by the NIH[2] and the DBS, that the DBS had used ***"dubious techniques"*** to test the flu vaccine and had ***"tampered"*** with the test results, permitting the vaccine labels to show higher potencies than the true value, thereby certifying and releasing watered-down vaccines to the public. They also stated that the DBS harassed many scientists whose research work affected any vaccine market and had forced them to leave the DBS, and actively discouraged pertinent lines of research relating to many vaccines. The Turner/Morris memorandum also

2 National Institute of Health.

charged that in 1966 and 1967 the DBS released at least three lots of potentially contaminated flu vaccine despite one of its scientists, Dr Casper Hiatt, putting a ***"hold"*** order on them.

The NIH set up a special committee in response, to investigate the ***"unsubstantiated"*** claims.

At the same time Dr Morris and some other DBS researchers took a copy of the memorandum to Senator Ribicoff, who initiated a General Accounting Office enquiry at the highest level, not just into the claims of Dr Morris, but into the regulatory responsibility of the DBS.

The GAO concurred with some of Morris's criticisms finding that scientific studies disagreed significantly on the effectiveness of flu vaccines.

Dr Morris said that the benefit of the flu vaccine had been overrated. In children it often induced fever; in some pregnant women it could endanger the fetus, and in all users there was a risk that vaccine ***"literally loaded with extraneous bacteria"*** will be injected. Further, he said that it had been impossible for him to test the product, known as bivalent influenza virus vaccine, for potency.

A former DBS scientist B. G. Young, who endorsed the criticism of the DBS management characterized the DBS attitude towards research as being one of:

> ***"Suppression, harassment, and censorship of individual investigators . . . I finally came to realize that you either had to compromise yourself or leave. Morris and Eddy are the real heroes in that place because they stayed and fought. The others voted with their feet and left."***[3]

There were repeated cases of potentially dangerous vaccines being authorized for release without adequate screening.

Another issue was the use of a Typhus vaccine developed in the 1940s. In 1969, the Armed Forces Epidemiological Board found that some vaccine lots were not giving good antibody responses even though DBS had passed the potency of them. It wasn't known for how many years before 1969 the army had been using useless vaccine. The incident simply added to the catalogue of DBS lack of diligence over the years.

---

3 Wade, N. 1972. "Division of Biologics Standards: The Boat That Never Rocked". *Science*, March: 1225–30. p. 1227.

Naturally enough, the public was never told any of this at the time. The twelve-member special NIH committee came back on 29 November with the astonishing findings that:

> ***"Only a few minor irregularities could be confirmed: however these did not involve any risk to the public."***

It was further stated that as a result of the committee's findings, NIH considered Dr Morris's charges were *"without merit"*.

Dr Morris and James Turner, in turn responded with a 30-page analysis, showing that the committee's report was so seriously flawed that the experts themselves should be investigated by the subcommittee. They presented voluminous data in support, pointing out that the committee had ignored issues they had raised, while responding to issues they had not mentioned, regarding Dr Bernice Eddy. However, they pointed out in reply, that both of Bernice Eddy's memoranda (which the committee had said didn't exist), in which she informed the DBS that the polio vaccine was contaminated, were handed to the committee chairman, and both proved that the conclusions drawn by this committee were at the very least erroneous.

Increasingly, American scientists were understanding that they were expected to be state scientists, not rocking the boat nor making independent findings.

In 1972 a Senate hearing was conducted at the highest level, with these, and other vaccine-related irregularities investigated. At one point Senator Percy asks a Dr Isacson what he thinks the monetary value would have been of the 32 other vaccines, discovered to be of no known protective value, which had been licenced for use by the DBS. The exchange,[4] was:

> ***DR ISACSON. Well, I think it must be astronomical. I do not think I could give you an actual figure. Since some of these appear from the investigation to have been on the market for 20 years, certainly it must add up.***
>
> ***SENATOR PERCY. But we are talking about a cost investment of hundreds of millions of dollars, maybe. Certainly I think that incident very dramatically indicated***

4 From the printed transcript of the Senate Hearings before the Subcommittee on Executive Reorganization and Government research (S.3419) April 20, 21, and May 3, 4, 1972, p. 346.

something was wrong . . . We are locking the barn now, after the horse has gone out . . .

Meanwhile, working for the Food and Drug Administration, Dr Morris was working on a new live flu vaccine to be administered as nose drops, which it was hoped would solve all the problems of the killed flu vaccine. It was reasoned that this vaccine would create immunity in the mucus membranes where it was most needed, and a trial had just been done in children. Dr Morris began testing the vaccine in mice – a precaution which had not been taken previously – and found that the live influenza vaccine accelerated the growth of tumours in test animals. This finding markedly increased Dr Morris's unpopularity among health bureaucrats, but little was said, and the live vaccine was side-lined. I wonder if the manufacturer of the new Flumist vaccine (sprayed up the nose) repeated that work?

In 1976 came the last straw as far as the bureaucrats were concerned. Something which made them determined to get rid of Dr Morris forever. It was the *"Swine Flu fiasco"*.

In February 1976, in Fort Dix in New Jersey, a swine flu strain had been found in a soldier who died on a march. It couldn't be identified in the public health laboratory in New Jersey so they sent it to CDC[5] Atlanta, who designated it as a swine flu virus and immediately started talking up a resulting worldwide pandemic. It was believed that the 1918 epidemic had been due to a swine flu virus, but Paul Brown and Dr Morris, as part of the work in the islands, had been able to prove that the 1918 Spanish flu epidemic wasn't caused by the swine flu virus. It was PR8, another strain of influenza, that was discovered in Puerto Rico many years before. So the CDC's assumption that this was a swine flu that would cause another worldwide pandemic was wrong from the start.

Unfortunately, powers that were, didn't check that out. No other swine influenza virus was recovered except the one at Fort Dix, which was sent to Fort Detrix (the biological warfare unit) who found it was an ordinary pig virus, and that there was no reason to be alarmed.

The virus was then given to Tony Morris's lab to look at, and he also found nothing to distinguish it from any other swine flu strain.

5 Center for Disease Control.

But it seems that the CDC decided that this would be an ideal opportunity to revive the ailing flag-ship of flu vaccination campaigns which had taken a bit of a public denting.

The next thing that was discovered was that they couldn't make a vaccine on that swine flu strain, because it grew too slowly and would take years. So the slow-growing swine flu strain was hybridized with PR8, which meant the swine virus took on the fast-growing properties of 1918 virus. So the viral antigen used in the Swine Flu vaccine wasn't the ordinary pig strain from the soldier, but a fast-growing hybrid.

They sold the vaccine by dramatic hard sell, insisting that a flu epidemic like the 1918 pandemic that killed millions worldwide was imminent unless everyone lined up for the swine flu vaccine. The estimated deaths throughout USA were put at one million. In terms of the chances of it being like 1918, estimates were ***"1 out of 2"***.

The only problem was Dr Morris. Because of what he and the other laboratories had found, he felt the public needed to know that there was no cause for alarm. When he told his then boss he was going to speak out, he was told, ***"I would advise you not to talk about this"***.

He continued to study the virus, and when sure of his facts, went public stating he could find no evidence that this strain was dangerous, or would spread from human to human, but that on the other hand, the vaccine was dangerous and might induce not only hypersensitivity but also neurological side effects; and that there was no precise way to measure the vaccine's potency and its efficacy appeared to be comparatively low.

When vaccine recipients started to experience Guillain Barre, amongst other reactions, Dr Morris's laboratory looked more closely at the vaccine, and publicly reaffirmed their feelings about the lack of effectiveness, and safety. The inevitable happened. The Federal Drug Administration fired Dr Morris for insubordination.

Tony worked out of his lawyer, James Turner's, small office, and his own home, continuing to carry arguments to the press, assessing case histories of side-effects and continuing to attend NIH flu meetings to argue the facts.

By October 1976, 33 people had died after receiving the Swine Flu vaccine, and by mid-December there were about 500 cases of Guillain-Barre. But even up to December all authorities were publicly stating that there was no relationship between any of the deaths or side-effects and the vaccine. In December of that year, at an urgent meeting, Dr Langmuir, one of the chief immunologists at the CDC said, *"We cannot look at these data and not conclude that it was this influenza virus vaccine that precipitated Guillain Barre in those who developed it, so we must consider stopping the programme."* The round-the-table vote was 13 to 1 to stop the programme.

On 16 December 1976 after 46 million shots had been administered, three vaccine-associated deaths were officially admitted to, and the programme was stopped. But the main message continued to be denial, and more denial.

Tony Morris said to the *Washington Post*[6] about flu vaccines:

> *"It's a medical rip-off . . . We should recognize that we don't know enough about the dangers associated with flu vaccine. I believe the public should have truthful information on the basis of which they can determine whether or not to take the vaccine." And he adds, "I believe that, given full information, they won't take the vaccine."*

In 1979, the Civil Service review panel ordered the FDA to reconsider their sacking of Dr Morris, firstly because he had been motivated by public welfare, and also because the Civil Service Reform Act of 1978 was designed in part to afford additional protection to whistle-blowers, or employees who exposed practices which they believed to be a violation of law, rule, or regulation, or to constitute among other things, a danger to the public health or safety.

Testimony given by Dr Morris to the Senate Committee on Ways and Means, on 5 March 1987 showed that by August 1982, there were 1571 lawsuits filed by individuals who had suffered serious adverse reactions as a result of the swine flu vaccination.

Of these 290 had been settled at a cost of $57,000,000 by 5 March 1987 and another 693 were still pending, with the amount requested by plaintiffs standing at $1,027,000.00. Dr Morris said:

> *"These figures give some idea of the consequences resulting from a program in which the Federal government assumes liability of a product known to produce in an indeterminate*

6 Cockburn, A. et al. 1977. "Scientist J. Anthony Morris – He fought the flu shots and the US fired him". *Washington Post*, 13 March: 22.

> *number of recipients, serious damage to health . . . when I left the Food and Drug Administration in 1976, there was no available technique to measure reliably and consistently neurotoxicity or potency of most of the vaccines then in use, including DPT vaccines.*
>
> *Today, 11 years later, the situation remains essentially the same."*

The really telling thing about the whole Swine Flu issue, is that health policymakers did not, and will not, learn anything from the fiasco.

For instance, at a meeting in 1996, Dr Peter Patriarca discussed a proposed Influenza Pandemic Plan. On page 2 of the briefing document handed out is this:

> *"The successes and failures of the Swine Influenza Program of 1976 have been reviewed in detail elsewhere. Perhaps the most important failure of the program was the lack of a preemptive and proactive plan, which could have addressed many of the technical, political and administrative issues that ultimately hindered program implementation. This experience, more than any other, has underscored the need for the development of a comprehensive, contemporary and action-oriented plan."*[7]

Think about that. The predicted swine flu pandemic didn't happen, and vaccination with a dangerous vaccine was stopped because of deaths and injuries. Miffed that they didn't have a plan to make an unnecessary vaccination campaign succeed, the authorities were using that disappointment to develop a much more successful, comprehensive, contemporary and action-orientated plan. But for when?

To ensure the world might be pre-emptively vaccinated with an untested vaccine using squalene as an adjuvant, to supposedly prevent a Bird Flu epidemic they say might also kill millions of people, but that also might not happen?

Have the authorities learned any real lessons from all this? When will they admit the truth, namely that the guts of the matter is that in

7 WP3.0\FLU PLAN\DRAFT #6, January 1996 discussed on Thursday, 29 February 1996, at the Advisory Commission on Childhood Vaccines.

1976, everything they said was wrong? Fortunately, they didn't have a plan then, for if they had, perhaps we would never have known the truth about the Swine Flu epidemic that never was.

It is important to know the background to issues. Without that background, statements like the 1996 one above become the foundation stones for medical myths ultimately enshrined in textbooks. Even today if you do an internet search, you will find medical people who truly think that those 46 million doses given, prevented a swine flu epidemic of the proportions of 1918 pandemic.

(All information relating to Tony Morris's work has been checked by him, and comes from published studies, newspaper articles, Senate records of the relevant hearings, either collected, or given to me by him, and public and private comments he has made.)

32 Of Vaccine Contaminants – Monkey Business

To understand Dr Morris's situation, we also have to understand the situation of Dr Bernice Eddy, since they were friends who worked on the same floor and had similar interests, and both later became the combined subject of the previously mentioned 1972 Senate enquiry.

Dr Bernice Eddy was a scientist who specialized in leprosy, pneumococcal pneumonia, influenza, adenovirus infections, and, in later years, the immune responses to oncogenic viruses. She discovered the polyoma virus in the late 1950s, which is capable of producing in its natural host, the mouse, more than twenty distinct cancers, and in unrelated mammalian species, a variety of distinct cancers. This work turned out to be crucial, because in the mid-1950s Dr Eddy had also discovered that there was something in the polio vaccines that cause cancer in hamsters, which turned out to be what we know today as SV40. Repeated experiments showed consistent results.

Administrative clearance to publish this work was denied until after her findings had been conclusively substantiated by others, a process that took many years.

So there was a time in 1959, 1960 and 1961, when government health officials were frantically trying to remove a tumour-inducing factor from polio vaccines, and at the same time, the same government health officials were vigorously conducting a campaign to inject the same contaminated polio vaccines into millions of people.

We in New Zealand were one of the countries hardest hit, because all our polio vaccine from 1956 was contaminated, though at the time, the New Zealand Government said they didn't know that. However, they did know by 1960, and even in 1962 they knowingly ordered SV40-contaminated vaccine, on the assurance from the manufacturers that SV40 was harmless.

The manufacturers knew before 1960 that their vaccines were contaminated with a cancer-inducing virus, because they were informed from 1955 in writing by Bernice Eddy that there was something in all the polio vaccines causing cancer.

In 1954 and 1955, Dr Bernice Eddy also discovered live virus, capable of causing paralysis in several lots of polio vaccine. She notified the DBS leadership of this in two memoranda, one dated 12 May 1955, but they released the vaccines anyway. In 1955 she was relieved of her duties as polio vaccine control officer.

In the late 1950s after a cold vaccine had been developed it was handed to Dr Eddy for testing. She discovered that it could cause cancer in hamsters.

The publication of all Dr Eddy's papers was blocked, and she wasn't allowed to attend professional meetings. She suffered the same sort of harassment as Dr Morris, with whom she sometimes collaborated.

Dr Eddy's work resulted in the eventual discontinuance of the use of adenovirus vaccines in children. This type of vaccine, too, was grown on the same substrate as the polio vaccines, and it was found that SV40 had succeeded in forming a type of stealth virus in the substrate, which hid from the then testing procedures. The vaccine, however, was continued to be used in the military.

Others within the NIH who understood how critical Dr Eddy's work was, spoke out in 1972. DBS scientist Kendell O. Smith, subsequently Professor of Microbiology at University of Texas Medical School, said:

> ***"There are inexcusable gaps in the DBS research program, specifically in regard to the safety of the viral substrates used to grow vaccines."**[1] **and***
>
> ***"To detect all possible contaminating viruses, you need to***

1 Wade, N. 1972. "Division of biologies standards: the boat that never rocked". *Science*, 17 March; 1225–30. p. 1226.

> *hold the cells for much longer than the 2 weeks specified in the DBS regulations. One of the chief ways I became obnoxious to the DBS management was in continuing to press for a longer incubations time. I think it is unforgivable that the DBS did not change their regulations."* (p. 1227)

It wasn't for lack of trying on the part of Dr Bernice Eddy. As Ribicoff stated in his speech to the Senate:

> *"She (Dr Eddy) was deprived of most of her testing animals and most of her testing facilities. Finally, on 8 March 1961, she was relieved of her job and reassigned."*

The issue of vaccine substrates was one which the head of DBS did not regard as important, yet history was to show that it was, and is still vital. The substrates on any of the vaccine cultures, be they monkey kidney, duck egg or whatever, were only screened in a cursory manner, for economic reasons.

For example: *"the DBS required the monkey kidney cells used in growing live polio vaccine to be held for only 28 days in order to ensure that they contain no SV40 virus. According to A. Girardi of the Wistar Institute, SV40 may remain latent for up to 35 days. Nor does the DBS require monkey kidney cells to be screened for chromosomal abnormalities – a possible indicator of cancerous tendencies – a test they would probably fail in large numbers."* (p. 1228)

Many substrate contaminants were identified in various vaccines not withdrawn from sale, and by 1968 these filled a hefty 608-page monograph.[2] In 1972 the DBS finally changed polio vaccine manufacture to using WI-38 (a cell line from a human aborted foetus). That decision wasn't as a result of scientific reasoning, but because[3] vaccine manufacturers said they would quit making polio vaccine unless allowed to do so in WI-38 cells.

So you have to ask yourself what it was that the manufacturers knew, and that DBS scientists had been saying, that DBS was refusing to allow publication of.

And what specific relevance does this have for New Zealand?

---

2 Merchant, D.J. (ed). 1968. "Cell cultures for Virus Vaccine Productions". *NCI Monograph*, 29 December. U S Department of Health, Education and Welfare.

3 1971. *Drug Research Reports*, July.

In 1999, a newspaper stated:[4]

"Waikato Hospital histopathologist Dr Fred Mayall and Waikato University PhD student Greg Jacobson have uncovered a link between asbestos exposure, the SV40 virus and mesothelioma . . .

"The research, published in the UK Journal of Clinical Pathology shows that the SV40 virus is linked with mesotheliomas . . . until recently, mesotheliomas . . . were linked primarily to asbestos. In the past few years, overseas studies have found that around 70 per cent of cases test positive for the SV40 virus DNA.

But until now, no one had investigated factors that could predispose people to SV40-related tumours.

Dr Mayall said the public should not be alarmed.

'One should remember that, at most, only a very small percentage of immunized patients have developed cancer as a result of SV40 virus . . . we need to find out much more about SV40 virus.'"

The asbestos/SV40 link was also discussed by Dr Michele Carbone in 1990, and later expanded on by Dr Fernanda Martini of the Institute of Histology and General Embryology in Italy, who found SV40 in 83% of choriod plexus papillomas, in 73% of ependymomas, in 47% of astrocytomas, in 50% of glioblastomas, and 14% of meningiomas. SV40 has been found in 61% of all new cancer patients too young to have received contaminated polio vaccine.

In March 2002, researchers led by Janet Butel of Baylor Medical College reported[5] that 42% of non-Hodgkins lymphomas they analysed contained genetic sequences from SV40. About half the cases had SV40, whereas no virus was detected in non-malignant lymphoid samples.

Another University of Texas study found the same. The lead author, Dr Adi Gazdar, said to the *San Francisco Chronicle*:

"'. . . data is very very solid.' He said it had to be more than coincidence that the four types of tumors found in hamsters

---

4 Garner, T. 1999. "Researchers show lethal cancer link". *New Zealand Herald*, 6 April: A3.

5 Wlichez, R.A. et al. 2002. "Association between simian virus 40 and non-Hodgkin lymphoma". *The Lancet*, 359: 817–23.

> *after injections with SV40 – brain, bone, mesothelioma and lymphomas – are now exactly the same tumor types in humans found with detectable levels of SV40. 'The chances are 10 million to 1 that it is a coincidence.'"*[6]

For those of us who have sat and watched these past 20 years it has been interesting to see from the start who the establishment favourites have been on the SV40 issue. Every time research threw a less than complimentary light on vaccine there would always be a flurry of studies pulled out of the hat to prove the opposite. It has been alleged that after Michele Carbone's work, the only people who have received USA government funding to study SV40, were those who said that there is no issue with SV40 even before they applied for research funding.

However, SV40 isn't new news. Otherwise there would be no discussion about Bernice Eddy. SV40-like particles were found in many different hybrid viruses in brain tumours and these research results have been published since the 1970s in various cancer monographs, away from public eyes.

At a medical conference in July 1998, Dr Michael Carbone explained how SV40 switches off a protein that protects cells from becoming malignant. This protein is not cancer-type specific, but cell-function specific. Not everyone who is infected with SV40 will get cancer, for the same reason that not every smoker gets lung cancer. A variety of assaults on the immune system usually combine to trigger malignancy.

In October 1998, the *Journal of Cancer Research* suggested that the reason many cancers are now on the rise (it included only three varieties, but commented that most others haven't been studied yet) is because SV40 is spread both sexually, and from mother to child *in utero*. So you don't need to have received an SV40 contaminated vaccine to have been exposed to SV40. In USA, SV40 is found routinely in 23% of blood samples and 45% of sperm samples from donors.

In order to discredit the findings, cases have been alleged of people who supposedly had SV40 long before the vaccine. For obvious reasons, similar to the supposed pre-AIDS HIV patients, the credibility of such cases is severely strained.

---

6 Carlsen, W. 2002. "Simian virus in polio shots tied to cancer". *San Francisco Chronicle*, 12 March: A1.

Professor Mauro Tognon of Italy's University of Ferrara's School of Medicine was the researcher who showed SV40 in the blood and semen of healthy study subjects. He also pointed to SV40 as one possible reason for the 30% increase in US brain tumours over the past 20 years. This means that SV40's effects cannot be limited to, as Dr Mayall says, "those few" who received the vaccine.

The journal *Cancer Research*[7] published a study showing that contamination of oral polio vaccine used in Russia, Eastern Europe, Asia and Africa with SV40 continued until the early 1980s, and was far more widespread than had been believed, exposing hundreds of millions more people to the virus than previously thought.

SV40 is a topic that the New Zealand Health Department remains clench-lipped on, as it has been from the start. Why?

Because if you classify Mesotheliomas and other cancers as SV40/ Polio-vaccine related, people might ask questions about long-term trade-offs. The importance of not talking about that, is shown in the Federal Register Volume 98, No. 107, Friday June 1st, ***"Rules and Regulations"*** on page 23007 where it says:

> "... ***any possible doubts whether or not well founded, about the safety of the vaccine cannot be allowed to exist in view of the need to assure that the vaccine will continue to be used to the maximum extent consistent with the nation's public health objectives.***"

In terms of New Zealand, what is the significance of the SV40-contaminated vaccine?

In the first place, the polio vaccines were not contaminated with just SV40. SV40 was only the fortieth monkey virus to be found in vaccines. After SV40 was found, many others continued to be discovered and studied.[8] Some other simian viruses are of significance, but they are not being discussed at all. One of these is called the Mason Pfizer Monkey Virus (MPMV) which causes AIDS-like disorders in monkeys in which MPMV isn't normally found. After the polio vaccine campaign, it will be interesting to see if anything comes out

7 Cutrone, R. et al. 2005. "Some oral poliovirus vaccines were contaminated with infectious SV40 after 1961." *Cancer Res.* November: 15;65(22): 10273–9. PMID: 16288015.

8 Hull, R.N. 1968. *The Simian Viruses.* New York: Springer-Verlag. Congress catalog Card Number 68-26921.

about MPMV in the future.

Health Department records of 1962 show that of 2,515,800 New Zealand people, over 2,000,000 received SV40-contaminated oral vaccine between August 1961 and December 1962. Most of the injectable SALK vaccine used from September 1956 onwards was also contaminated with SV40. It isn't known how many New Zealanders received contaminated vaccine after 1962, but it is known that contaminated vaccine was ordered and bought after 1962.[9]

Records show that New Zealand had a theoretical upper limit of 50,000 SV40 *"uncontaminated"* citizens. However, given that SV40 is spread via blood and semen, and handed down, mother to child, the chances of this country having any segment in the present population without SV40 is virtually zero.

It should therefore be routine that all cancers in this country are studied for SV40 DNA integration. But that hasn't happened, and isn't likely to happen, because the government doesn't want you to know this now, any more than it wanted you to know this in the past.

(All information on Bernice Eddy comes from her own monographs, other medical articles, newspaper articles, the Senate hearing record which included all memoranda and evidence, and the eulogy presented at her funeral by Dr John Anthony Morris.)

9 Data pulled from the Report to the Minister of Health of the Special Committee to Investigate the Safety of Poliomyelitis, 7 March 1983. This report focused solely on SV40 contamination, and gives numbers of injections from start of campaign.

33 Talking of Vaccines and Treatments of No Worth

The *"worthless vaccines"* item in the Senate record sent me off at a tangent, to see if there were other vaccines which most people have no idea about, used in this country. One example is our parliamentary records of 1912, which show that in New Zealand in 1912, the following vaccines and serums were used:

> ***Vaccines and Sera purchased and sold at the Vaccine Station for the Year ending 31st December 1911:***
>
> *Acne Vaccine (Mixed)*
> *Acne Bacillus vaccine*
> *Coley's Fluid*
> *Coli Bacillus Vaccine*
> *Combined Vaccines for colds.*
> *Catarrhalis Micrococcus Vaccine*
> *Dipth. Anti Sera,*
> *Friedlander Bacillus Vaccine*
> *Gonococcus Vaccine*
> *Influenza Bacillus Vaccine*
> *Meningococcus Anti Serum.*
> *Plague (Haffkine's Prophylactic)*
> *Pituitary Extract (Valporole)*
> *Pneumococcus Vaccine*
> *Staphylococcus vaccine (mixed)*

Staphylococcus Vaccine (Aureus)
Staphylococcus Anti Serum, (Polyvalent)
Staphylococcus Anti Sera, Puerperal Fever
Staphylococcus Anti Sera, Pyogenes
Staphylococcus Anti Sera, Rheumatic Fever
Staphylococcus Anti Sera, Erysipelas,
New Tuberculin T.R. (Koch)
New Tuberculin T.R. (Azoules)
New Tuberculin T.R. (Koch), (Lucius and Bruning.)
Tuberculin for Von Piquet's reaction.
Tuberculin (Old) Human (Koch)
Tuberculin (Old) Bovine (Koch)
Tubercle Emulsion (Lucius and Bruning)
Tubercle Vaccine 0.0005 mgm
Tubercle Vaccine 0.0001 mgm.
Normal Horse Serum.
Tubercle, Moist, for opsonic estimation.
Staphylococcus Albus Vaccine,
Tubercle for conjunctival test.
Typhoid Bacillus Vaccine
Tetanus Anti Serum.[1]

Another example was the report in 1919[2] that a Mr P.L. Hickes had, for the year 1918, supplied all hospitals with plenty of the mixed-catarrhal vaccine *"used with considerable success in the New Zealand Expeditionary Force in England and France during the influenza epidemic."*

Funny how, in the discussion of the 1918 epidemic, no mention of a vaccine is ever made. Today, historians say that the epidemic happened because there was no vaccine.

No one talks about Scarlet Fever either, preferring people to think that it declined on its own. The facts are that there was a vaccine against Scarlet Fever, first used in 1912 by Gabrischewsky in Russia, and later used widely in America, Hungary and Poland.[3] It wasn't

1 House of Representatives. 1912. *Appendices to Parliamentary Journals*, Sess 2 V. iv. Page 108 of the Director General of Health's report.
2 House of Representatives. 1919. *Appendices to Parliamentary Journals*, Sess VI, V.II, Page 19 of the Director General of Health's report.
3 Professor Friederman, 1928. "Epidemiology of Children's infectious Diseases". *The Lancet*, August :218.

much used in the UK, because where it was, it was usually followed by serious reactions and death. No-one talks about the haemolytic streptococcal vaccine[4] that was used for a while either.

When reading this, it pays to also know that orthodox treatment in those days, of most of the diseases we know of today, was not just laughable, it was plainly ridiculous. For example, a common treatment of measles[5] was to

> ***"withdraw 25 c.cm. or so of blood from the parent's arm and inject this intramuscularly into the child's buttock, putting half into each side."***

Similar treatment[6] was used for polio. Worse than this was a different letter[7] commenting on the use of:

> ***"anti-measles serum from the placentas of normal women, which had been tried out on 4000 children, and was found to be quite as good as, if not indeed better than, convalescent serum."***

Until 1928, another universally useless method of treating disease was the use of alcohol for diphtheria. It was only in 1927, when a British hospital decided not to use alcohol, and found that the mortality rate became much lower, that doctors realized alcohol increased myocardial degeneration.[8] Yet very few listened. In 1935, standard alcohol-infused treatment was still pretty appalling:[9]

> ***"Every case of diphtheria is put on to a mixture of digitalis and squills . . . and also given calcium by mouth or intramuscularly . . . with the sudden onset of cardiac arrest camphor oil given intramuscularly . . . acts like a charm. In regard to toxaemia the solution is the administration of Pituitrin . . . brandy too is valuable both by mouth***

---

4 Summer meeting of Association of Clinical pathologists: Dr Shera. The *Lancet*, August 3, 1935, page 251

5 Porteous, A.B. The *Lancet*, March 23, 1935, Page 700 "Attenuation of measles by adult serum".

6 "Serum treatment of poliomyelitis" *British Medical Journal*, June 8, 1933, page 71.

7 The *British Medical Journal*, April 27, 1935, p. 899.describing a treatment detailed in a note in the *British Medical Journal*, April 6 1935 quoting Dr Y. A. Finkelstein (*Sov. Pediatr*, 1934(iii): 34.)

8 Hewat, A.F. 1928. "Prevention and treatment of diphtheria". *The Lancet*, Sep 8; p. 516.

9 1935. *British Medical Journal*, p. 852.

> ***and intramuscularly. Post diphtheritic paralysis . . . port wine and other such stimulants, even in children, give apparently valuable results."***

At the same time, four separate studies found that Vitamin C had the power to neutralize, inactivate and render harmless, diphtheria toxins.[10,11,12,13] This and more literature was known about in the USA particularly, where Dr Frederick Klenner published a lot of articles on his successful use of sodium ascorbate in the treatment of Tetanus, Poliomyelitis, diphtheria and snake bites. He published usually in the *Tri-State Medical Journal*, or *Southern Medicine and Surgery*. As with other innovators of the past and present, Dr Klenner was ignored except by patients who flocked to him in droves. As he said when recounting his successes with Vitamin C:

> "***. . . there are some physicians who would stand by and see their patient die rather than use ascorbic acid – because in their finite minds it exists only as a vitamin.***"[14]

Why is that people today automatically assume that mainstream disease treatment then, was actually of any use or that it was responsible for the substantial mortality decreases which occurred before vaccines arrived on the scene?

Or that there are no modern counterparts? Only recently has the medical profession[15,13] admitted that ***"growth failure and malnutrition are iatrogenic complications of cystic fibrosis."*** Iatrogenic meaning that for decades, cystic fibrosis children suffered, because doctors got it wrong.

---

10 Harde, E. et al. 1934. "Observation on the antigenic activities of combined diphtheria toxin and Vitamin C". *Comptes Rendus Hebdomadaires des Séances de L'Académie des Sciences*, Vol. 199: 738–9.

11 Jungeblut, C.L. et al. 1935. "Inactivation of diphtheria toxin *in vivo* and *in vitro* by crystalline Vitamin C". *Proceedings of the Society of Experimental Biology and Medicine*, Vol. 32: 1229–34.

12 Sigal, A. et al. 1937. "The influence of Vitamin C deficiency upon the resistance of guinea pigs to diphtheria toxin". *Journal of Pharmacology and Experimental Therapeutics*, Vol. 61: 1–9.

13 Kligler, I.J. et al. 1937. "Effect of Ascorbic Acid on Toxin Production of C. Diphtheriae in culture Media". *Journal of Pathology and Bacteriology*, Vol. 45: 414–429.

14 Klenner, F. 1957. "The Black Widow Spider". *Tri State Medical Journal* December. This child, according to the rules, should have died. She lives, in our opinion, because we elected to use this powerful therapeutic agent. But, then, there are some physicians who would stand by and see their patient die rather than use ascorbic acid – because in their finite minds it exists only as a vitamin.

15 Colombo, C. et al. 2005. "Growth failure in Cystic Fibrosis:a true need for anabolic agents?" *J. Pediatr*, March: 146(3): 303–5. PMID: 15756206.

34 One Thing Leads to Another

There were several families in the district who were home schooling, all within easy walking distance of each other.

It was when one of the mothers, Ngaire, badly twisted her ankle, that I became involved in an interesting few days. Ngaire, accompanied by her daughter Ruth, and a close friend, had gone to the medical centre to check that there was no fracture. There wasn't, but Ngaire's mobility was going to be limited for a few days and as a result the families rallied around to ease Ngaire's load especially the "school" studies. These families often combined for educational experiences and opportunities, and frequently called on other "resource" people willing to help out.

I was asked to take a short, integrated thematic unit of work with a small group of 12 to 14 year olds. The next morning we set about finding an answer to this question-topic:

"How far can you go on a sprained ankle?"

Ruth started the ball rolling by telling the group what had happened at the medical centre the previous day. Her friends asked all sorts of questions and from this we compiled the following list for language work – vocabulary, dictionary skills and further individual research:

What is the difference between a physician and a surgeon?

The doctor's "bible" – what is it?

Do "drugs" and "medications" mean the same thing?

What are pharmaceuticals?

Are pharmaceutical companies and vaccine manufacturers the same?

Why do doctors need pharmacies?

What is a "guaranteed market"?

What are profits?

Do doctors and the drug companies make a lot of money? Why? How?

What is an agenda?

What are mergers? What use are they?

It was quite amazing how all these things emerged from the children's interest, curiosity and observations!

Each student was given the task of finding out the answers to the questions in whatever ways they could – dictionaries, visiting the public library, on the internet, or talking things over with their parents, or other contacts and resources they could refer to.

The following morning the "theme" was continued.

What a lot they had learned overnight!

Once the flow of information they had gained, started, there was no stopping it! For example: "I know why pharmaceutical companies, vaccine manufacturers, vested interests, profits and mergers all go together," said Gerry whose father was an accountant. "I've got it all written down here."

"I learnt a lot when I went down to the chemist's to get Mum a crepe bandage," said Ruth. "The lady who served me spent a lot of time answering my questions. I know why doctors have to have a handbook on their desks. It's how the drug companies tell them what to prescribe for their patients. She showed me how they use it."

"Dad showed me on the internet just how much money these pharmaceutical companies make," added Gerry. "He says the shares in these companies can be worth a lot of money."

Alison had been doing her maths and explained to the group

how the medical system guaranteed the drug and vaccine makers the markets they needed by making the patients dependent on the products they produced. "My parents showed me an old newspaper article from the Sydney Morning Herald[1] *where a doctor is reported as saying that because the medical system is a monopoly, 'we can get away with murder whenever we want'. That's really scary."*

"So why has a sprained ankle caused us to be talking so much about 'vested interests'?" I asked the group. "Matthew could you tell us what 'vested interests' means?"

Matt looked at his notes. "It means a strong personal interest someone has in a matter because he or she might benefit from it."

"You have to pay so much when you go to a doctor," said Ruth, "and then usually you have to go off to the chemist and pay more money for what has been prescribed."

"Yeah, that's right," said Gerry. "Dad showed me a report in the New York Times[2] *about a lady who paid $77.50 for a prescription lasting two weeks, and when she went back for a refill, she had to pay $548.01! The same article talks about another drug that went up in price from $230 a dose to $1900 a dose. I couldn't understand why that was such a big increase, until he explained that the old accountant's way of working out how to price something sometimes no longer applies. Now, drugs and vaccines can be given a 'value-added' price, which he said means that if people value staying alive, they will pay as much money as it's worth to stay alive."*

"So you can see what I was saying about a guaranteed market," said Alison. "If the doctor says you need a certain drug you either pay

1 "WHO leader says doctors are most alienated group" *Sydney Morning Herald*, 21 June 1977. Dr Halfdan Mahler, Director General of WHO speaking at NSW Medical school: "'Doctors are the most alienated group in society although they regard themselves as a small group representing God' . . . 'I expect most of you are firm believers in the open market system' Dr Mahler told the audience. However, in medicine it simply doesn't exist. We are absolutely just a monopolistic organization, that is why we can get away with murder whenever we want.'"

2 Berenson, A. "A Cancer Drug's Big Price Rise Disturbs Doctors and Patients." March 12, 2006 Available from <http://www.nytimes.com/2006/03/12/business/12price.html?_r=2&th=&oref=slogin&emc=th&pagewanted=print>

through the nose or you do without it. Is that what that doctor meant by 'getting away with murder'?"

"That's a good question," I said. "We need to dig deeper."

Gerry had brought along some websites to go to, and these were given to the group to continue their study.

Would you like to join them?

Berenson A. "A cancer Drug Shows Promise, at a Price that many can't pay." February 15, 2006. <http://www.nytimes.com/2006/02/15/business/15drug.html?ex=1142485200&en=c93c499564af0695&ei=5070> (accessed 15 March 2006)

Hirschler, B. "Vaccines to stay hot for research and M&A" (Reuters) February 24, 2006. <http://today.reuters.com/summit/summitarticle.aspx?type=summitNews&summit=BiotechnologySummit06&storyid=2006-02-24T155451Z_01_L24568878_RTRUKOC_0_US-SUMMIT-VACCINES.xml&archived=true> (accessed 15 March 2006)

I wonder if you'll come to the same conclusions that we did! The sprained ankle was in much better shape by the time we had finished, even though we used "it" to traverse a lot of "ground"!

35 On Flu Epidemics

"The only sin this season is to leave vaccine on the shelf." [1]

In March 2005, my father rang me in a total panic. He's 94, with a long memory. "Darling," he said, "I don't want you to die. There's something you have to do!"

I cut in and said, "Oh Dad, what ARE you going on about?!!" "It's this bird flu from Taiwan, Darling," he replied, "It's all over the news. They are saying it will kill everyone soon, so you've got to disinfect your telephone every day."

Choke . . . "My telephone??! . . ." I gargled . . . (I was at the computer and my early morning coffee disappeared where it shouldn't. My keyboard survived but my lungs took a little longer.) "Well, what about all the other door knobs, the taps, the whole bathroom, the fridge handle . . . and maybe I shouldn't kiss anyone either?"

Silence.

"But it's ON television Dear!"

Dad's funny sometimes. Right up until 2004, he'd never had a flu

1 Associated Press. 2004. "Rationed flu shots may go to waste". *St Petersberg Times*, 17 December. Retrieved on 18 September, 2005 from <http://www.sptimes.com/2004/12/17/Worldandnation/Rationed_flu_shots_ma.shtml> "Many of us are now concerned we will not use vaccine supplies. The only sin this season is to leave vaccine on the shelf," said Dr. William Schaffner.

vaccine in his life. He had a reputation, in his previous home of being feisty, and telling the nurse she could have his dose, or "stick it you know where!" In 2004, I happened to ring him and he was a bit under the weather. "Why are you sick, Dad? You never get sick." And it came out that he had caved and had the flu vaccine, and then got sick.

"Why Dad? What on earth possessed you to do that after all these years. You had the flu in 1918, and lived through it, and have never wanted a shot."

"Well Dear," he said, "she was such a nice girl, and I did it because I liked her."

What can you say? Especially when he's been saying for years that he's only marking time, and wants to "go"! Maybe he did want to go.

But it reminded me of something else. Dad wrote his memoirs years back, at our prompting, in written form, and on audio tape. So I went and got them.

Dad's father was a Yorkshire man working for the British Hongkong/ Shanghai Bank, and his mother, a quite unconventional and very resourceful, knowledgeable woman from Surrey.

During one posting to India there was a Typhoid outbreak in Calcutta. Dad's mother got typhoid, and survived, but all her hair fell out and grew back auburn. Other postings were Singapore, Malaysia, and China where there was an outbreak of cholera, and his mother took many of the local sick into her house to nurse them. She did not get cholera herself. Then they spent time in Japan, where my father was born, and migrated with their young family to New Zealand in 1917, for the duration of the First World War.

They were living on Kawau Island in 1918 when the flu epidemic struck. Governor Grey's old large house had been turned into a hotel, and the gardens and grounds were fantastic. My father was in kids' heaven surrounded by beaches, fish, gardens, wallabies, and kookaburras. A coastal ferry brought supplies twice a week. The main occupation for the children was fishing from the pier. The sting rays were huge and the children always watched out for either sting rays or sharks.

When the flu epidemic hit, Dad's mother turned the hotel into a hospital, with the help of the maid. The men were nursed upstairs, and the women downstairs. Dad clearly remembers getting it. He was at the pier, and simply buckled. By the time he managed to crawl up the steps of the hotel he was exhausted. By the end of the epidemic, only two people on the whole of Kawau Island had not had the flu. They were Dad's mother, and the maid, who between them, with help from others when they could, had nursed the whole Island back to health with not one death.

Why was it that no one on Kawau Island died? Could it be that deaths are often caused because people either don't have the care, or the knowledge to look after themselves and one another? And why was it that the two people who had maximum exposure to the virus, never got it themselves?

This story is worth telling, because it is stories of that time which people recount to this day, often forming the basis of future scare-mongering about the flu. Good news, it would seem, is no news. We only get told about how many people died in 1918, not the ones who survived because of the skills of the people who looked after them.

Because of the current ramping up of fear about a potential bird flu epidemic, it's a good idea to talk about some of the epidemic propaganda that passes for history, starting with the 1976 "Swine flu".

Perhaps it's best called HOGWASH AND GUANO.

No Known Vaccine Available To Halt the Deadly Menace

World Is on Brink of Killer Flu Epidemic[2]

A flu that normally affects only hogs may wipe out millions of people beginning next year.

So read the first paragraph, and further along to make the point, readers were told that

"In 1918, the killer disease was preceded by a milder epidemic such as the U.S. is experiencing now . . . ONE BILLION people fell ill – one of every three persons in the world," . . . and ". . .IF THE swine virus is as deadly as some scientists believe it to be, it already may be too late to prevent an epidemic – even if a vaccine is found tomorrow."

Sound familiar?

---

2 Small, P. 1976. "No known vaccine available to halt the deadly menace. World is on brink of killer flu epidemic". *The National Insider* 11 April: Front Page.

Literally thousands of articles predicting a fate worse than Black Plague appeared in the USA in 1976. It's no different in 2005. Nationwide US TV broadcast two doctors saying:[3]

> ***"Michael Osterholm: We would expect between 1.5 and 1.7 million Americans to die . . . Irwin Redlener: We could have a billion people dying worldwide."***

Have these experts read "The Boy Who Cried Wolf"? (Aesop's Fables.) We know, though they don't appear to, that this bird virus was first noted in 1959[4] forty-seven years ago. USA had a two-year outbreak in 1983.[5] This virus is nothing new. The history of bird flu shows it's not likely to become a human to human epidemic.

In 1976 death on its own, though, was not enough. Having scared people witless, the experts suddenly announced that there was going to be a shortage of swine flu vaccine, because one major manufacturer had got the wrong virus in it, and were going to have to start again.

So, the headlines read:

"Kids" flu shots in short supply

Vaccine's availability will be limited at first

The strategy in 2005 in New Zealand was no exception, even with regard to the normal flu. Looking back through my collection of newspaper clippings from 1977, I find that one of the most skilful manipulators of propaganda of the "crying wolf" story has always been the *New Zealand Herald.*

Taking just a few of its headlines over the years, we find that they all build a long-term picture which ramp up, and misrepresent a situation that actually does not yet exist.

Flu vaccine flaws boost epidemic fears 12 March 2005

Study warns of grim toll if bird flu hits NZ 11 March 2005

---

3 ABC News. 2005. "Are we ready for the bird flu?" *Primetime*, Sept 25; available from <http://www.abcnews.go.com/Primetime/print?id=1170177>

4 WHO. 2006. "Previous outbreaks . . ." Table. Available from <http://www.who.int/csr/don/2004_03_02/en/#world "1959-Scotland-chicken-H5N1">

5 Wood, J.M. et al. 1985. "Host range of A/Chicken/Pennsylvania/83 (H5N2) influenza virus". *Avian Dis*. Jan–Mar; 29(1): 198–207.

Feather pillows may carry Asian bird flu 7 March 2005

Bird flu shots coming – in winter 25 February 2005
(That winter has been and gone . . .)

Repeated flu injections save lives 5 March 2004

Vaccine readied to ward off killer flu strain 25 July 2004
(Which one was that?)

Killer lurking in our midst 3–4 May 2003

Complacency deadly with chameleon virus 25 March 2002

Elderly to be vaccinated as "big one" looms 11 January 2000
(Did that even happen?)

Flu potential killer of millions 2 June 1999

HORROR on the home front 10–11 October 1998

These headings catch the eye, so that the reader reads the body of each article which ramps up emotional responses even further to scare people – into having a vaccine.

In my opinion, health authorities feed and encourage such hysteria. Hysteria certainly creates stress, suppresses the immune system and is another risk factor that can MAKE you sick. Although a study in the past[6] showed that Vitamin C reduces the flu's severity, you never hear about that. You are only told that you can take the vaccine. Studies indicate that the selenium and Vitamin E status of a person could determine whether and how badly they get influenza.[7] This country's soil is chronically selenium deficient, but has anyone studied the implications of that on the health of New Zealanders?

6 Chamberlain, J. 1996. "Viral vileness the flu and you". *North and South*, June; pp. 92–97. Dr Lance Jennings "conducted at the University of Wisconsin in 1988 which demonstrated that a daily dose of 2000 mg of Vitamin C reduces the severity of a cold by one half, and alleviates influenza symptoms."

7 Nelson, H.K. et al. 2001. "Host nutritional selenium status as a driving force for influenza virus mutations". *FASEB J*, August:15(10): 1846–8. PMID: 11481250.

Sometimes, media hype unravels on medical authorities, and events in America in 2004 provided a very interesting lesson: 40 million doses of its flu vaccine were found to be contaminated and had to be ditched. The vaccine was rationed, but no great epidemic happened.

The CDC stated, as they do most years, that ***the big epidemic*** was going to happen in 2004. The vaccine available made antibodies the authorities knew wouldn't stop the new viruses very well.[8] But because the manufacturers hadn't even been able to isolate a reference strain to the 2004 new variant of influenza A, they couldn't put the new circulating strain in the vaccine.

They had tried military labs, the Hawaii labs, and other WHO collaborating centres, but no one could get the new virus to grow. Instead of the usual egg culture, they even tried using primary monkey kidney cells, an attempt that was also unsuccessful.

Authorities knew that from October 2002 to 2003, 25% of all USA isolates were this fujian strain. So chances of any protection from the old vaccine were moot.

But the public was not told any of that. What they then said publicly was that that the current vaccine should be used, even though it wasn't totally compatible with circulating strains, because some protection was better than none.

This caused Dr Walter Royal to raise a question at an FDA meeting, addressed to a Dr Decker. The answer is very interesting. He declared that[9]

> ***"Everyone has to take it on faith that the strains selected, if grown properly and inoculated, will produce the relevant antibodies and they will not only work against that strain, but they will, hopefully, work against whatever circulates.***
>
> ***All that has to be taken on faith, because by the time you produce it, there's no time left to do any testing. Were***

8 Retrieved on 18 September, 2005 from <http://www.fda.gov/ohrms/dockets/ac/03/transcripts/3922t1.doc> 20 February, 2003. FDA Meeting ". . . just to reiterate, it shows that current vaccines produce antibodies that don't really inhibit many of these new viruses very well". "It has not been possible to isolate a reference strain in eggs from of the new variant strains . . ." "Work has been proceeding at other WHO collaborating centers . . . and it has just not been fruitful, and none of us really understand why. But I think there are probably some answers in the receptor binding area."

9 Retrieved on 18 September, 2005 from <http://www.fda.gov/ohrms/dockets/ac/03/transcripts/3922t1.doc> 20 February, 2003. US FDA Vaccines and Related Biological Products Advisory Committee 94th meeting.

there any time to do testing, there would be no time left to manufacture anything."

So from the manufacturer's point of view, their obligation is to produce whatever this Committee tells them to produce. So, how can there be any scientifically valid assurance in the statements of the past twenty years that said, *"Go and get the flu vaccine, it will protect you"?*

A few paragraphs later in the meeting's report we read:

". . . further to the clinical side of things, we don't really ever know how immunogenic any particular strain is going to be before a vaccine is manufactured, and there really isn't time to do the kind of clinical trials you would anticipate for any other kind of vaccine. Influenza virus vaccine is different from every other one in that it is changed almost every year and it's a new experience with each one."

Those given the available vaccine, just assumed that it would prevent the flu. The rest of the public seemingly stopped thinking about it even though predictions of deaths had been dire. If you aren't allowed to have vaccine there is nothing you can do. Contrary to the CDC crystal ball predictions, it turned out to be the mildest flu season for years.

Near the end of the flu season the government suddenly realized they had all this flu vaccine that hadn't been used, so the newspapers ended up running stories telling people to line up for jabs, because it would be wasteful not to use vaccine supplies that were good for one season only.[10]

CDC, FDA and WHO may find it harder in the future to say: *"The reason we didn't have the terrible flu epidemic we predicted was because we had a good, safe, and effective vaccine which stopped you all being sick."*

Being proven wrong is not a good look when it comes to persuading people that you know what you are talking about in advance. However, the new strategy is now in place, to try to avoid a similar situation. You could call it *The Plan*. It's here for all to see:

10 Dainie, Y. 2004. "US weighs easing flu shot restrictions". Retrieved on 18 September, 2005 from http://aolsvc.news.aol.com/news/article.adp?id=20041216131609990007&_ccc=4&cid=842>

www.ama-assn.org/ama1/ pub/upload/mm/36/2004_flu_ nowak.pdf

In terms of New Zealand, the 2005 flu vaccine shortage here suddenly resolved itself after many months. The company had made a mistake and tests in Australia found that the vaccine was potent. Which means that the vaccine provokes the formation of antibodies. Whether it protects is another matter.

But the question has to be asked, "Was it just an error in a worker's notebook?" The reputation of the vaccine was now redeemed. Was the worker smacked over the hand with a wet bus ticket and given bonus shares in the other, for providing publicity that money couldn't buy? After all, for weeks, lots of people who wouldn't normally pay attention to flu vaccine propaganda, followed the not-enough-vaccine, we-might-all-die saga, like *Days of our Lives*.

36 Flinging off the Bed Covers

Before flinging off the bedcovers and arising to a new day, Hilary and I had been talking. At that time of the day it's not such an unusual activity, even though it's often nice just to enjoy each other in relative quietness. However, Hilary was in writing mode, and had been for some days, so the topic would have to be . . .?

You've guessed it!

Vaccination!!

So it was Hilary doing the talking while I did my best to keep up with the flow. It had to do with some articles she had been looking at before coming to bed the night before. Yes, she did actually make it to bed before midnight!

When I sat down to my breakfast, my lovely wife presented me with a little bit more reading matter. A few (?) pages from a CDC PowerPoint presentation dealing with planning influenza vaccination campaigns. Groups who have the vaccine, those who don't, and what they can do to up the numbers. That sort of thing.

Because it was a different format to the usual full pages of type – and in colour!! – I was not too depressed by such an early offering.

However, my breakfast is always eaten slowly, as I savour each mouthful while I think my own thoughts and prepare myself for whatever the new *day may bring. The PowerPoint pages would have to wait. Several hours later and three jars of preserved apples for the coming winter behind me, I sat down to study the CDC material, before returning it to Hilary's "desk". Then stepping carefully over the piles of files and folders covering the sitting room floor, I sat down to have a breather.*

A few minutes later: "Well, Darling, what did you think of it?"

"Um," I replied, "that depends which side you're on of course, but I'll try to be fair. If your job is to convey to the audience the concern the public health providers have for the well-being of the population, then I suppose it does set out the background for the vaccination programme and the likely responses from various sections of the community, as well as strategies to achieve a good acceptance rate."

At this point I went over some of the comments we have tossed around before, relating to why people so often succumb to receiving a vaccination. "If you ask people if they are going to get their jab there will be those who say yes, and those who say no. If you ask them why, especially those who say "no", how many will be able to give clear, precise, well-thought out reasons? It's certainly easier to go with the flow and mumble something about what the Health Department says."

"And what would you say?" said Hilary.

"Well, that would depend on a number of factors including how much time the person asking me had, and if they were really interested! I would probably say that I don't agree with it, then if they really want to find out more, they will have to ask more questions."

"And what would you say then?"

"Okay, I would talk about not wanting poisons put into my body; not wanting to interfere with a marvellous immune system which God has given me; about my responsibilities to treat my body with respect and in accordance with the provision my Creator has made for eating a good balanced diet, and the confidence I have in Him to keep me well. If I had the opportunity I would also say, that if for some reason I was to die as a result of the 'flu then I am ready to die, and I know where I am going to spend eternity."

I would ask them: "Do you?"

37 So, Does the Flu Vaccine Work?

You all know, don't you, because we've been told since the 70s, that when the flu vaccine is given to the elderly it protects them against the flu, and stops them dying?[1] In fact, it doesn't work at all. To fix the problem doctors say that all we have to do is vaccinate 70% of school children[2] as well as still vaccinating all the grannies and grandads in whom the vaccine doesn't work.

Just stop and think about this for a minute. For 35 or more years, we've been told that this wonderful flu vaccine will solve all the problems for the elderly. Newspapers extol its virtue, and everyone sticks to the party line.

The authorities don't want to JUST tell you that flu vaccine doesn't work very well, so AT THE SAME TIME they come up with a new "solution".

A question for you all. On what scientifically accurate basis do

1 Roos, R. 2005. "Flushots in elderly don't cut mortality". Retrieved on 18 September, 2005 from .http://www.cidrap.umn.edu/cidrap/content/influenza/general/news/feb1605elderly.html. "Researchers who tracked national data on influenza vaccination rates and mortality in elderly people from 1968 through 2001 say they could find no evidence that flu shots reduced death rates."

2 CIDRAP News. 2005. "Immunising children a better way to fight flu". Retrieved on 18 September, 2005 from <http://www.cidrap.umn.edu/cidrap/content/influenza/general/news/feb2205flushots.html> Emory University: "The idea that vaccinating schoolchildren is the best way to prevent influenza throughout the US population received a boost last week with the publication of a commentary and a Texas study in separate journals . . . 'If the 70% threshold can be reached, then high-risk people are protected even if they are not vaccinated,' the authors assert."

you think their new idea of lining up 70% of schoolchildren as well as still vaccinating the elderly, is any better than vaccinating the elderly, which doesn't work?

To understand the whole mess, let's look at the so-called facts, and start with this oft repeated so-called statistical baseline:

"Influenza is the sixth leading cause of death for older Americans and infects 5% to 10% of elderly Americans every year. The flu leads to 300,000 hospitalizations and kills 30,000 to 40,000 Americans every year."[3]

The CDC says[4] that:

"Every year in the United States, on average:

- ***5% to 20% of the population gets the flu;***
- ***more than 200,000 people are hospitalized from flu complications, and;***
- ***about 36,000 people die from flu."***

These are interesting figures. Here are the CDC's own statistics. In 2002: 753[5] people die of flu. In 2001: 267.[6] In 2000: 2175[7] and in 1999: 1685.[8]

If you research it, it's very hard to find out where the 36,000 figure comes from. The question is, even if we could trace the 30,000 deaths, would the vaccine prevent them?

Then we read:[9]

---

3 American College of Physicians. 2004. "Should vaccinations be required for health care workers?" *ACP Observer* [Internet] Available from <http://www.acponline.org/journals/news/jul-aug04/vaccinations.htm> Accessed 18 September, 2005.

4 Retrieved on 18 September, 2005 from <http://www.cdc.gov/flu/keyfacts.htm>

5 Kochanek, K.D., and Smith, B.L. 2004. "Deaths: preliminary data for 2002". *National Vital Statistics Reports*, February: 52(13): 16. Available from <http://www.cdc.gov/nchs/data/nvsr/nvsr52/nvsr52_13.pdf>

6 Kochanek, K.D., and Smith, B.L. 2004. "Deaths: preliminary data for 2002". *National Vital Statistics Reports*, February: 52(13): 16. Available from <http://www.cdc.gov/nchs/data/nvsr/nvsr51/nvsr51_05.pdf>

7 Kochanek, K.D., and Smith, B.L. 2004. "Deaths: preliminary data for 2002". *National Vital Statistics Reports*, February: 52(13): 15. Available from <http://www.cdc.gov/nchs/data/nvsr/nvsr49/nvsr49_12.pdf>

8 Kochanek, K.D., and Smith, B.L. 2004. "Deaths: preliminary data for 2002". *National Vital Statistics Reports*, February: 52(13): 28. Available from <http://www.cdc.gov/nchs/data/nvsr/nvsr49/nvsr49_08.pdf>

9 2005. "Flu efficacy in Doubt Study questions saving elderly", *Washington Times*, 15 February: A9.

"A new study based on more than three decades of U.S. data suggests that giving flu shots to the elderly has not saved any lives."

Led by National Institute of Health researchers, the study challenges standard government dogma . . .

However, the US Center for Disease Control and Prevention in Atlanta plans no change in its advice on who should get flu shots, saying the NIH research isn't enough to shift gears.

'We think the best way to help the elderly is to vaccinate them,' said CDC epidemiologist William Thompson. 'These results don't contribute to changing vaccine policy.'"

No articles on this topic made it into New Zealand newspapers. For the whole 2004–2005 flu season, the CDC said[10] that only 14.9% of influenza cultures submitted since October 2004 were positive. Of these, 75.4% were Influenza A. Out of the 157,759 individuals nationwide who had gone to the doctor and been diagnosed with the flu, only 23,549 people actually had the flu.

In the study[11] mentioned in the *Washington Times*, Dr Simonsen developed 'a cyclical regression model' which carefully and methodically estimated influenza-related deaths, and all deaths, among the elderly in the United States during thirty-three consecutive flu seasons between 1968 when Tony Morris's work found the flu vaccine was of no use, to 2001.

The study found that mortality didn't change at all through those years, and that in the age group 65–74 years, mortality had remained the same between 1970 and 2001. In other words, her results were the same as Dr Morris's results. Flu-related mortality in the elderly was always less than 10% of the total number of winter deaths. So the current flu vaccine isn't much better than when Dr Morris got fired for saying the pre-1970 flu vaccine didn't work.

In an interview,[12] Dr Simonsen said that the dramatic increase

---

10 2005. U.S. Influenza Season Summary: 18 Jun, 2005. Available from <http://www.cdc.gov/flu/weekly/weeklyarchives2004-2005/04-05summary.htm>.

11 Simonsel, L. et al. 2005. "Impact of influenza vaccination on seasonal mortality in the US elderly population". *Archives of Internal Medicine,* 14 Feb; 165(3): 265–72. PMID: 15710788.

12 Boyles, S. 2005. "Do flu shots save lives?" *MD Medical News* [Internet] Available from <http://webcenter.health.webmd.netscape.com/content/Article/100/105852.htm?printing=true>

in vaccination coverage should have led to a dramatic drop in flu deaths. ***"This is not what we found,"*** she said. ***"Certainly if this intervention really does reduce winter deaths in the elderly by 50% we would expect to see it. So the mortality benefits are probably very much overestimated."***

Dr Simonsen then commented on the 1997/1998 flu season where the vaccine contained totally different strains from those cultured in the fifty states and therefore the vaccination of over 60% of eligible elderly was useless. Yet there were approximately 5000 fewer excess deaths in this age group than there were the following flu season, when the same percentage of people were vaccinated with the correct strains.

But in some strange twist of logic, Dr Simonsen then said that their study argued in favour of vaccinating everyone: ***"We totally agree that influenza is a major cause of serious illness, hospitalization, and death,"*** she says. ***"Vaccinating the elderly is a major tool, but our findings suggest that there is more that can be done."*** How can something that has no impact, be a major tool?

This sort of statement seems to be mandatory when criticizing any vaccine. In 1995, Dr Jenkinson wrote a whole article showing that the medical profession's assertions that whooping cough was always serious and always had major complications were totally wrong. Yet in the key messages and final paragraph he says:

> ***"it is important to emphasize the vaccine's major role in maintaining herd immunity."***[13]

That's not what the body of Jenkinson's article says at all. My guess is that if he hadn't said something supporting the vaccination of everyone, he wouldn't have been allowed to say all the rest showing the whooping cough vaccine doesn't work for most people. I believe it's the same with Dr Simonsen. Is she being tolerated, because her recommendation to vaccinate the kids as well, at least doubles the amount of useless flu vaccine dished out?

Even more interesting is other discussions on this study[14] in *Infectious*

---

13 Jenkinson, D. 1995. :Natural course of 500 consecutive cases of whooping cough: a general practice population study". *British Medical Journal*, Vol. 310: 299–302. [Internet]. Available from <http://bmj.bmjjournals.com/cgi/content/full/310/6975/299>

14 Reichart, T.A. et al. 2005. "Enhance the national influenza vaccine strategy; Researchers defend influenza vaccine study; and Should we question the benefits of influenza vaccination for the elderly?" *Infectious Disease News*, August. Available from

Disease News. Simonsen et al. said:[15]

> ***"There is a void of evidence from randomized, placebo-controlled clinical trials in the elderly for influenza . . ."***

And they point out the statistical fallacies and manipulations by CDC of cases and death numbers which they politely call ***"the vast disconnect"***.

For Americans, this vast disconnect is the statistical baselines rolled out every year to justify the vaccinating of everyone over 65.

Dr Fedson[16] in response, discusses every possible ***"ecological fallacy"*** to attempt to discredit Simonsen's comments, then amazingly reiterates the dogma, saying:

> ***"Greater efforts to improve the vaccination rate for the elderly, including eliminating disparities in the vaccination rate among different groups, will help prevent more influenza-related hospitalizations and deaths. Nonetheless, whatever the 'obvious implications for influenza vaccination policy' of Simonsen's results might be, we should not doubt the benefits of current policy to vaccinate all elderly people, over 95% of whom still live in the community."***

When you read anything by Dr Fedson, it's important to take into consideration very creative remarks he has made in the past like this one:

> ***"'The failure to use pneumococcal vaccine can no longer be attributed to limited protection of the vaccine itself,' said Fedson. 'It is the result of limited imagination regarding the burden of pneumococcal disease and the limited understanding of the protection afforded by vaccination. The effectiveness of pneumococcal vaccination is firmly established and requires no further demonstration.'"***[17]

<http://www.infectiousdiseasenews.com/200508/frameset.asp?article=guested3.asp>

15 Simonsen, L., Ward, C., Blackwelder, W., Taylor, R., and Miller, M. 2005. "Researchers defend influenza vaccine study". Available from <http://www.infectiousdiseasenews.com/200508/frameset.asp?article=guested2.asp> accessed 18 September, 2005.

16 Fedson, D.S. and Nichol, K. 2005. "Should we question the benefits of influenza vaccination for the elderly?" Available from <http://www.infectiousdiseasenews.com/200508/frameset.asp?article=guested1.asp> Accessed 18 September, 2005.

17 Fedson, D.S. 1998. "A commentary on the report of the Swedish pneumococcal vaccination study group". National Adult Immunization Conference (Atlanta), March 3–4.

Actually, the effectiveness of the Pneumococcal vaccination is debatable and repeated Cochrane reviews[18] have shown that:

> *"polysaccharide pneumococcal vaccines do not appear to reduce the incidence of pneumonia or death in adults with or without chronic illness, or in the elderly (55 years and above), . . . the evidence from non-randomized studies suggests that the vaccines are effective in reducing the incidence of the more specific outcome, invasive pneumococcal disease, among adults and the immunocompetent elderly (55 years and above)."*

To make the debate on flu vaccine more interesting, Reichert chimes in and after saying that the result was a misinterpretation of the conclusions, and having stated that influenza vaccine is of great benefit to the elderly, strangely says this:

> *"The only national vaccination program that has produced a decrease in excess mortality in the elderly population on a national basis was the schoolchildren vaccination program in Japan."*[19]

Apparently, between 1962–1987, 50–85% of Japanese schoolchildren were vaccinated annually.[20] Supposedly the death rates in the elderly fell, then when they stopped vaccinating, it rose again. Reichert, Fedson, and Simonsen as authors of the Japanese study,[21]

---

18 Dear, K.B.G. et al. "Vaccines for preventing pneumococcal vaccines in adults". Issue 2, 2005. Available from <http://www.cochrane.org/cochrane/revabstr/AB000422.htm> Accessed 18 September, 2005.

19 Reichart, T.A. et al. 2005. "Enhance the national influenza vaccine strategy; Researchers defend influenza vaccine study; and Should we question the benefits of influenza vaccination for the elderly?" *Infectious Disease News*, August. Available from <http://www.infectiousdiseasenews.com/200508/frameset.asp?article=guested3.asp> "An enhanced strategy will be critically important in the event of a pandemic when vaccinating those who are most likely to spread the disease will have a multiplier effect in reducing total population deaths. Results from studies on selected subpopulations that cannot be extrapolated to the total population to be protected must not distract us." "We suggest . . . that to overcome this lack of progress, the national strategy should be enhanced. Evidence from studies of multiple types indicates that significant reductions of mortality in the elderly as a whole can be achieved by expanding the vaccination program to include not only risk groups, but also transmission groups, specifically schoolchildren."

20 Isaacs, D. 2005. "Should all Australian children be vaccinated against influenza?" *MJA*, 182(11): 553–554 [Internet] Available from <http://www.mja.com.au/public/issues/182_11_060605/isa10175_fm.html>

21 Reichert, T.A. et al. 2001. "The Japanese experience with vaccinating schoolchildren against influenza". *N Engl J Med*, March: 22;344(12): 889–96. PMID: 11259722.

postulate that: *"When most schoolchildren were vaccinated, it is possible that herd immunity against influenza was achieved in Japan. If this was the case, both the incidence of influenza and mortality attributed to influenza should have been reduced among older persons"*.

Is the influenza vaccine in the elderly in Japan any use? A Japanese study[22] looking at elderly in the 2003–2004 showed that the influenza vaccine over there *"was 20% effective, although this effectiveness was not statistically significant."* So the *NEMJ* study is the sweetener to the unpalatable fact that the flu vaccine doesn't work in the elderly. In the UK, a Cochrane review looking at vaccines in the elderly made some blunt comments in Pulse,[23] saying:

> *"Researchers on the Cochrane Vaccines study said Government claims that the flu vaccine was 70 per cent effective were 'a total fantasy'. The review of 64 international studies in patients aged 60–65 and over found community vaccination had no effect on rates of influenza, influenza-like illness or pneumonia."*

What the New Zealand media was concentrating on in February 2005 was the Health Department statements that *"vaccinating the elderly against the flu spares lives, and giving the shot yearly prevented the deaths of about one out of every 200 patients."*[24]

The same paper went into greater detail in March 2005[25] saying that, in patients above 65 *"a single flu vaccination reduced the risk of death by about 10 per cent . . . those who were vaccinated again the following year had a 24 per cent lower risk of death."*

However, that article says[26] that the vaccine may prevent 1 death

---

22 Ozaka, K. et al. 2006. "Retrospective assessment of influenza vaccine effectiveness among the non-institutionalized elderly population in Japan". *Vaccine*, March: 24(14): 2537–43. PMID: 16417955.

23 Wright, E. 2005. "Flu vaccine efficacy warning". *Pulse*, 1 October. [Internet] Available from <http://www.pulse-i.com/search/default.asp?issuedate=1128121200000> Accessed 4 October 2005. "Government claims that the flu vaccine was 70 per cent effective were a total fantasy . . . But Dr Jefferson insisted the study included fit, healthy individuals and not just the old and frail. 'The vaccine was ineffective in the younger elderly as well as those in their 80s,' he said. He criticised officials for failing to take responsibility for the fact figures on the vaccine had been distorted and patients misled." (no longer available).

24 2005. "Repeated flu injections save lives". *New Zealand Herald*, 5 November: A17.

25 Editorial. 2005. "Flu vaccine debacle puts many at risk". *New Zealand Herald*, 17 March: A16.

26 Voordouw, A.C.G. et al. 2004. "Annual Revaccination Against Influenza and Mortality

for every 302 vaccinees . . . BUT it also said ***"a first vaccination was associated with a non-significant annual reduction of mortality risk."*** But . . . vaccinate again the next year and the protection rate is 28%. Was that result any better than those from Dr Morris's original work from the 1950s which showed a 20% rate, which was considered statistically insignificant? I sent the study to him. His reply to me[27] reads: ***"If this claim is valid, then the authors of the paper will be nominated for the next Nobel prize in medicine. It's validity is not established in this paper."***

Yet the author of this study said:[28]

> ***"Both patients and physicians should be convinced about the benefits of annual influenza vaccination, and no opportunities should be missed to have all patients recommended for vaccination against influenza," Hak tells WebMD.***

Using the criteria use by Dr Fedson to criticize the US study showing no efficacy in the elderly, you have to wonder about the evidence for using it in children. A recent Cochrane review[29] found: ***"limited evidence that vaccines reduce the burden of school absences . . . Vaccination of very young children is not supported by the evidence . . . at present we could find no convincing evidence that vaccines can reduce mortality, hospital admissions serious complications and transmission of influenza"***

However, a member of the American Academy of Pediatrics committee on infectious disease said[30] that while the Cochrane Review was exhaustive, and meticulous, it was unpersuasive, and had ***"failed to account for variation in the quality of vaccines and research methods. The review . . . also fails to account for the fact that much of the efficacy data on vaccines is gathered by drug companies that***

Risk in community-Dwelling Elderly Persons". *JAMA*, 3 Nov; 292(17): 2089–95. PMID: 15523069.

27 Personal Correspondence, 20 March 2005.

28 Boyles, S. 2005. "Do flu shots save lives?" *MD Medical News* [Internet] Available from <http://webcenter.health.webmd.netscape.com/content/Article/100/105852.htm?printing=true> Accessed 18 September, 2005.

29 Smith, S. et al. 2006. "Vaccines for preventing influenza in healthy children". *The Cochrane Database of Systematic Reviews*, Issue 1. Art. No.: CD004879. DOI: 10.1002/14651858.CD004879.pub2. Available from <http://www.mrw.interscience.wiley.com/cochrane/clsysrev/articles/CD004879/pdf_fs.html> Accessed on 18 September, 2005. PMID: 16437500.

30 Mott, G. 2006. "The Toddler Debate". *Washington Post*, 31 January. Available from HE02 <http://www.washingtonpost.com/wp-dyn/content/article/2006/01/30/AR2006013001253_pf.html>

may choose for business reasons not to publish their findings." Really? CDC chimed in by saying that because kids make antibodies and the vaccine is safe, it was a reasonable thing to recommend.

So, the flu vaccine will be given to the children when according to the Cochrane Review there is ***"no convincing evidence that vaccines can reduce mortality, admissions, serious complications and community transmission of influenza of children either."*** Will that too, be exposed as another item on a wish list in 35 years' time?

Another risk group to whom the flu vaccine is already recommended is asthmatic children to prevent asthmatic exacerbation, because studies done by authors like DeStefano F, Chen RT who have conflicts of interest, had found it protected against asthma. A new study has found the opposite:[31]

> ***"RESULTS: After adjusting for other variables, the vaccine group had a significantly increased risk of asthma-related clinic visits and ED visits (odds ratios 3.4 and 1.9, respectively)."***

Another unrelated study in Turkey confirmed this.[32] Yet another concluded ***"that influenza vaccination did not result in a significant reduction of the number, severity, or duration of asthma exacerbations caused by influenza."***

All this talk is academic because it has never been the intention of the Influenza policy planners to aim for anything other than vaccinating everyone against the flu annually no matter what the efficacy isn't. The only thing holding them up was the lack of manufacturing technology to make enough vaccine to do it. Growing flu virus for vaccines in chick eggs is a very slow process, but cancerous cell lines grow flu viruses rapidly. So the FDA has decided it's time to seek permission to use them.[33] New Zealanders were recently used in a trial by Chiron,

---

31 Christy, C., and Aligne, C.A. et al. 2004. "Effectiveness of influenza vaccine for the prevention of asthma exacerbations". *Arch Dis Child,* August: 89(8): 734–5. PMID: 15269071.

32 Abadoglu, O. et al. 2004. "Influenza vaccination in patients with asthma: effect on the frequency of upper respiratory tract infections and exacerbations". *J Asthma,* 41(3): 279–83. PMID: 15260460.

33 "FDA To Seek Input On Safety Of Flu Vaccine Produced In Tumorigenic Canine Cells". 2005. Available from <http://www.fdaadvisorycommittee.com/FDC/AdvisoryCommittee/Committees/Vaccines+and+Related+Biological+Products/111605_FluVaccine/111605_MadinDarbyP.htm> Accessed on 18 September, 2005. "'The agency appears comfortable that potential risks associated with tumorigenic cell substrates can be mitigated . . .' Although there is a perception that highly tumorigenic

of a flu vaccine made on a tumorigenic dog kidney cell substrate.[34]

Whatever technology is around, the USA CDC is likely to recommend vaccinating everyone with the flu vaccine yearly[35] with major vaccine proponents being very enthusiastic: *"This is long overdue,"* said Dr Paul Offit, *". . . Influenza is an infectious disease that can be prevented easily and safely, and it should be."*

Even before childhood studies were completed, on 13 May 2005, Lindsey Tanner was reporting that within five years, every person in the USA would be vaccinated yearly, with Dr Herb Young of the American Academy of Family Physicians saying that recommending flu shots for everyone would ease the confusion and that his group would support the idea.

The response to the ongoing debate about how useful the flu vaccine is has also resulted in some USA medical centres trying to make the flu vaccine compulsory for staff, because of another statement by Gregory Poland:[36]

> ***"At an Annual Session presentation on immunizations, Gregory A. Poland, FACP, made a case for requiring – not merely recommending – annual flu vaccinations for all health care professionals. 'That's because data have shown that health care workers aren't stepping up and getting the vaccine,' he said. Despite recommendations from organizations like the CDC, only about 36% of health care workers are immunized against the flu."***

Some medical centres tried to make 'failure to receive flu vaccine' grounds for dismissal. One medical centre rebelled and the workers took the issue to Arbitration, where the arbitrator found against the

---

cells may carry greater risks than less tumorigenic cells, we are proposing that such risks can be mitigated by careful testing of the cells, validation of the production process for its capacity to remove adventitious agents, and limitation of residual DNA in the final product," FDA said . . . FDA is also asking the committee to discuss whether the agency should take additional steps "to address issues associated with the use of MDCK cells or neoplastic cell substrates."

34 NZPA. 2005. "NZers in flu vaccine trial". *New Zealand Herald*, Nov 28: p. A11. "New Zealanders have been used by a big British Drug Company to test a new way of making flu vaccines using animal cells which may also have the potential to trigger tumours in humans."

35 "Should vaccinations be required for health workers?" Available from <http://www.ajc.com/news/content/health/0204/20flu.html> Accessed on 18 September, 2005.

36 2004. "Should vaccinations be required of health care workers?". *ACP Observer*, July–August. Available from <http://www.acponline.org/journals/news/jul-aug04/vaccinations.htm> Accessed on 18 September, 2005.

medical centre,[37] not on the basis of staff's autonomy of choice, but because the centre didn't negotiate it with the union! So the medical centre now hopes that it can use financial incentives or other incentives to get staff to comply. In 2005 the Virginia Mason Medical Centre did the job properly. They simply said, "Have the shot or leave". Most of the staff capitulated without a whimper.[38]

Meanwhile, Medicare and Medicaid applied to the Federal Register[39] on 15 August to force nursing homes to vaccinate the elderly with influenza and pneumococcal vaccines, or lose their funding. If the elderly who don't want to be vaccinated live in the community, their right to choose is more easily defended. But if they live in a nursing home, their choice is no longer theirs. Expect this to become mandatory in New Zealand sometime soon!

If you as a New Zealand parent are soon told that vaccinating yourself, your babies and children every year will help protect your vaccinated Grannie from the flu because her vaccine doesn't, what will your response be?

There is nothing quite like a new scare tactic to divert people from thinking about FACTS. Even though the evidence is quite clear that the flu vaccine does not work for the flu, experts declared that the flu vaccine, by stopping the flu, (which we know it doesn't), will stop a bird flu pandemic.

The best hype story I've seen appeared in the *UK Times*:[40]

> ***"'MORE than a million children in Britain must be vaccinated against flu as soon as possible,' senior health officials said last night as the deadly avian form of the virus reached Europe . . .***
>
> ***Scientists are concerned that, if the bird virus were to infect anyone already suffering from ordinary flu, the victim could then act as a "mixing vessel" in which the***

---

37 Galloway, A. 2005. "Virginia Mason nurses can shun flu shots". Available from <http://seattlepi.nwsource.com/pqa/wlocal_story.asp?id=236097> Accessed on 18 September, 2005.

38 Rusk, J. 2006. "Mandatory flu shots boost health care worker immunization rate at Virginia Mason". *Infectious Disease News*, March. Available from <http://www.infectiousdiseasesnews.com/200603/frameset.osp?article=mandatory.asp>

39 Retrieved on 18 September, 2005 from <http://www.regulations.gov/freddocs/05-16160.htm>

40 Elliott, V., and Henderson, M. 2005. *The Times*, 14 October, [Internet] Available from <http://www.timesonline.co.uk/article/0,,2-1825271,00.html> Accessed on 18 September, 2005.

germ could adapt to spread more easily from person to person. This would be the key mutation that could trigger a devastating pandemic."

There is one big stick that most people in this country didn't hear. The influenza vaccine manufacturers, in the face of evidence that their vaccine has never been any real use from Dr Morris's era to now, have threatened that unless the government of the UK[41] expands the mandated use of the ordinary flu vaccine, they will not produce enough bird flu vaccine. Have similar verbal bazookas been delivered in the ears of other governments as well?

In the USA, potential bird flu vaccine manufacturers demanded the identical indemnity that they got when they manufactured the swine flu vaccine.[42]

It was therefore a relief to read in the *New Zealand Herald* one person who hadn't lost their head. Dr Peter Curson, from MacQuarie University Australia, described our Government's bird flu preparation as *"over the top"*,[43] and *"getting into a flap over nothing"*. He said that the country would be better off declaring a pandemic on real issues like diabetes and obesity.

British experts now realize that you have more chance of winning the lottery than getting bird flu[44] and research teams have figured out why, in the last decade, bird flu has only hit people who play with, spend all their time with, or eat sick birds. The receptors in people's lungs are too deep to cause infection human to human.[45]

41 West, M.R. 2005. "'Firms' threat to limit bird flu vaccine". 26 October. Available from http://www.telegraph.co.uk/news/main.jhtml?xml=/news/2005/10/26/nflu26.xml> "Richard Stubbins, of the UK Vaccine Industry Group, told a House of Lords select committee that it was 'unreasonable' for the Government to expect the industry to build new plants to produce enough vaccine for a pandemic then mothball them. He called for the Government to vaccinate everyone aged over 50 and possibly children against common flu as a matter of routine. That would guarantee that the extra capacity would be used"

42 November 1, 2005 Available from <http://news.yahoo.com/s/ap/20051101/ap_on_go_pr_wh/bird_flu_liability_2> Accessed on 18 September, 2005. "Two weeks ago, the Senate's health committee approved a bill that said the "manufacturer, distributor or administrator" of a pandemic product shall be immune from lawsuits caused by the dispensing of that product."

43 "Australian academic mocks our bird flu 'over-reaction'". 2006. *New Zealand Herald* [Internet] Available from <http://www.nzherald.co.nz/section/print.cfm?c_id1&objectid=10364832> Accessed on 29 March, 2006.

44 Henderson, M. "Lottery win more likely than bird flu". *The Times*, March 3. Available from <http://www.timesonline.co.uk/article/0,.25149-2067213,00.html>

45 Price, H.J. 2006. "Bird flu too deep in human lungs to spread easily". *The Washington Times*, March 23. Available from <http://www.washtimes.com/functions/print.php?StoryID=20060322-111957-5097r>

And it doesn't help the hysteria promotion when the proposed bird flu vaccine only produces antibodies in half the people[46] given huge doses (12 times the normal flu shot).

Furthermore, the bird flu strains circulating now, are quite different[47] from the 1997 Hong Kong strain which killed six people. Another pointer to the fact that a bird flu outbreak is unlikely, is a study[48] which showed that a strain of bird flu that had been circulating for 12 years in 1992, hadn't killed anyone, and had given millions of Chinese antibodies. It could be that Peter Curson was right. All the New Zealand panic mongering and buying of drugs could have been a total waste of time, drugs, and millions of dollars, while the real health needs of this country have to wait.

It's a shame the New Zealand experts have been conspicuous by their silence on all this.

One final thought. Why is it, do you think, that the New Zealand Government is proceeding to invest $27 million in a drug called Tamiflu, which does not work on the bird flu virus?[49]

---

46 Health Day News. 2006. "Experimental bird flu vaccine falls short". *Forbes Magazine*, March 29. Available from <http://www.forbes.com/lifestyle.health.feeds.hscout/2006/03/29/hscout531823.html>

47 Grady, D. et al. 2006. "How serious is the risk of Avian flu?". *New York Times*, March 27. Available from <http://www.nytimes.com/2006/03/27/health/28qna.html>

48 Kolata, G. 2005. "Hazards in the hunt for flu bug". *New York Times*, November 8. Available from <http://www.nytimes.com/2005/11/08/science/08flu.html?ex=1144123200&en=0e90a913f6003e71&ei=507> "Peter Palese of the Mount Sinai School of Medicine in New York said the H5N1 viruses are a false alarm. He notes that studies of serum collected in 1992 from people in rural China indicated that millions there had antibodies to the H5N1 strain. That means they had been infected with an H5N1 bird virus and recovered, apparently without incident."

49 "Bird Flu resistant to main drug". [YEAR?]. *CNN News*, [Internet] Available from <http://www.cnn.com/2005/WORLD/asiapcf/09/30/birdflu.drugs.reut/> Accessed on 18 September, 2005. A strain of the H5N1 bird flu virus that may unleash the next global flu pandemic is showing resistance to Tamiflu, the antiviral drug that countries around the world are now stockpiling to fend off the looming thread. Experts in Hong Kong said on Friday that the human H5N1 strain which surfaced in northern Vietnam this year had proved to be resistant to Tamiflu.

38 Owls and Roosters

"East is east,
And west is west,
And ne'er the twain do meet."

One of the fascinations of magnets is that like poles, when brought together, repel each other whereas when the unlike poles are brought together, they attract each other.

How often in marriage, husbands and wives can be opposites. Is that what attracts them to each other in the first place?

Hilary is an owl.

I am a rooster.

For me the best time of the day is the early morning, when the energy levels are high, and the day has not had a chance to be derailed by the interactions of people, circumstances and situations.

I need my eight hours' sleep.

My normal bedtime is ten o'clock and I wind down as that hour approaches, and avoid unnecessary mental stimulation.

I will now be ready for the proverbial cock crow of the new day.

Hilary, on the other hand, comes to life as the darkness deepens! So while I slumber and snore, she will be busy reading, writing, and doing all those other things which come with being wide awake and functioning on all cylinders.

When she is "ready" she will come to bed.

Usually this will be after midnight and can on occasions be at three or four am.

"Ah ha!" you say. "Problems."

Yes, there can be, especially when lack of sleep begins to catch up with her. And this can be aggravated when the telephone starts ringing early the next morning.

There are some things with which I will not compromise. There are priorities which I will jealously guard, to protect our marriage.

We discovered early on, and especially in our homeschooling lifestyle, how fragile relationships can get when an owl and a rooster live in the same nest, and as so often is the case, the kidlets seem to be more young roosters than owlets!

The closeness and intimacies of marriage are essential. Full stop!

Over the years as we have had to adjust to the fine-tuning of our lifestyle, we have developed "strategies" designed to maintain and enhance our personal privacy. The best laid plans of mice and men – sorry, of an owl and a rooster – can sometimes come unstuck. But we learn from them and try not to get caught out a second time!

Now let's see. Wednesday.

Rooster went to bed 10.00 pm.

Owl arrived about midnight.

Rooster got up at 6.20 am to talk to the birds, etc.

Rooster came back to bed about 7.00 am.

Owl still dozing.

Rooster has perfected soothing caresses to keep Owl's feathers from getting ruffled, and to allow whatever doziness there is to remain. Deep steady breathing, the hint of a snore, indicates the gentle touch is working its magic.

At 8.00 am Rooster again slides out into the new day.

Rooster begins the day's chores.

Owl has flown out from her roost and is now tapping away on the computer and consulting her files.

Owl and Rooster embrace. For the time being they have assumed human form!!

And the day ahead of us?

Whoooo knooows!

39 The Fever-Pitch Bandwagon

***"The fear of fever is deep-seated and is mainly historic, having been passed from one generation to another. Changing that perception will be a mammoth task."*[1]**

Health Professionals appear to have a love affair with paracetamol. It features not just in their recommendations to have on hand for the bird flu, but paracetamol products appear to be the automatic[2,3] reflex advice given to parents for fever, illness of any kind, teething, and sometimes, unidentifiable grumpiness.

Why would anyone recommend paracetamol for any influenza, when it is known[4] to considerably prolong the duration of influenza? An online newspaper[5] once quoted Dr Karen Plaisance, Associate

1 Blumenthal, I. 1998. "What parents think of fever". *Family Practice*, Vol 15(6): 516. PMID: 10078789.

2 Styrt, B., and Sugarman, B. 1990. "Antipyresis and fever". *Arch Intern Med*, August: 150(8): 1589–97. PMID: 2200377.

3 Isaacs, S.N. et al. 1990. "Antipyretic Orders in a University hospital". *The American Journal of Medicine*, January: 88: 31 "Antipyretic orders are routine and correlate more strongly with hospital service than with individual patient characteristics . . . we found antipyretic ordering to be routine, imprecise and rarely noted or commented upon in patients' progress notes." PMID: 2294763.

4 Plaisance, K.I. 2000. "Effect of antipyretic therapy . . .". *Pharmacotherapy*, Dec; 20(12): 147–22. PMID: 11130213.

5 Burke, A. 2001. "Health Scout" "Take Two aspirin and Prolong the Flu", Fever-reducers may hinder infection fighting" URL now inactive.

Professor at the University of Maryland School of Pharmacy and one of the study's authors as saying:

> *"an elevated temperature may actually help the body fight the infection quicker or better than if you don't have a fever.' . . . 'Influenza A sufferers who were treated with aspirin or acetaminophen extended their illness from five days to about 8 1/2 days."*

Six years ago Dr Pascale Allotey from Australia spoke out against mothers using paracetamol and other sedative drugs to sedate unruly children.[6] In the article, one mother said, *"These medications save children's lives because it stops mothers from throwing them against the wall."*

Quite apart from the lack of parenting skills this attitude exhibits, paracetamol is potentially highly toxic. The only reason no action has been taken on this very contentious issue worldwide (not that most parents would know about it) is to avoid offending the pharmaceutical industry[7] for whom paracetamol and like products are financially lucrative. We are talking about a drug that every year in the States causes[8] *"more than 56,000 emergency room visits, 2600 hospitalizations, and an estimated 458 deaths due to acute liver failure"*.

What relevance is this to children? Starship Hospital[9] used to have a pdf on its website about paracetamol poisoning, which said: *"Paracetamol is the most common single agent involved in poisonous ingestion in young children."* I wonder why, at the time of writing, the pdf has disappeared?

6 The *Dominion*, Wednesday 29 November, 2000; *New Zealand* Herald 4 December 2000.

7 "FDA fails to reduce accessibility of paracetamol despite 450 deaths a year". 2002. *British Medical Journal*, [Internet] Available from <http://bmj.bmjjournals.com/cgi/content/full/325/7366/678> Accessed 18 September, 2005. PMID: 12351357.

8 Lee, W.M. 2004. "Acetaminophen and the U.S. Acute Liver Failure Study group: lowering the risks of hepatic failure". *Hepatology*, Jul; 40(1): 6–9. PMID: 15239078. ". . . 700 patients with acute liver failure across the United States implicates acetaminophen poisoning in nearly 50% of all acute liver failure in this country. Available in many single or combination products, acetaminophen produces more than 1 billion US dollars in annual sales for Tylenol products alone. It is heavily marketed for its safety compared to nonsteroidal analgesics. By enabling self-diagnosis and treatment of minor aches and pains, its benefits are said by the Food and Drug Administration to outweigh its risks. It still must be asked: Is this amount of injury and death really acceptable for an over-the-counter pain reliever?"

9 http://www.starship.org.nz/docs/paracetamol.pdf. Inactive URL The title is there as of December 2005, the pdf is not.

Most parents automatically reach for a paracetamol product whenever their children have a fever, because doctors don't tell them that the medical literature makes it quite clear that painkillers, used to reduce fevers, can make all infections of any kind worse.[10,11,12,13]

Why do doctors give out painkillers to reduce fevers? Because[14]

> ***"physicians often treat fever to alleviate anxiety in patients, their families, or medical personnel, and that such treatment often lacks a compelling medical rationale."***

The World Health Organization states quite clearly that the use of paracetamol for fevers is undesirable:[15]

> ***"Fever represents a universal, ancient, and usually***

10 Saper, C.B. 1994. "The neurologic basis of fever". *The New England Journal of Medicine*, June: 30(26): 1880–6. PMID: 7832832.

11 Roberts, N.J. 1991. "Impact of temperature elevation on immunologic defenses". *Reviews of Infectious Diseases*, May–June; 13(3): 462–72. PMID: 1866550. "Overall, it appears that temperature elevation within the physiologic range most effectively enhances the processes involved in initial antigen recognition and support for immunologically specific response to challenge." Pg 470: "Accumulated direct and indirect evidence suggests an overall beneficial effect of physiologic temperature elevation or fever on host defense mechanisms." "Paracetamol may prolong infection and reduce the antibody response in mild disease, and increase morbidity and mortality in severe infection . . . there is no evidence that antipyretics prevent febrile convulsions . . . Antipyretics may be harmful. Conclusion: There is little evidence to support the use of paracetamol to treat fever in patients without heart or lung disease, or to prevent febrile convulsions. Indeed paracetamol may decrease the antibody response to infection, and increase morbidity and mortality in severe infection."

12 Shann, F. 1995. "Paracetamol: use in children". *Aust Prescr* Vol. 18: 233–234. Available from <http://www.australianprescriber.com/index.php?content=magazines/vol18no2/paracetamol.htm> "It should be explained to parents that fever is usually a helpful response to infection, and that paracetamol should be used to reduce discomfort, but not to treat fever".

13 Russell, F.M. et al. 2003. "Evidence on the use of paracetamol in febrile children". *Bull World Health Organ*, 81(5): 367–72. Epub 2003 July 7. PMID: 12856055. "Fever represents a universal, ancient, and usually beneficial response to infection, and its suppression under most circumstances has few, if any, demonstrable benefits. On the other hand, some harmful effects have been shown to occur as a result of suppressing fever: in most individuals, these are slight, but when translated to millions of people, they may result in an increase in morbidity and perhaps the occurrence of occasional mortality. *It is clear, therefore, that widespread use of antipyretics should not be encouraged either in developing countries or in industrial societies*."

14 Styrt, B., and Sugarman, B. 1990. "Antipyresis and Fever". *Arch Intern Med* August: 150(8): 1589–97. "The decision to administer antipyretics is frequently made *without a documented rational*. Current understanding of the mechanisms and pathogenesis of fever suggests that the febrile process has a role in host defense and that *routine antipyretic therapy for fever is generally unnecessary and conceivably harmful*." PMID: 2200377.

15 Eichenwald, H. F. 2003. "Fever and antipyresis". *Bull World Health Organ*, [Internet] December: 81(5): 372–374. PMID: 12856056. Available from <http://www.scielosp.org/scielo.php?script=sci_arttext&pid=S0042-96862003000500012&lng=en&nrm=iso>. ISSN 0042-9686.

> ***beneficial response to infection . . . widespread use of antipyretics should not be encouraged either in developing countries or in industrial societies. Unfortunately though, just as fever represents an ancient biological response, an emotional effect is embedded deeply . . . parents have seen that when fever begins to diminish and disappears, the child feels better and recovers from the illness — whatever it was. Thus, the fever has become synonymous with the illness. This flaw in logic has persisted in parents' and physicians' minds, and they are seduced by the thought that if they "make the fever go away, the patient will be well. "No amount of scientific discourse will change this attitude, and antipyresis will continue to be used in children with low-grade fevers, or even no fevers, in the home as well as the hospital."***

Perhaps more forceful than the World Health Organization's, is this comment:[16]

> ***"Paracetamol may prolong infection and reduce the antibody response in mild disease, and increase morbidity and mortality in severe infection."***

I disagree with the WHO.

If parents knew that paracetamol has no benefit in the treatment of fevers, and is a risk factor for the development of asthma,[17] eczema and rhinitis[18] in children, I think they might think long and hard before acting on that oft-heard automatic response "Just use p___l, dear."

---

16 Shann, F. 1995. "Paracetamol: use in children". *Aust Prescr*, 18: 233–234. [Internet] Available from <http://www.australianprescriber.com/index.php?content=/magazines/vol18no2/paracetamol.htm>

17 Beston, A. 2004. "Early paracetamol use linked to asthma: study". *New Zealand Herald* 17 Sept: A3.

18 Cohet, C. et al. 2004. "Infection, medication use, and the prevalence of symptoms of asthma, rhinitis, and eczema in childhood". *Journal of Epidemiology and Community Health*, 58: 852–857. PMID: 15365112.

40 1989 – The Battles Begin

I didn't see the storm clouds coming in 1989 because part of me yearned to be optimistic about intelligent medical people talking sensibly about vaccine issues. Looking back at a letter Tony Morris sent me dated 26 June 1987 I didn't see that maybe it also applied to New Zealand. A paragraph read:

> ***"At the 23–24 June 1987 Atlanta meeting of the Immunization Practices Advisory Committee ACIP chairman Sam Katz and other ACIP members heard a Navy spokesman report that Marine recruits were not given typhoid vaccine before basic training, but rather after basic training, because when given typhoid vaccine '. . . the recruits dropped like flies . . . ' and that the severity and frequency of adverse reactions to typhoid vaccine interfered with basic training. This report evoked not concern, but laughter from (some of those[1]) at the conference table."***

In January 1988 both our children had measles for the second time. David had Koplik spots and all the things he had had the first time, but the diagnosis exempted itself in my mind, because I was conditioned enough to believe that measles doesn't happen twice.

1 The names that were provided have been deleted in this text for legal reasons.

When David hit rock bottom I was coming down with something myself. David let every man and his dog know that life was the pits for 24 hours a day. I admit, I had had enough, so I took him to the doctor. Big mistake. My husband tagged along, worried, as I was slightly past reason. David didn't like the attention, was totally uncooperative and shut up, sullenly retreating under his father's chin. After a while he let the doctor look in his ear, then hid it. The ear was very red and "bulging", according to the doctor.

We didn't want to use antibiotics, but agreed to try nasal decongestant, which might ease the ear-drum pressure. This child had never felt the sting of decongestant squirting up his nose before, and greeted it with screaming. When he had worked himself up to a frazzle I rang the doctor, to ask if he thought it was just a tantrum, or ear ache. The doctor said he thought meningitis was the problem.

The word *meningitis* brought me up with a start. The doctor wanted us to take David to hospital for blood work and a lumbar puncture, but the diagnosis didn't fit, so I refused. He spoke to Peter who just thought one little boy was reacting out of all proportion to the problem, and also didn't want him to go to hospital.

After we refused to take him to the hospital, the doctor said he would be ringing Social Welfare, mentioning the Young Person's and Children's Act.

Hmmmm . . .

That afternoon, once David had calmed down, I was able to have a good look at him. By this time, the rash was looking different, and the light came on. It had a brown stain. Only one type of rash had that, and that was measles. But you can't get it twice. Or can you?

Six week prior to getting pregnant with our oldest, I had returned a high good positive rubella antibody test. Yet at eight weeks' pregnancy, I had come down with rubella again, confirmed by two blood tests four weeks apart which showed rising IgM titres. I thought . . . well . . . very odd, but if I could get rubella a second time, unlikely though it sounded, why couldn't the children get measles again?

That night, admittedly quite late, I rang the doctor who was asleep, and agreed to take David through to hospital. The doctor asked why I wanted to go now, not in the morning. I said, "Because I don't believe he has meningitis; I believe he has measles. And he's never been to hospital before, so it will be quiet at night, and far less stressful for him." More than anything else, I wanted to pre-empt anything that the doctor might do in the morning, which might mean we didn't have control of the situation. I now felt confident that it was measles, therefore I felt that any sensible medical person would see that.

The doctor rang ahead supposedly to organize an emergency team for a seriously sick child with meningitis, who arrived at the hospital bright-eyed and bushy-tailed about such an extraordinary adventure in long, dark echoey corridors. He spotted a giraffe on the wall: "Can I see the top, Mummy?"

The emergency team melted away, and left us with two paediatricians, who were great. I wasn't quite so great. Somewhat defensive actually, and straight away said I believed he had measles, and they could even take a blood test if they wanted to check for measles, but not a lumbar puncture. I couldn't get out of my head, the memories of one event, six years before.

After extensive goings over, which lasted two hours, they agreed that there were absolutely no clinical signs of meningitis. On seeing a few residual Koplik spots as well as a browning rash; an ear, which was apparently no longer red or bulging, and slight bronchitis symptoms, they too pronounced measles. Until they saw in his file that he had had measles two years before, with ironically, identical though not as severe symptoms. They scored out measles, and put instead, ***"morbilli-like illness"*** explaining that "lots of other viruses" could cause measles-like symptoms.

Then they checked his immunizations, to find he had had none. Surprisingly, they grumped that, had he been immunized, we wouldn't be at the hospital. I pointed out they had just said it wasn't measles. "Would you like to take that blood test and look for rising titres to make sure?" No, we were told, since he wasn't dying, and it would be a waste of money. But because they were both annoyed at us for not immunizing, it became a matter of honour for me to pursue this issue further.

I asked them, "So how would a doctor, before the measles vaccine, have known the difference between what you see here today, and classical measles? You have the files there yourself. His symptoms are classical measles, again. Doctors didn't know pre-vaccine, that lots of viruses cause measle-like diseases. So how is it then, that you say that the measles vaccine wiped out measles, if you don't know whether those cases were actually measle-like illnesses or not?" They didn't know. "If you don't know, then why are you criticizing me for not vaccinating, particularly as you now say he hasn't got measles, and you won't check for it?" Silence.

A few days later, we got a rather large bill from the GP, and a contractual agreement which we were supposed to sign, or the doctor would terminate family care. The agreement stated that parental rights regarding children's treatment were not absolute, and any future decisions by the doctor would be non-negotiable. There were other clauses that were unacceptable as far as we were concerned, particularly in the light of the fact that we had been right, and he had been wrong.

I decided that I needed to challenge both the validity of contractual agreements, and the size of the bill. The doctor gave his point of view, and we gave ours. The actual process of going to a formal hearing not only became time consuming and intimidating, but also expensive, so we gave up, which left just the bill. My husband and the doctor negotiated that, and we just walked away from the situation, returning to our old doctor miles away, assuming that was that.

But that was not that. More was to follow a few months down the line.

41 1989 – More of the Same

Later that year, a wee girl in Taranaki who had received the plasma-based Hepatitis B shot, went downhill a few days after the shot. Her mother took her to the doctor who pronounced the flu, and sent her home with Paracetemol. The mother's instincts told her that this diagnosis didn't sit right, so she kept going back to the doctor and being serially fobbed off. Then another doctor thought maybe it was glandular fever. The mother by this time was tired, and reacting on a tightly coiled level. I sympathized with her, as not long before, I'd been there, done that.

After the little girl's distraught grandmother contacted me, they both took the girl to the hospital, and insisted on her staying, but tensions ramped up, as the staff became more and more convinced that the mother was the problem, not the child. The staff had just got to the point where they were ready to bounce the mother when the child instantly, and dramatically collapsed. Within five minutes she was on life support. At 2.00 am the next morning, the grandmother rang to say that though the girl was on life support, the hospital said they didn't know what the problem was.

When the grandmother had mentioned earlier extreme sensitivity of the legs, pins-and-needles, the child hurting when touched and not wanting to be touched, I felt it might be vaccine-induced Guillain Barre and sent her the vaccine manufacturer's data detailing it, and some other articles, explaining Guillain Barre in easier language.

Because the hospital continued to hold out on them saying they didn't know what was wrong, I suggested that the grandmother go and see the paediatrician, and instead of asking him anything, to place the manufacturer's International Physician's circular on his desk, with the part underlined in front of him, and simply say: "Why did you not tell us she had Guillain Barre?"

She did. His head whipped up, and he retorted, "How did you find out?" She just stuck to the broken record, and repeated the question, "Why didn't YOU tell us?" with the emphasis on *you*. He admitted that it was Guillain Barre, but that he didn't think it could possibly have anything to do with the vaccine. "Then why is it written here in the vaccine manufacturer's leaflet? She's got it within the stated time frame." The grandmother asked.

It turned out he'd never read the leaflet, and had no idea about side-effects, other than that he'd heard that there had been a few rare anaphylaxis issues.

The grand-daughter stayed in hospital for some time. She eventually got ACC, and the case was eventually reported after the grandmother had confronted the paediatrician for the umpteenth time. And even then, it was reported as a reaction following the yeast-based vaccine, rather than the plasma-based shot.

This child represented the seventh possible Guillain Barre case from the Hepatitis B vaccine whose parents had come to me that year. I also had a long list of other conditions arising after the vaccine which upset parents greatly, so started prolonged written communications with the Medical Assessor, Dr Ralph Edwards in the Centre for Adverse Reactions Monitoring (CARM) at Dunedin Medical School. He turned out to be another man who was a thinker, and really did care.

We had had written and phone conversations when the Menomune A campaign had turned messy, so there was a tenuous link already established.

He turned out to be seriously concerned and started to get frustrated himself, as some of the serious reports I put his way involved hospitalized children, but hospitals were sometimes obstructive when he sought relevant information.

At the same time, two GPs approached me, who had vaccinated their own children, in their own practices, and had had to watch their own children struggle with serious reactions. I think the only thing harder than being a parent watching a reaction, is being a doctor having given it to your own child, then watching. Other doctors also approached me, who were starting to see things in their patients that worried them. Being the "face" of the other side, and out there a bit more, perhaps they came to me, because they couldn't talk to their own. While I knew about the brick walls people like Tony Morris faced, I hadn't realized that ordinary doctors would face problems just as daunting.

In 1989, another questioning voice arose out of the blue about ME* in particular. One morning while listening to *Morning Report*, and attempting to wake up with a cup of coffee, and reading the paper, a Professor of something was going on about ME patients having compromised immune systems and suggesting that antibiotics and immunizations might be causing chronic malfunction of the immune system. I nearly choked.

Having missed the first volleys in this debate during the preceding days, I listened with great interest, as a lilting Scottish voice coursed the airways, quite clearly stating concerns.

Then someone said that the Christchurch Polytechnic had held an audiotaped public talk on 31 May 1988 with Dr Nigel Ashworth, this Scotsman, another doctor and a homoeopath on the topic of the Hepatitis B immunization during which these concerns were elaborated on more fully. Listening to the tape was a revelation. Here was a Professor of General Practice being right out there?

I wrote to Professor Murdoch expressing surprise at his stance, and offering to help him out in terms of medical literature he might be interested in looking at should he have the need. I also mentioned that I also had ME, though thought it was mild most of the time. The hardest thing was periods of tiredness, where my blood pressure dropped so low that I had to be really careful standing up quickly, but most of my tiredness was self-inflicted from spending long hours at the medical library, which wasn't always conducive to family life or good health.

*ME - otherwise known as myalgic encephalomyelitis, or chronic fatique syndrome (CFS).

42 1989 – Silenced

Interesting correspondence with a lot of medical articles, passed down Professor Murdoch's way, and a few this way. Then, in September that year, I accepted an invitation to join an all-day meeting in Christchurch at which various speakers, including Professor Murdoch, would air their concerns. The day was very interesting because of just how far out there Professor Murdoch was prepared to be, which had me worried. As he was doing a study of ME patients and red cells, he asked for a blood sample from me. I tensed a bit, as doctors aren't normally very good at drawing blood, but it's one of the few times I've never even felt the phlebotomist's needle, and he did not say, "It's just a little prick."

Before catching respective night flights the speakers congregated at the sponsor's house, where I buttoned Professor Murdoch, and said that I wondered if, in terms of his own safety, he was perhaps being a bit out there, and that I foresaw a day when the wrath of his Masters would descend upon his head even more than it already had.

With a broad smile, he leaned forward and said that he was very important, and very brave with broad enough shoulders to cope with whatever came his way.

A few weeks later, I got two calls, the first about the red cells which, he said, were "pretty atrocious" and "what we would normally see in patients with pretty bad ME". I was feeling fine by that time, so when the results arrived in the mail, they were filed in my medical records as being an interesting finding.

The other call was far more intriguing. My ex-doctor had decided to write a theoretical article about the ethical problems of families who prefer alternative care and had asked Professor Murdoch to be a referee, who had declined on the grounds that on reading it, he immediately figured it was us, and told the doctor that since he knew us, and the events that had taken place, and that he didn't consider it ethical for him to referee an article that was not theoretical.

Another referee was found, and the article was subsequently published. I wrote a rebuttal which might have been published, had not the editor of the journal changed, and I ran out of steam.

Every now and again at the end of that year, I would say, "I feel like my head is fit to bust." It was like a tight band. I became very sensitive to light, even on overcast days. I felt tired, tired, and more tired. My husband had been going on, for some time, about me not being able to say "no", talking to too many people, helping too many people and burning the candle at too many ends. Now, he said, "Be careful, you are about to crash."

One Saturday, we were collecting pinecones, and as we returned home with sacks over our shoulders, I felt as though someone collected me across the stomach with a bar, and I buckled, my head wanting to split at the seams. The right cheek was numb yet felt as if it had spider webs on it, and the right arm had gone suddenly heavy and numb, yet hurt amazingly. When I opened my mouth to speak, nothing came out. My husband saw I was a mess, and carried my sack home.

I can't remember how I got home but remember coming inside, and with my left hand grabbing the Arnica. I don't know why; it just felt like my head was massively bruised and that's all I could think of to do. My right hand was useless, so I jammed the bottle between my legs and got the lid off with my left hand. What was going on here?

I could think just fine, apart from struggling with incredible pain, which wasn't like a headache, just . . . something I can't describe. When Peter asked me if I was okay, I shook my head. He said, "Say something". It was too hard. Though my arm was limp and numb, it was so painful, I would have been happy to have chopped it off. The right leg was also weak and wouldn't take my weight without hurting.

For the next week, I was waited on hand and foot and did nothing. Simple words were there, but if I tried to say anything complicated, absolute garbage came out.

During that time, I took Arnica, and massively increased supplements like vitamin C, omega-3's and other things. When I had reasonable control on linking simple words, I went to see my doctor, who wasn't happy with the fact that the pin-prick tests showed I had reduced sensation on parts of my right side, so sent us to the neurology department at Auckland hospital.

Blood work was apparently somewhat suspicious, so they did a cat-scan looking for a stroke, but that came back clear. Also, my blood pressure was 125/65, which was normal for me, except when I had ME when it would go even lower . . . The neurologist said that 30% of scans in strokes came back clear, so he wanted to do another scan with dye. Trouble is, that had a 1% mortality rate, and not liking those odds, I declined.

He decided it was a migraine, and prescribed me antibiotics despite a large red heading in the file saying that I was allergic to it. He also prescribed warfarin, anti-migraine tablets, and more incredibly, medication he said was for "blood pressure".

I discharged myself, as I couldn't see any point in staying, and took the prescription and the discharge letter to my doctor who looked at the prescription, rolled his eyes, and ripped it up.

Earlier that year, my embroidery had taken a new tangent, as I had started an embroidery apprenticeship by mail, with a school in Japan. Just before the pine-cone-collecting day, I had stretched up fabric for a brightly coloured rooster.

As the days passed I got bored and frustrated. Reading was difficult. Tracking with my eyes hurt. However, I decided that even though my right hand wasn't working very well, that embroidery was going to get done. I plonked the semi-attentive hand on the frame, and made it do what it could, using the left hand to do what the right hand couldn't. It took six weeks to complete the rooster, and was an exercise in sheer stubbornness. But at the end of that time the right hand was starting to behave itself.

It took a year before I could whisk eggs without the whole arm seizing up in agony. A year later, I did the same embroidery in different colours and it took five days.

It was three more months before I could confidently talk on the phone, and read with ease. My self-confidence had taken a dent, and I was scared to talk publicly in case stress reduced my words to rubbish, so I concentrated on research, writing, and embroidery for much of the next year.

But when Maggie Barrie asked me to do a programme on Radio New Zealand I had enough confidence to undertake it. It was to be about influenza. Someone from the Health Department would oppose me, but the name given meant nothing.

Just before the programme, Dr Edwards had mentioned in passing during a discussion that his three-year contract with CARM was being renewed.

On arrival at the studio they said that, at the last minute, Dr Edwards had been brought in. From my point of view, it was a fair programme, something that doesn't happen that often. I told the truth, and so did he, and it seemed that discussing the blindingly obvious was useful. Perhaps things were looking up.

Apart from that I continued to avoid public discussion, because it was too draining on energy.

Most people wouldn't have known much had happened, as they thought I was just having a break. There were various theories amongst doctors I knew as to the problem, but migraine wasn't one of them, though for a while, when stressed I got what I called aurora blotchialis in the eyes, for about 20 minutes. Something had definitely happened up there but we never found out what.

In October 1989, I had made contact with Dr Robert Reisinger, who was later to provide me with another piece of the puzzle. He was also a colleague of Tony Morris. A summary of his work had previously been sent to me by Glen Dettman years before, when I started researching SIDS. By the time Bob had finished with me over the years, I understood *E-coli* endotoxin fairly clearly, and had a large library of information solely on endotoxaemia. Since then, I've kept an eye on the medical literature for anything to do with SIDS or *E-coli* endotoxin, which I believe is implicated, not just in SIDS but in other metabolic conditions as well, including some types of vaccine reactions.

In November 1989 the *Medical Journal of Australia* published an article called "Toxigenic Escherichia coli associated with sudden infant death syndrome". I sent a letter to the authors enclosing Dr Robert Reisinger's work, and a paper from Bendig and Haenel, and suggesting that they might profit from talking to Dr Reisinger. Neither of the authors, Bettelheim or Goldwater, replied, nor did they contact Dr Reisinger, but in early 1990, a follow-up medical paper by them contained the two references.

In June 1990, I went to America to take up a month's scholarship with the American branch of the Japanese Embroidery School. It was selfish of me, and neither the kids nor my husband were happy with my decision to go, but it seemed an ideal opportunity to get away, get myself together and to think ahead.

It was also an interesting time because the US media was zeroing in on supposedly appalling national vaccination rates, and vaccine controversies seemed to stare out from every newspaper, magazine and television.

While there, I spent one Saturday with Dr Morris and Dr Reisinger. Robert had always thought it natural to call me Hilary, but Tony had not. I'd also been too scared to call Dr Morris, Tony. Over desert I watched intently as two scientists carefully debated the etiquette of personal address, and whether or not it was gentlemanly to use a person's first name. Bob debated that Tony was being stuffy, and Tony expounded that Bob had forgotten a gentleman's code of manners. In the end, they asked me what I thought. It's a double-edged situation. Being addressed as Mrs Butler, denoted profession distance, but also respect and manners, and is the way of a certain generation. On the other hand, using a first name without invitation, can also be presumptive and intrusive. But I felt a decade on surname terms was enough, if that was acceptable. Since that time, Dr Morris has called me Hilary, and I have called him Tony. It's a weekend I will always treasure.

After finally meeting two people I respected very much face to face, I went home in December to start the beginning of new tangent of research.

The first piece of news to greet me was that not only was Dr Edwards now in Europe, but that Michael Soljak had also gone overseas as well.

I thought, "What's with this? Why do all the people who are open, prepared to think, and prepared to discuss things with me, stop talking to me, then either up and go, or seemingly are turfed out of the country?"

Who was it, who said, not so long ago, 'You are either with us, or against us?'

Others were to pay a lesser price as well.

43 Getting it Right

What goes up must come down. Right? You know – gravity and all that.

What goes in, must come out. Right? I mean, even a baby knows that. Disposable or washables, makes no difference. They still need an awful lot of them.

But hang on a minute.

We decided to go visiting. Hadn't been there before so we rang up to check things out. Would it be OK?

Yes. Love to see you.

Would there be somewhere to park the bus?

Yes. No problem.

How do we get there?

The instructions seemed straightforward enough.

"There's just one thing though," said Graham. "When you turn in at the gate you'll have to do it right, first time. You probably won't be able to have a second go. It can be a bit tricky; you know . . ."

That sounded ominous but I decided not to ask any more questions in case my ignorance showed through.

Well, we got there, no trouble. Certainly couldn't mistake their place. Graham had described their big white gate. It was one of those old-

fashioned solid timber affairs. Tall square posts with shaped pointed tops. We soon saw what the "getting it right first time" was all about. The gate way wasn't over-wide, and it was quite a bit below road level. Between the two, on that steepish slope, was a fair bit of loose metal. If the turn wasn't right, there would be no traction for reversing. So I guess you'd have to shift the gate!

We made it – just right, you know. Sailed down the driveway as if we did this sort of helmsmanship all the time.

The next stage was the "no problem" parking. It was just a matter of leaving the garage in one piece and making sure you didn't drive into the kitchen or take away the corner of the house. Simple – says he, remembering the sore arms after tugging so long on the steering wheel, and the raised blood pressure.

But we got in.

Would we get **out** *though?!*

I'll let you into a little secret. Every day that we stayed enjoying the family's hospitality I went for a lot of leisurely walks. Strangely enough they were all in the same direction. All very casual and with the right amount of nonchalance. But always with only one purpose in mind. Getting OUT. I reckon I knew the shape of just about every stone on that metalled entrance. The exit campaign was being planned in meticulous detail! The right strategy was crucial. The approach had to be right. The speed had to be judged correctly. Couldn't afford to stall. Not too fast either. Once the front wheels were on the road, knowing when to turn so that we didn't land up in the ditch on the other side or clip the gate post with the rear end. But there was just one other little detail that remained unpredictable. Traffic on the road at the wrong time! There was limited visibility. A car passing at the wrong moment would wreck the whole operation; or the car, or the bus, or all of them put together!

Time to go.

The mental rehearsals paid off.

Other road users stayed away.

The "getting it right" was achieved for the second time.

We got out. Our Guardian Angel chalked up another successful assignment.

But I'm not so dogmatic about this business of what goes in MUST come out. Maybe "what goes in SHOULD come out," would be better.

Yeah. Come to think of it, that's right.

The pages of the book are before you.

What you read is going **IN** *– or should be!*

Now we come to the crunch.

What will come **OUT***?*

Anger?

Indifference?

Frustration?

Incredulity?

Involvement? (But how?)

Excuses? (To do nothing?)

Something has to come **OUT**. *Or should do.*

The Jordan River flows **IN** *to an inland "sea".*

Always flowing **IN**.

But there is no flowing **OUT**.

There is a limit to how much IN this sea can take before its use is restricted.

It becomes a **DEAD SEA**.

It **is** *the* **DEAD** *Sea.*

44 When is a Reaction a Reaction?

A friend of mine who had had a stroke came to see me. She had reacted to an anaesthetic, then had serious delayed allergic reactions to subsequent drugs which ruined her gut, causing food absorption problems and chronic diarrhoea. She wore two medic alert bracelets.

She had come to talk because her son had had a tetanus booster, and had had a reaction. The doctor wouldn't accept that it was a reaction, and she couldn't understand why it was that they could see that immediate drug reactions after her stroke, were reactions, and that delayed reactions were reactions but then said that her son's vaccine reaction couldn't possibly be caused by a reaction from the vaccine, yet could give her no other cause for the problem.

We talked about my own medic alert bracelet, because I'm allergic to most major antibiotics, which is a big deal if you get sick and have an immunodeficiency, because what medical people have to offer is somewhat limited.

My recall of the first penicillin episode is hazy, because I was 16, and it happened so fast. I was given the tablet by the doctor one evening. Fortunately, he stayed because he didn't have television, we did, and Jacqueline du Pre was performing Elgar'sCello concerto in E minor with her husband, Daniel Barenboim. As a classical music lover, who loved Jacqueline's passion for her playing, he wanted to watch it.

As I drifted off to sleep to the music, all hell broke lose in my body. I was being choked and everything mentally disintegrated; a needle come from somewhere, my heart went berserk and I don't remember much else.

At the next doctor's visit a bracelet was put on my wrist, he waggled his finger, and said very earnestly, "You mustn't ever have penicillin again. Next time you could die. You were very lucky I was there!"

I know.

Now, *that's* a reaction caused by the body deciding *no more of that stuff*. Correct?

Next time I got sick he tried Tetracycline. Bad move. Broncho-oedema, and though that's not as scary as anaphylaxis, it comes close.

The bracelet was sent away to have another allergic reaction engraved on it, and replaced on my wrist after another finger-wagging intonation.

When I was 26 years, a doctor tried Bactrim Drapsules. Not a good idea either. My face swelled up, my jaw locked and he had to use large doses of a bronchodilator to keep me breathing until things settled back to normal.

A third allergic reaction was added to the bracelet list.

I haven't had antibiotics since, and have found other ways to support my somewhat crock immune system when I'm sick.

But the question I still have, and my friend had, is still relevant.

Why is it that the medical profession will accept reactions of some sorts, and not others?

When it comes to anaesthetics, other drugs and antibiotics, it's self-evident.

When it comes to vaccines, its usually *coincidence.*

Or as I witnessed in the doctor's surgery when some parents of a vaccinated child were unhappy about a red, hot hard lump the size of a twenty-cent piece at the injection site, and hives on his arms and body. "Oh no," said the nurse. "That can't possibly be from the vaccine."

"What caused it then?" said the mother.

"Must have been the sticky plaster . . ." was the reply.

45 Why do Vaccine Reactions Happen?

During 1991, exercise book after exercise book was being filled with name after name of babies, children and even adolescents having vaccine reactions. I felt I was swamped. Time after time, the medical profession said that the vaccine reactions parents talked about were all coincidental.

A pattern was emerging, which was fascinating, but frustrating.

Parents wanted to know *Why?* but the medical profession said there was no need to know why, because it doesn't happen. With the DPT vaccine reactions, there seemed to be a common thread. Most of the babies who had reactions were formula fed. Some of those babies had died, and their deaths were labelled as SIDS. There was also usually a history of parental illnesses such as epilepsy, asthma, drug allergies, or immune dysfunction.

Some parents, who were convinced their babies were not SIDS victims, said that doctors were of the view that anything abnormal in parental medical history was not relevant, and neither was the vaccine.

One doctor gave the mother a then "recent" medical article, which she gave to me. Ironically it said:[1]

> ***"A family history of asthma, urticaria, food allergy and skin disease was a significant factor."***

---

1 Williams, A.L. 1990. "Sudden infant death syndrome". *Aust NZ J Obstet Gynecol,* May; 30(2): 98–107. PMID: 2205194.

These parents thought there was a link between family history and SIDs. I thought there was a link between bottle feeding and SIDS too. But doctors thought none of that was relevant. I pointed out to the mother two other interesting comments, which showed how unscientific this study really was:

> *"Feeding – intention not to breast feed is a risk factor."*

As if a mother's intention is relevant? Action is important to study. Not intention. The bit I liked best was right at the end when the authors were discussing why babies die.

> ***"We seem to be no nearer to being able to answer the question which every SIDs parent asks, namely, 'Why did my baby die?' Perhaps as John Emery believes, we have not found the right answers because we have not asked the right questions."***

That the medical profession has no answers, but then say that family history, vaccines and bottle-feeding have no relationship to SIDS or vaccine reactions, defied logic then, and still does now.

Yet in 2005 we are told,

> ***"Children who are not breast-fed may have a greater risk of a drug reaction . . . the relationship between the (lack of) reactions and the breastfeeding has never been observed before and therefore cannot really be explained."***

Here I was in 1989 *observing* and *discussing* this 2005 observation with doctors and immunologists, and asking, "Why?" . . . yet they said it was all co-incidental? It had been observed, but they have spent decades denying this very phenomenon.

Why is bottle-feeding a common feature in SIDS? Why does SIDs sometimes follow a vaccine shot? Most thought it totally unrelated. It's mentioned in the literature but thought to be irrelevant.

Maybe to doctors the "why" didn't appear to be relevant because other vaccinated, formula-fed babies, some with family histories of allergies, didn't react or die. So, perhaps they reasoned that the vaccine couldn't possibly provoke anything that would lead to SIDS. Not everyone is allergic to antibiotics either, but that doesn't make antibiotics irrelevant to reactions.

They were not interested in asking the question:

> ***What is it about the babies who DO have a vaccine reaction or die, that is "different" to babies who don't react to vaccines?***

This became my research focus and was again both fascinating, and frustrating.

I quickly discovered that most of that information on the difference between bottle-fed and breast-fed babies, and how that affects the gut and the immune system, had suddenly stopped being published about the time vaccine research started, and formula had become the favourite modus operandi of paediatricians. In the light of the incredible research done before that, showing the amazing differences between bottle-fed and breast-fed babies, I was left totally floored as to how any medical person could consider formula an option, as opposed to a last-resort necessity, let alone comparable in either nutrition or function to breast milk. The nutrition in, and immunological function of breast milk are not synonymous.

The attitude seemed to be that there was no need to continue to look at the role of gut flora and how it affected health and disease, because vaccines and antibiotics were going to be the saviours of mankind, and bowel flora are irrelevant. Vaccines and antibiotics are patentable, and profitable drug ventures. Gut flora isn't a golden goose . . . yet. But its time may come.

Dr Reisinger's work became a very important link, because his life had centred around studying animal and human gut flora. His veterinary focus had been calf scours, resulting from calves being deprived of their mother's colostrum. He had amassed huge amounts of information on the topic of colostrum and breast milk in a very broad way, by also studying cows, horses, monkeys, humans and humans and humans.

His study of the human aspect was sparked when a relative's baby had a severe vaccine reaction and nearly died. The baby was bottle-fed, but the connection made no sense at the time. As he saw more cases, he started asking questions, and looked at the composition of human breast milk in comparison with formula, and how that affected the gut. That's when he saw the similarity between *E-coli* and SIDS in babies, and fatal scours in calves being fed powdered milk and no colostrum. The two looked very similar in pathology and outward symptomatology. Back in the medical library he found the early literature which so clearly showed the *E-coli*/SIDS connection in humans.

I had asked him to look at some of the baby cases I had been involved in, who had died after the DPT shots. He studied them and then rang me to say, "I've put some 'stuff' in the mail to you . . ." It arrived, and then he elaborated on the points he had already made. He said, "Most of these babies in these studies were bottle-fed. Even your own experts know that bottle-feeding is a risk factor for SIDS." He included in the 'stuff' a copy of a presentation given at a SIDS symposium in 1974.

Titled "Epidemiology of SIDS in Auckland, New Zealand", by Shirley Tonkin (Appendix E-6).

> ***"Of the 86 cases of 'cot deaths' occurring in these three years, 83 were artificially fed and only three breast-fed at the time of death."***

My reply was, "Well, what has that to do with vaccine reactions?"

He said that what I had to understand was the difference between the metabolism, immunology and biochemistry of breast-fed and bottle-fed babies saying, "They are from different planets."

First he defined *"breast-fed"* because some medical people think that "breast-fed" also can include babies who receive occasional bottles of formula as well. He raged against people who had no idea that, ***"Any breast-fed baby receiving one bottle of formula has such significant gut flora change that they must be classified as formula fed for two weeks."*** Another medical article winged its way to me, with the relevant passage underlined, showing that just one bottle of formula changes the gut flora and ph so dramatically that it takes two weeks of breast-feeding to return it to ***"normal"***.[2] As far as he was concerned, any baby receiving any formula, was NOT breast-fed.

"Rather old study don't you think?" I said. "Yes," he replied, "but it was replicated not that long ago with modern formula and the results were the same." "So where's that study?" I asked. He snorted, "It was never published. The journal said the work 'had no meaningful application'."

Not much help in a world that considers up-to-date references

2 Gerstley, J. et al. 1932. "Factors influencing the Fecal Flora of infants". *Amer J Dis Child*, 43: 555–565.

more valuable than common sense, and references as the only way to prove the credibility of information.

The term old research in many doctor's minds means it's not relevant. In a sense they are right, because nutrition these days is in some respects much worse than it was up to the 1950s.

Tissier in France did the first studies on gut flora in babies in 1900. Books came out on the subject steadily after that, but Erik Olsen's 1949 book should be mandatory reading even now.[3] These form a vast resource showing the normal baselines for societies with little junk food, where a bottle was rare, and antibiotics nonexistent. The old knowledge of appropriate gut flora bacteria is reasonably up to date, with the bacteria types seen today the same, but the balance of bacteria in the gut markedly changed.

Many recent studies (seemingly done by people who haven't read the early studies) include babies who have formula in the breast-fed section, which nullifies the relevance of the findings. Nor is the current rampant indiscriminate and repeated use of antibiotics in babies, which radically alters gut flora, thus encouraging dangerous bacteria, factored into their thinking.

The recent *clostridium difficile* outbreak in England[4] brought this into sharp focus with recommendations given to adults as to the foods they should eat for eight weeks after antibiotics to return the gut flora to normal. How is it that this is never considered necessary for bottle-fed babies?

What is the difference between formula-fed and breast-fed babies, which might lead to a bottle-fed baby being more susceptible to drug reactions, including vaccines?

One of the studies done in 1963 has a table[5] showing that the intestinal pH of a breast-fed baby is 4.5–5.8 (acid), and while that of a formula-fed baby is 7.2–8.0 (alkaline). pH is crucial as to which bacteria will grow where. Good probiotic bacteria like the pH of a breast-fed baby, but the more dangerous gram-negative and bad bacteria like the higher gut pH of a bottle-fed baby.

Gut flora in breast-fed babies have a lot of *lactobacillus* and *bifidus*

---

3 Olsen, E. 1949. *Studies on the Intestinal Flora of Infants*. Copenhagen: Ejnar Munksgaard.

4 June 2005.

5 Dubos, R. et al. 1963. "Alteration and effects of the intestinal flora". *Ped Proc*, November/December: 22: 1322–1329.

bacteria and other probiotics, which is another name for good bacteria, like the stuff you find in Easiyo Biolife yoghurt, only more so.

Compared with breast-fed babies, bottle-fed babies have 1000 times the numbers of a bacteria called *E-coli* which likes the alkaline environment. Every time one *E-coli* bacterium divides into two, it drops off a bit of its envelope (lipo-polysaccharide), which is an *endotoxin* in itself, though some medical people have the illusion that only certain strains of *E-coli* can cause this problem. The other name for this *E-coli* envelope particle is *curlin*. Curlin has to be chomped up (degraded) by the liver, because curlin is very dangerous. Bottle-fed babies also have high levels of other gram-negative bacteria, some of which can also produce similar toxins.

Because of the difference in acidity and nutrients received, the gut flora of a bottle-fed baby is very different to that of a breast-fed baby, and has different influences on the baby immunologically, physiologically and biochemically.

E. Coli bacteria love the higher than breast milk protein concentration of baby formula. There are also other crucial nutritional imbalances and bioavailability issues with formula, which put a bottle-fed baby's metabolism and biochemistry under far greater stress than that of a breast-fed baby.

Sleeping metabolic rates and body temperatures are higher in formula-fed babies. Total daily energy expenditure is significantly greater, which is understandable, since the ingredients in formula puts the body under a lot of physiological stress, a problem known to doctors for decades.[6] Again, *E-coli* both thrives in heat, and because it is potentially pyogenic, creates heat.

Heat itself also changes the pH of gut flora, and both conditions encourage even more *E-coli* growth.

I can hear a lot of great-grandmothers at this point say, "But our babies were on formula and didn't have vaccine reactions." There is a simple answer to that. Those babies got far fewer vaccines and were given them when they were a lot older. Most babies now finish a large primary vaccine schedule at five months. Prior to the 1950s the uptake of the diphtheria vaccine was about 9%, and whooping cough vaccine was only given on request. Babies born in the 1950s

6 Miller, M.J. et al. 1990. "Casein: a milk protein with diverse biologic consequences". *Proc Soc Exp Biol Med*, Nov; 195(2): 143–59. PMID: 2236098.

didn't get their first single vaccine until 6 months, if then, and in the main polio years, all vaccines except polio were discontinued. The DPT was first introduced in 1961 at the age of three months. Also, the vaccine take-up was very slow, and for many years, less than 50% of babies had the full series. There were still reactions, but far fewer opportunities to have them at a really early age. That is why grandmothers didn't know too many babies who had vaccine reactions.

Dr Reisinger also explained that breast milk isn't just a food. Naturally his expertise was from the cow, horse and monkey perspective, but he saw no reason why human milk shouldn't have similar protective functions. He talked about how vital animal milk is to the priming of baby animals' immune systems, and again, couldn't see how it could be any different in humans. Neither could he see the value of feeding milk from one species with specific needs, to a different species with different needs. It turned out he was right about that too. An article in *Discover*[7] about Dr Catharina Svanborg's breast-milk research shows clearly just how amazing an immune system breast milk is.

Breast milk is designed to form an immune system bridge between the baby's immature immune system and the world out there. Breast milk teaches the baby's immune system how to function the right way. Breast milk also steps in and fills the maturity gap between a baby's immune system and that of an adult by providing lots of anti-bacterial and antiviral substances, as well as other vital fighting organisms to help a baby cope with what comes into its mouth, and through the digestive tract. Even better, breast milk vastly reduces the chances a baby will have cancer later on.

By the time a baby is two years old, its immune system is still only 80% of that of an adult, and becomes comparable to that of an adult at the age of eight. Even then, puberty years and the mad rebellious teens stage puts a different strain on the immune system, so it isn't until a child becomes an adult, that you get some sort of immune system stability at times when life ticks over evenly. And maybe with some adults' lifestyles, that never happens.

Breast-feeding is crucial:[8]

---

7 Radetsky, P. 1999. "Got Cancer Killers?" *Discover*, Vol. 20(6). [Internet]. Available from <http://www.discover.com/issues/jun-99/features/featcancer/> Accessed 18 September, 2005.

8 Hanson, L.A. 1998. "Breast feeding provides passive and long-lasting active immunity".

"Breastfeeding may, in addition to the well-known passive protection against infections during lactation, have a unique capacity to stimulate the immune system of the offspring possibly with several long-term positive effects."

Breast milk includes protection against different sorts of cancers, Crohn's disease, coeliac disease, diabetes . . . the list goes on and on, and the more you know, the easier it is to understand why formula-feeding a baby puts the whole immune system under considerable strain.

Breast milk patrols the gut like a sentry, destroying anything dangerous, priming the baby's immune system, and seems to teach it things that formula-fed babies don't learn.

The *Globe and Mail* in Canada on 16 January 2001, commented on a paper[9] and interviewed the lead author who said:

"It's a really good idea to breast-feed; we already knew that, but the key advance is that now we know why . . . the babies of mothers who do not breast-feed will still develop active immune systems, but breast-fed babies are more robust."

He was discussing a molecule in breast milk called sCD14, which has the power to ***"switch on the immune system"***. Formula can't do that.

It's important to talk about breast-feeding here because of all the babies with vaccine reactions whose parents come to me, the babies who recover the quickest, and the most completely, are fully breast-fed.

The other question, then, is:

Why don't the formula-fed babies recover so well?

Bottle-fed babies don't have any of the immune protection that breast milk gives. At times of stress, the breast milk is working as part of the baby's immune system, rather than just food, whereas bottle-fed babies have to rely on their own resources.

Given that formula-fed babies have 1000 times more *E-coli* than breast-fed babies; have an alkaline gut that favour gram-negative bacteria and a higher base temperature to start with, bottle-fed babies

---

Ann Allergy Asthma Immunol. Dec; 81(6): 523–37. PMID: 9892025.

9 Filipp, D. et al. 2001. "Soluble CD14 enriched in colostrum, and milk induces B cell growth and differentiation". *Proc Natl Acad Sci USA.* Jan 16; 98(2): 603–8. PMID: 11209057.

are disadvantaged during times of stress.

The key research to understanding the reactions I was seeing from the whole-cell pertussis vaccine is that in some babies, that vaccine partially shuts down a very important part of the liver for between 7–14 days.[10] The very system the baby relies on to denature (chomp up) curlin is slowed down. That same enzyme function is used to denature toxins in the vaccines as well. If that *E-coli* endotoxin manages to get through that part of the liver which the vaccine slows down and gets into the blood, it can cause trouble, leading to an excess of serotonin and deep sleep.

This was first reported in humans in the medical literature in 1955,[11] and then confirmed in animal studies in 1990 when Sherry Ansher and William Habig showed that the whole cell DTP vaccine, or the Tetanus toxoid alone, could suppress the P-450 liver system and increase the hexobarbital induced sleep time for 7–10 days in mice.[12] They pointed out that other vaccines could do it as well, and speculated that it could have been the endotoxin in the vaccines that created this reaction, but that it was apparently "not the only cause of inhibition". But they didn't say what "other" causes there might be.

A subsequent study testing acellular vaccines as well has found that the acellular vaccine increased the sleep time by only 15% which indicated that the new pertussis vaccines[13] have a lower toxicity level. However, another hospital study showed shock and induced sleep time in babies with both whole-cell and acellular pertussis, and a group that wasn't given pertussis vaccine at all.[14] The babies given whole-cell pertussis vaccines showed exactly the same breathing and heart instabilities and other signs you would expect to find with *E-coli* endotoxaemia. And some of the babies given only Haemophilus

10 Ansher, S. et al. 1992. "Role of Endotoxin in Alterations of Hepatic Drug Metabolism by Diphtheria and Tetanus Toxoids and Pertussis vaccine Adsorbed". *Infection and Immunity,* Sep; 60(9): 3790–8. PMID: 1500188. (There are two other papers as well.)

11 Caps, R.B. 1955. "Hepatitis in infants and small children". *Amer J Dis Child,* Vol. 89: 701–716.

12 Sixth International Symposium on Pertussis, 1990. Abstracts and Program, p. 124.

13 Fantuzzi, G. et al. 1994. "Depression of Liver Metabolism and Induction of Cytokine Release by Diphtheria and Tetanus Toxoids and Pertussis vaccines: Role of Bordetella Pertussis Cells in Toxicity". *Infection and Immunity,* Jan; 62(1): 29–32. PMID: 8262641.

14 Pourayrous, M. et al. 1998. "Interlenkin-6, C-Reactive protein, and abnormal cardiorespiratory responses to immunization in premature infants". *Pediatrics* March: 101(3): e3. PMID: 9481022. Available from <http://www.pediatrics.aapublications.org/cgi/content/full/101/3/e3>

B, Hepatitis B vaccine and Injectable Polio vaccine also showed similar signs, including moderately severe signs of cardiorespiratory disturbance, which confirms that other vaccines may affect the liver detoxification centre in the same way as do the whole-cell pertussis vaccine. Ironically, the researchers seemed to know nothing about the consequences or origins of *E-coli* endotoxaemia, or didn't appear to understand what they were seeing in either group and reported the results as ***"incidental findings"***.

Since then, I have not found anyone looking at what vaccines do to any functional aspect of the inate or cellular immune system of babies.

The fact that doctors first "observed" in 2005 that bottle-fed babies are more likely to experience "drug reactions", is because, as John Emery said, "They haven't been asking the right questions". Or should I say, "Looking at the right symptoms". Had they been looking at what was in front of them, in particular, the role of gut pH and flora, in comparison with the protective and priming effects of breast milk on the immune system, susceptibility to drug reactions while being bottle-fed should have been self-evident long ago.

Any baby with high levels of gram negative bacteria such as gut *E-coli*, whose liver is shut down by a vaccine, runs a potential risk of going into endotoxic shock and could die very quickly, but the picture the doctor sees is usually called SIDs.

If doctors knew how to do autopsies related to endotoxaemia they would soon pick up that in bottle-fed vaccinated babies, a death shortly after vaccination isn't SIDs at all, even if it looks like it from the outside.

To complicate the picture, what you see happening to the baby depends on how long the curlin takes to build up. If the levels of gut endotoxin are lower to start with, and the baby's liver is less shut down, the levels of curlin build up more slowly, and the temperature rises slowly as the liver tries to denature it. Viruses can also take advantage of the situation where the immune system is struggling and the baby might also show only symptoms that look like a cold a few days later. Perhaps a parent then takes the baby to the doctor who prescribes antibiotics. The baby might seem to get better, yet suddenly die.

Why? There are several biologically plausible reasons. One is that, gradually, over a few days, the antibiotic might kill all the *E-coli* or other gram-negative bacteria in the gut. All the killed *E-coli* bacteria envelopes then become endotoxin (curlin) and the liver suddenly has to deal with a whole mass of endotoxin over a short period. If the liver cannot keep up, there comes a point where the curlin gets through into the blood supply.

SIDS babies show very high levels of *E-coli* curlin, whereas non-SIDS babies don't.

That has been shown in several medical articles by Dr Karl A. Bettelheim and Paul N. Goldwater in Australia. But their research implies that their interest in *E-coli* seems primarily towards making an *E-coli* vaccine to give to babies, to prevent SIDS.

Which is strange when the ideal solution is feeding the baby using the two mammary glands on the front of every mother's chest, unless the mother has had a bilateral mastectomy, or is physically unable to breast-feed.

Breast-fed babies have *E-coli* as well, but in very small numbers. Breast-fed babies have an acid gut of 4–5 pH. *E-coli* doesn't like or grow well in an acid gut. Heat, such as from an infection-based temperature can quickly change the gut pH to alkaline, which *E-coli* likes and this will help *E-coli* to divide and drop off lots of curlin. But breast milk helps return the gut to an acid pH, has immune factors in it, which act as an outside neutralizer and the breast milk quickly helps destroy any increase in the *E-coli* and other toxins produced by other bacteria.

Sick breast-fed babies feed a lot more often than usual, if only for comfort, so they get that anti-bacterial dose on tap, on demand when they are sick, which is when they really need that immune system the most.

Bottle-fed babies are also more at risk from SIDS than breastfed babies, *whether or not* they have had a vaccine. Formula as it is currently made cannot supply gut protection or immune system support. A baby whose system has high levels of gram-negative bacteria, can be right at that precipice anyway, so if that baby is given a vaccine it runs the risk of immediate severe shock.[15] Without any breast milk immune system to help neutralize the bacteria which happily multiply in hot formula-fed intestines, if the liver is shut down for any reason, those babies have to rely on themselves.

A further confounding factor is babies with a family history of allergies and other health problems. The way their immune systems

---

15 Pourayrous, M. et al. 1998. "Interlenkin-6, C-Reactive protein, and abnormal cardiorespiratory responses to immunization in premature infants". *Pediatrics* March: 101(3): e3. PMID: 9481022. Available from <http://www.pediatrics.aapublications.org/cgi/content/full/101/3/e3>

work may be completely different to those of other babies. Just as these babies may be more at risk of disease and allergy, they are also the ones I see as more at risk of vaccine reactions because their immune systems are different. Enough is known to show that these babies really need to be breast-fed.

You cannot say, though, that the immune system is the problem.

I'm not about to try an antibiotic, or another rubella vaccine to see whether I'd have anaphylaxis or arthritis again. I'm fine just as I am. It is antibiotics, not my immune system that are the trigger for my allergic reactions. The rubella vaccine, not my immune system, was the trigger for my arthritis.

In 2000, I was invited to speak at an International SIDS conference. I put a lot of this information together in a 30-page position paper in medical language, which was put into the bags of all participants.

For a variety of reasons, I flubbed my verbal presentation, but most of the audience "said" they had read the paper beforehand. I stayed for the rest of the conference, yet everyone I spoke to considered that the literature I presented had nothing useful to contribute to the issue.

All SIDs experts seem to think that their idea is the best idea of them all, yet they still argue amongst themselves as to what causes SIDS. And they all refuse to look at the biggest piece of evidence right in front of their eyes, which is the immune system and the gut flora of every baby they are talking about. They don't seem to want to talk about what biochemical or immunological factors make SIDS baby's different. They'd rather talk about long QT intervals, genetic influences or maternal Munchaussens.

When I am rung about babies with vaccine reactions, there is usually one common factor. Babies with vaccine reactions can produce the most horrible smelling, strange looking poos you will ever see, which is the first, and best, sign that a baby's gut flora has changed for the worse, and that baby is potentially in endotoxaemia-type trouble.

Usually, but not always, the baby is bottle-fed. Quite often, there is a history of allergies and chronic health problems in one, or both, parents' families.

To the medical profession, all that is irrelevant. To Bob Reisinger, that was the crucial starting point.

46 Ready-Made for the Family

The Auckland Domain.

I was first introduced to this delightful place in the 1940s. A place for family outings during holiday periods when we came from New Plymouth to stay with my grandmother in Auckland. In 1946 we moved to live in this city and I attended Auckland Grammar School for the next four years before going to Auckland Teachers' College. I played rugby in the Domain. I watched (and fed) the ducks in the pond near the tearooms. I spent a month or more at the educational unit attached to the Auckland War Memorial Museum as children from many Auckland schools, and class levels, studied a wide range of topics from the displays in this wonderful museum.

This 75-hectare park, developed around the cone of a volcano, is a place which can satisfy the needs and moods of people in so many different ways. A place you can return to time after time after time.

Never in my wildest dreams would I have thought that forty years later I would be reliving so many of my boyhood memories with another generation of my own children.

So how did this come about?

Well, next to the Domain, on one side, is the Auckland Hospital, and across the street from the main gates of the Domain, in Park Road, is the Auckland School of Medicine Medical Library.

So if your maths is good, you put two and two together and you get: **research**. Throw in Hilary and you get: **need to go and study in the medical library**. Throw in a husband and two children and you get: **a place to occupy them**. Throw in home schooling and you get: **an open-air classroom**. Throw in convenience, location, interests, variety, fresh air and sunshine, and plenty of space and you get: **the Domain**.

Consequently, on many occasions over a number of years we would head off for a day in Auckland. We would take the car, and park in the Domain. Then we would walk with Hilary to the Medical School Library, kiss her goodbye and retrace our steps.

Maybe four or five hours to fill in.

That was always a challenge, because although there were plenty of things to do, there is a limit to that thing called "attention span".

What would we do?

Well it might go something like this.

During the day we would visit the Museum at least once. It was best to go there fairly early on because it was the place furthest away.

Whilst in that vicinity the big guns in front of the museum would be given the once-over. Various targets would be identified and "destroyed" by accurate gunfire!

We might then go over to the Winter Gardens, where we could enjoy the flowers, and other breath-taking displays – or Dad might find himself alone, suddenly talking to thin air, whilst his two sons were investigating the goldfish or hunting for the little frogs that had long since learned that survival was dependent on keeping as still and quiet as possible.

Next might be a walk through the fernery – usually at high speed with Dad trailing behind.

The ducks were always a drawcard. So off we would go and have a talk with them – in duck language of course. Our most practised "quacks" would be greeted with quizzical, bemused looks. Ducklings in tow were always a highlight.

Maybe a loo stop next.

Now what shall we do?

"Can I go back to the guns Dad?"

"No, I want to go and catch the frogs."

"I'm hungry."

Sometimes Hilary would come and join us for lunch at a time we had agreed upon.

Consult watch. Too early.

"Okay, we'll go back and look at the guns and while we're there we might see some of those big tourist buses. But this time, let's go a different way."

Off we'd go again, with the kids probably running on ahead.

"Look out for any cars," I would call after them.

Lunch was always eaten near the duck pond. It was geographically convenient for Hilary and we were sure of an attentive audience in the form of our feathered friends. Well fed they were too.

Hilary would leave us for another stint in the Med Library, and the rest of the family would hold a pow wow. More likely than not, the morning agenda would be repeated but at a more subdued pace and very much in random order, and always open to flashes of inspiration!

As the time for going home approached, we would wend our way back towards the Med Library and if Hilary wasn't in sight, we might cross the road and sit down on the seats in front of the library, until once again we were a complete family.

"What took you so long Mum?"

"Can we go now Mum?"

"Mum, Dad made us walk a long way."

Or it might be a recital about anything and everything.

"Darling, am I sure glad to see you. My feet are killing me!"

"And my head's in a spin. Come on then, let's go home."

About an hour and a half later, all going well, we would be back in our own backyard – until next time.

47 Hepatitis B – Alaska

In August 1988 a letter had arrived from Bernadine Atchison, a Dena'ina Indian from the Kenai Peninsula asking for information on the Hepatitis B vaccine. The elders from the combined council of native tribes had become more concerned about the use of the vaccine in their country when children started being pulled out of class and vaccinated against their parents' wishes under instruction from the Indian Hospital in Anchorage. There was a huge, sudden increase in depression and suicides amongst Alaskan indigenous teenagers, which doctors blamed on increasing alcohol and drug culture, but was seen quite differently by the elders. It wasn't as if the supposed new alcohol and drug culture appeared at the same time as the vaccine.

Previously, when Native Hospital teams had gone around the villages, vaccinating babies, babies would get sick, and no explanation was offered. In Bethel over 100 babies got sick and some died after the ***"Hep B at birth"*** team had been through. American doctors and some from other countries were sent to investigate, but no-one was ever told the results, yet word went around that it was nothing to do with the vaccine, but was the ***"respiratory syncytial virus"*** that killed the children. The trouble was that this coincidental RSV followed everywhere the team went.

These stories were very reminiscent of the stories that I had heard from Africa where, as credible evidence showed, sickness, death and higher incidence of AIDS also followed behind vaccination programmes, especially those carried out with insanitary reusable needles.

To the Alaskans, because of their feelings about being fobbed off regarding both baby and adolescent deaths, such rumours assumed huge proportions.

The other anger behind their desire for knowledge, was that native people had repeatedly complained that under the Unites States Arctic Research Plan, that not only were they *"subjects"* of experiments, but that often they were not told what the research being carried out was, or the results.

Some aspects of the Alaskan Hepatitis B campaign didn't make sense. Why did the authorities only target the 60,000 isolated indigenous Inuit people, instead of the much larger 400,000+ group of other Alaskan inhabitants? Where did this Hepatitis B come from, anyway?!

Until the mid-1940s no such disease as hepatitis had even been known amongst the indigenous people in Alaska, just as there had been no smallpox or tuberculosis until Russia, then America, stole their country. The elders told me that the only clue they had was that it seemed that the first cases of hepatitis appeared amongst indigenous men in the 300,000 military personnel both in the USA and overseas who had been vaccinated with Hepatitis B contaminated yellow-fever vaccine in 1942.

A very small study 45 years later on 392 people who had received the contaminated vaccine found that a strikingly high proportion of that group, even amongst those without clinical jaundice, had antibody values usually only found in populations at highest risk, such as drug addicts, homosexual men, and haemophilia patients, but a very low carriage rate.[1] They did admit that given that carriage can resolve at an annual rate of 1 to 1.5%, the low carriage rate might be partially explainable. They also hypothesized that being injected with a hepatitis B contaminated vaccine which also contained live yellow fever virus, might have altered the outcome of the epidemic. The case fatality rate for those with icteric hepatitis was 2 to 3 per 1000. Interestingly the article described the recipients as *"healthy young white men"* when in fact the mix was across all the races.

1 Seeff, L.B. et al. 1987. "A serologic follow-up of the 1942 epidemic of post-vaccination hepatitis in the United States Army". *N Engl JMed,* April: 316(16): 965–70. PMID: 2436048.

As far as the Alaskan indigenous people were aware, the contaminated vaccine was the index source for the introduction of Hepatitis B in the first place. It seemed a shame to me that an isolated population was now the study cohort for a vaccine supposedly needed because of a contaminated military vaccine administered decades previously. There was no study of Hepatitis B in the Alaskan community until 1981, and nowhere has there been acknowledgement that contaminated vaccine was probably the cause, though one elder showed me a letter from an Anchorage doctor admitting that it might have been, but that they thought any Alaskans in the National Guard might have only enlisted after the vaccine was used.

Over the years, I sent them information, but I learned far more from them than they learned from me.

In October 1993 I went to Alaska to attend the International Health and Alternative Medicine Conference. There I had a chance to listen first hand to accounts from parents and native workers, detailing what they saw from vaccines, to the mysterious problems they had had for decades around Point Hope on the North Slope. Strange cancerous growths wiped out not just whole families, but animals too. Rumours had circulated for years about people coming in and burying stuff while the community was away at summer fishing camp.

CDC, and all the authorities denied it, and said the rates of cancer weren't anything out of the ordinary, and all the native health workers believed them, but many people didn't. Authorities chose excuses like ***"Western diet, alcohol and smoking"*** to dismiss the murmurings in the community.

Nearly a year before the conference, the truth had surfaced. Fifteen thousand pounds of radioactive soil had indeed been transported from Nevada and spread out and buried near the village while the people were at summer fishing camp. The authorities wanted to see how far it would travel by river and in the rain. All those years, when denial was the modus operandi, the Inuit people had been part of yet another experiment without their knowledge or permission. No one had suggested they not hunt or graze animals or camp there. People had come and gone, looked at them, hummed and ha'd, and said nothing. For years the native health providers didn't listen to the people, or reminded them that the Federal Government had clearly stated that nothing had been buried near Point Hope, and while the people stopped complaining, they didn't stop thinking.

In 1992, some Inuit people found the documentation they needed to prove that they had been lied to. Most disillusioned of all were the health workers who ended up having to admit to their own people[2] that it was true, and were devastated that they had been suckered into believing their own government.

As I looked around me and listened to everything being talked about, I could understand why it was that the indigenous people of Alaska had absolutely no faith in the assurances of their Government, the CDC, or even of the doctors when they listened to platitudes about the Hepatitis B, particularly when it was now found that Point Hope people carry more radioactive elements in their bodies than anyone on earth except the survivors of Hiroshima and Nagasaki.

As I write this, and consider the parents in the USA, UK, New Zealand, Australia and many other countries of the world who consider their children are being damaged by vaccines, I wonder about the reality that the system operates in. As I look back at all these stories, the cases I've done, the misleading information, persistent and deliberate obstructiveness that officialdom has often put in the way of many of these people, there is part of me that still can't believe how authorities continue to turn blind eyes.

How is it that every country on the face of this earth has a dedicated group of people who only want the medical system to be honest, and accountable about vaccines?

How is it that in most countries the medical authorities characterize groups demanding real choice as misinformed and dangerous and use these groups as a reason to try to make vaccine uptake compulsory?

The latest term for people who question vaccines is ***"scientific terrorists"***. I wasn't surprised to see this line of thought continue on from 1988, when the wandering finger of the Health Department here, had accused supposed anti-vaccination campaigners of indulging in terrorism during the Hepatitis B campaign. But since 9/11, it has become more fashionable to call anyone who disagrees with the status quo, a terrorist. A few of the well-known historical figures who might be given the same label would be Copernicus, Gallileo, Marconi, and Barnes Wallace, all considered rabble-rousers of their era. Copernicus sensibly died not long after publishing his heretical view of the sun's

---

2 Patkotak, E. 1992. "Radiation lies ensnared this health worker". *Anchorage Daily News*, (Alaska, USA) September.

position in the universe, saving himself the agony of the normal punishment for heretics.

At a conference in 2002, Dr Jonathan Jarman[3] headed his presentation, *"Fighting Scientific Terrorism – Practical Advice for Vaccinators"*.

Another of like mind is Dr Glen Buchan,[4] who at the same conference gave a presentation which had this in the abstract:

> ***"On the other side is a small but vocal group who are not constrained by lack of facts and have little respect for logic."***

Sandy Milne once said that there was ***"a galaxy"*** of medical evidence that immunization against hepatitis B is a positive move in preventive health care. Then he said;[5]

> ***"The alternative view assumes that we are evil men and women up to mischief. Now, is that likely?"***

It's no more likely that those who denied that there was anything buried near Point Hope, Alaska, were evil. Or those who told Marconi that his ideas were stupid because of course radio waves would just keep on going out to the stars.

---

3 Jarman, J. 2001. "Fighting Scientific Terrorism – Practical Advice for Vaccinators". Available from <http://www.imac.auckland.ac.nz/resources/confer_2002/abstracts/jarman_ab.htm> Accessed 18 September, 2005. "The objectives of this talk are to look for the parallels between bioterrorism and the publications of the anti-immunization movement, *examine the reasons why 'scientific terrorism' is so successful*, and to make practical suggestions on *how vaccinators can reduce the hysteria of the anti-vaccination lobby*."

4 Buchan, G. "I think, therefore I vaccinate". Available from <http://www.imac.auckland.ac.nz/resources/confer_2002/abstracts/buchan_ab.htm> Accessed 18 September, 2005. "These groups appear to be irreconcilable. At stake is the silent majority who try and gather information as best they can. Unfortunately this is often presented in an indigestible form by the professionals while the sensationalist rhetoric of the anti-lobby, which is seldom informed, is widely reported and difficult to counteract."

5 Calder, P. 1988. "Campaign aims to cut hepatitis risk". *New Zealand Herald* 12 March: Section 2: 3.

48 Hepatitis B Reactions – a Saga of Lies?

"Worldwide sales of hepatitis B vaccine exceeded $1 billion in 1995, making it the first vaccine product of any kind to reach the billion dollar mark."[1]

On 30 April 1992, Dr J. Anthony Morris and I submitted a co-authored report in response to an invitation by the National Institute of Health, Bethesda, Maryland to submit evidence on or before 4 May 1992, for consideration by the Vaccine Safety Committee in its review of adverse events that followed injection of some commonly-used vaccines for babies and children.

The report on Hepatitis B, which fills a quarto folder, is called *"Nature and Frequency of Adverse Reactions following Hepatitis B vaccine injection in Children in New Zealand, 1985–1988"*.

Included in this lengthy report were:

1) Several memoranda from the New Zealand Health Department to all Hepatitis B co-ordinators advising the delay of the newborn H-B vaccination because minor side-effects may be confused with more serious ill health, and other memoranda reporting reactions, one of which

1 1998. "Biotechnology, the Promise is now". *FORBES* 4 May. A special report written by the Biotechnology Industry Organization.

reported 10 cases of anaphylactoid reactions occurring in children receiving hepatitis B vaccine.

2) The Medical Assessors 97-page report, called *"Analysis of Adverse Events reported after hepatitis B vaccination in pre-school children, amongst 166,757 children"*.

3) A report from a doctor on observations from their practice that newborns injected with Hepatitis B vaccine had prolonged jaundice in comparison with those who were not injected and that enquiries to the vaccine manufacturers about the etiology of this problem resulted in unsatisfactory responses.

4) A background paper discussing the Menomune A and the Hepatitis B campaigns.

The report also contained various medical articles dealing with many different aspects of Hepatitis B vaccine, including Guillain Barre and other potentially auto-immune responses.

Amongst all the Government paperwork included with the report, the key points in terms of New Zealand side-effects in the school catch-up campaign, which it seems was the only issue the committee was interested in, were that there were two cases of anaphylaxis, which required adrenaline, and:

Bronchospasm occurred on 70 occasions in 60 children.

47 cases of angioedema
107 cases of urticaria (or hives)
42 cases of convulsions.
22 cases of Ataxia or leg weakness.

And a whole range of other adverse events.

Our conclusion read:

"The New Zealand experience would indicate that all Hepatitis B vaccines carry a side-effects rate in excess of that admitted to by the manufacturers. It would also appear that the administration of the Hepatitis B vaccine to neonates has greater risks than presently recognized owing to the difficulty in recognizing what are considered side-effects mimicking illness.

The reasons for this are:

1) The refusal of the vaccine manufacturers to implement studies which would provide a sound basis for diagnosis.

2) Therefore chronic non-recognition and consequent under-reporting of adverse events following vaccine administration.

3) The practice of administering several different vaccines at the same time, therefore clouding the issue of which vaccine is the problem.

4) The uncertainties involved, of extrapolating results of one age group to another."

In January 1994 I received the final book-version of the Vaccine Safety Committee's report from its editor, Dr Katherine Stratton. It misrepresented the data we had presented and the report we had submitted, falsely claiming that anaphylaxis was not observed in New Zealand children vaccinated with a plasma-derived vaccine. Our attempts to have this misinformation corrected met with failure.

The same thing happened with some evidence presented to an enquiry into Hepatitis B Vaccine held in 1999 by the American Senate Subcommittee on Criminal Justice, Drug Policy and Human Resources. Our data was again incorrectly cited several times in different submissions to deny any negative effects at all in children vaccinated in New Zealand. I sent the Subcommittee's chairman, Senator John L. Mica, the 1992 report and more recent information on more serious reactions in New Zealand to the Hepatitis B vaccine:

Hives (urticaria), 36
Bronchospasm (difficulty breathing), 5
Anaphylaxis, 3
Anaphylactoid reaction, 2.

I posed a question in a written submission to the Committee which was this:

"QUESTION: . . . This blue and red book has consistently been upheld since then, as the 'gold standard' in scientific accuracy and review of vaccine reactions in children . . . If I know and can prove to you as co-author of this

submission that (a specific piece of data in this book is false, do you think that everything else in the book is error free?)”[2]

I never had any acknowledgement of receipt of the letters to Senator Mica, or the outcome of the enquiry.

The story doesn’t end there. I received e-mails from all around the world, from people who had had serious reactions to the Hepatitis B vaccine. Doctors were starting to get worried about this vaccine, in particular about auto-immunity. Dr Bonnie Dunbar started to get concerned about the vaccine, after her brother developed severe rashes, joint pain, chronic fatigue and degenerative disorders including lupus-like syndrome and multiple sclerosis-like symptoms.

Dr Dunbar said in testimony to Congress:

“. . . now he has further been diagnosed with POTS (an auto-immune, cardiovascular, and neurological problem) and subsequently with chronic inflammatory, demyelinating polyneuropathy. His problems have been attributed to the Hepatitis B vaccine by over a dozen different specialists around the United States of unquestionable medical expertise. He has now been rated permanently and totally impaired at greater than 90%. His health care has already cost the state of Texas about a half million dollars in the Texas Worker’s Compensation Program to date, and that figure will continue to rise given the severity of his health condition.

My other student went partially blind following her first booster injection, a medical condition that was markedly exacerbated by her second booster that resulted in hospitalization. Personal communications are that her eyesight is continuing to deteriorate. Because she is in medical school she has been, understandably in my opinion, afraid to pursue investigation into her medical problems because of her concern that they might affect her medical career.”

2 The section in brackets has been amended for legal reasons.

Dr Dunbar maintains that in certain people

"a genetic component sets off an explosive chain of events after they receive the vaccine. Within a month, most of these people have completely debilitating lifestyle changes."

Her testimony to congress, and her thoughts on the matter are widely available. Yet her colleagues continued to ignore her, because this is another vaccine that must be seen to be clean. Here is an example of what happens to people who question.

I received an e-mail on 7 December 1998 from a doctor in the UK who was studying these issues: In it he said:

"The information . . . made me more sure about the results that we have about the aminoacid sequence similarities between hepatitis B surface antigen and human proteins and how these could trigger – by molecular mimicry mechanism – autoimmune reactions seen in multiple sclerosis, optic neuritis, polyneuropathy and other demyelinating diseases. It may also be the case for other autoimmune reactions such as lupus, Guillain-Barre uveitis, retinopathies, vasculitis, arthritis, diabetes mellitus, fatigue, purpura and retinal epitheliopathy.

The reasons I am talking about these diseases is that we have found similarities amongst all these diseases and many others, strongly suggesting a molecular mimicry mechanism for hepatitis B virus . . . the mechanisms for these 'new' adverse reactions might also be explained by the similarities that I found. Since we are also studying the autoimmunity triggered by hepatitis B virus, we expected to find similar phenomena amongst the post vaccination hepatitis B adverse reactions, hepatitis B carriers, and chronic infected patients.

. . . If we do not have experiment results to prove the hypothesis, all these will remain as theories. That's why it is very important for us to collect as many sera and data as possible for our study. We would like to investigate separately all reported reactions and examine if there are any cross-reactions between particular proteins and particular autoimmune diseases associated to hepatitis

B vaccine. We are also interested in the HLA type of the patients because for us it is wrong to say that the risk of the vaccine is this and that when it is compared with the population vaccinated. The comparison should be based on the population with similar genetic background. In addition, we would like to know what the real risk facts are, when you vaccinate susceptible subjects."

I then put him in touch with other doctors and researchers overseas, and gave his contact details to the UK medical personnel who had contacted me with autoimmune problems following Hepatitis B vaccine. Suddenly everything went silent. E-mails went unanswered. The medical people with these autoimmune conditions told me that he became unavailable and disappeared off the radar screen.

I can only assume that he was told to shut up, and back off, or his future in the medical profession would be limited, a pattern I have seen repeat itself over time, and continues so to this day. In the meantime, other doctors like Dr Burton Waisbren were also finding demyelinating conditions.[3]

Over in France, life for people who speak out is even worse as related by Dr Marc Girard, a French drug specialist, in a paper repeatedly rejected by French medical journals but now posted at the Red Flags site.[4] The French Government was persuaded to commit to a Hepatitis B vaccination programme in September 1994, without even knowing what the rates of Hepatitis B in the country were;[5] the rates of Hepatitis B complications, which part of the population was most at risk, or how Hepatitis B was spread in France. Even in 2001, when the head of the French Centre for Disease control was asked about this by a medical journal, the answer was that it would help to answer these questions raised by health insurance policies if the French CDC were able to measure the Hepatitis B incidence.[6] An article published in 2000 (no less than 6 years after the campaign was launched) actually stated that: ***"This is the first epidemiological***

3 Retrieved on 18 September, 2005 from <http://www.waisbrenclinic.com/>

4 Girard, M. 2005. "Hepatitis B universal vaccination: learning from the French experience". *Red Flags,* Available from <http://www.redflagsdaily.com/articles/2005_aug10.html> Accessed 18 September, 2005.

5 1995. "The epidemiological surveillance of hepatitis in France remains insufficient". *Guide des vaccinations,* p.107.

6 Brucker, G. 2001. *Le Quotidien du Médecin,* January 29.

study of Hepatitis B in France."[7] Even worse, in 2003 it was admitted that not only was there no centralized collection of Hepatitis B cases amongst staff in hospitals, but that neither had cases been differentiated by type until 1997.[8]

As cases of vaccine induced autoimmune disorders such as multiple sclerosis started to skyrocket, and people vaccinated voiced discontent, the French health authorities went into data management mode, and performed 3 case/control studies, only 2 of which were published.[9,10] Even though all of them showed a relative risk of serious reactions to be more than one, the authorities convinced the public that there was no causal role of the vaccination, because this increase wasn't statistically significant. In fact, the recurring lack of statistical significance was simply a result of the French authorities' stubborn refusal to properly research why it was that thousands of people, previously healthy, may have been severely affected by the Hepatitis B vaccine.

As you look through the medical literature you can see how, by extensively duplicating, and selectively quoting two studies across a vast spectrum of other articles (a process known as ***"expert mongering"***), it is possible to then point to a body of information that says a vaccine is safe. As everywhere, the health authorities tried to explain away the new problems by saying they were due to latent predisposition, yet even the studies sponsored by vaccine manufacturers didn't support this excuse.[11]

According to Dr Girard 10 to 15 years ago, there were so few people in France with multiple sclerosis, that many doctors would never have seen a case in their practice, but that now, everyone, including non-professional lay people knows several cases. The same doctor also noted that at a 2004 meeting on Hepatitis B supposedly called to find consensus after a new study had shown significant increases in multiple sclerosis, that French neuropaediatricians stated

7 Minello, A. et al. 2000. "Epidémiologie de l'hépatite B dans 2 départements voisins. Résultats de 5années d'enregistrement en Côte d'Or (94–98) et de 3années dans le Doubs". *Gastroenterol Clin Biol,* 24:A153.

8 Antona, D., and Levy-Bruhl, D. 2003. "Epidemiology of hepatitis B in France at the end of the 20(th) century" [French]. *Médecine et Maladies Infectieuses,* May: 33(Suppl A): 34–41.

9 Touzé, E. et al. 2000. "Hepatitis B vaccination and first central nervous system demyelinating event: a case control study". *Neuroepidemiology,* 21:180–6.

10 Touzé, E. et al. 2000. "The first episode of central nervous system demyelinization and hepatitis B virus vaccination". [French]. *Rev Neurol* (Paris) March: 156(3): 242–6.

11 Confavreux, C. et al. 2001. "Vaccinations and the risk of relapse in multiple sclerosis". *N Engl J Med,* February: 344(5): 319–26.

that they were following a cohort of several hundreds of paediatric multiple sclerosis cases. This comment shocked the doctor, because multiple sclerosis in children has long been known to be the exception, and so rarely seen as to hardly ever be written about. One of the cases reported was 25 months old. There was also discussion of an AFSSAPS (Agence française de sécurité sanitaire de produits de santé) study which showed problems in the thyroid as well as a risk of lupus, but these studies have not been published.

However, the French social security system, Caisse Nationale d'Assurance Maladie (CNAM) does keep data of what they called severe neuromuscular diseases[12] which shows this:

Naturally enough when a medical study in 2004[13] finally proved what everyone in France knew, namely that the Hepatitis B vaccine was linked to a threefold increase in Multiple Sclerosis[14,15], it wasn't surprising to read the lead author state that because Hepatitis B was *"such a devastating disease"* this small risk would be outweighed by protection offered by the vaccine, and therefore the vaccine policy should remain as it is. The French Authorities continued to back the vaccine by saying that no such complications had been reported outside France, and that no causal link has been established by either expert panels, or the regulatory authorities.

To put things in proper perspective, Dr Girard says[16] that:

> ***"in the whole of France, there are fewer than 10 patients per year who develop a fulminant liver disease due to hepatitis B virus. Almost all of them come from populations at risk (immigrants, drug abusers . . .); but by way of comparison, a 3-fold increase in the risk of MS would translate to some 100,000 new cases if the WHO recommendations of universal immunization were applied (from the CNAM data above, it is plain that this horrific estimation is quite consistent with available data after less than half of the French population was vaccinated)."***

12 Graph provided by Dr Marc Girard. Dr Girard's website is http://www.rolandsimion.org.
13 Hernan, M. et al. 2004. "Recombinant hepatitis B vaccine and the risk of multiple sclerosis". A prospective study. *Neurology*, 63: 838–42.
14 Retrieved from <http://www.waisbrenclinic.com/> Accessed on 18 September, 2005.
15 "Jab linked to multiple sclerosis". 2004. Available from <http://news.bbc.co.uk/2/hi/health/3651782.stm> Accessed on 18 September, 2005.
16 Personal communication Dr Girard to Hilary Butler, 26/02/2006.

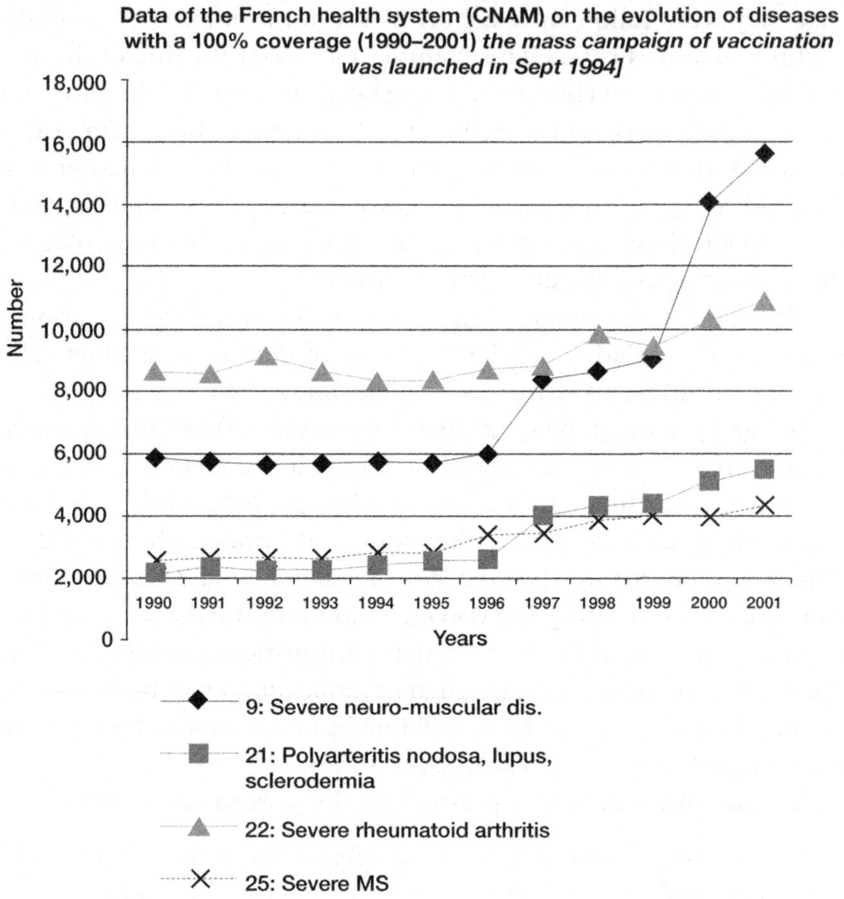

It will now be interesting to see what happens in India, where it was recently announced that the Hepatitis B vaccine would be introduced there because Hepatitis B was a bigger problem than AIDS. This was in part, a recommendation made after an American expert working for WHO claimed that 250,000 people die of Hepatitis B in India based upon a model stratified for geographic region and income groups. However, Indian scientists claimed that the alleged model never existed and the figures were far to high. Nonetheless, the Indian Government proceeded to implement the WHO ideas. That decision was met with fury and dismay by many doctors:[17]

17 "Government misleading country on Hepatitis B vaccination". 2005. Available from <http://www.newindpress.com/Newsitems.asp?ID=IE120051013110422&Title=Bangalore&Topic=0> Accessed on 15 October, 2005.

"A ridiculous impression has been created that Hepatitis B is a more serious problem than AIDS. The government's claim that 4.7 per cent of the Indian population is chronically infected with Hepatitis B virus is a gross overestimation. The actual hepatitis B carrier rate works out to only 1.42 per cent," says Dr Anant Phadke of SATHI-CEHAT, a Mumbai-based NGO working on public health issues. "The average fatality rate even among chronic carriers is around 5 per cent and not 25 per cent as has been claimed," he added.

The doctors then accused the Indian government of caving in to pressure from vaccine companies and international bodies, when it couldn't afford syringes to give the vaccine. One doctor, Dr S L Pawar who has worked in public health and rural development for a very long time, said that if the money was spent on providing drinking water and sanitation that *"will automatically wipe out a majority of the diseases."*

When the Government was asked to comment on the above the Union health minister Anbumani Ramdoss rubbished the allegations saying that a few jobless NGOs were just making senseless allegations, and that the decision followed WHO and UNICEF advice following "very successful" three year 13 district, 15 city pilot projects.

How did it get to the point where so many countries in the world have implemented universal mass Hepatitis B programmes based on data that might only reflect a tiny minority of high-risk people?

Perhaps a pointer to that is in an interview in a widely circulated French magazine[18] with a salesman of the company that manufactured the Hepatitis B vaccine. In it, the Business Manager claimed:

"We started increasing the awareness of the European Experts of the World Health Organization about Hepatitis B in 1988. From then to 1991, we financed epidemiological studies on the subject to create a scientific consensus about hepatitis being a major public health problem. We were successful because in 1991, WHO published new recommendations about Hepatitis B vaccination."

What the French people didn't know was that once the campaign

18 Labbe, C. et al. 1997. "L'habile stratégie d'un labo". *Sciences at Avenir,* January: 27.

was in full swing, the French official experts, including those in the French CDC didn't hesitate to co-author articles with this man, which could best be described as post-marketing hype.[19] But the Business Manager had it wrong. In 1981 the then head of Merck[20] said, ***"Eventually the World Health Organization will take this on as a new quest. And that could enable Merck to sell its vaccine to as many as 50 million people a year."*** Which is all part of what America calls ***"A Delicate Fabric of Public and Private Collaboration"***.[21]

And if a reader wishes to go and study a country's Hepatitis B vaccination programme that puts one's logic faculties into overdrive, they need look no further than the USA.

The pattern appears to be consistent worldwide, that the scientific basis for mass immunization in most countries is questionable, and vaccine reactions are consistently ignored, denied or minimized. And all the really important problems are left rotting by the roadside.

---

19 Carnall, D. 1996. "Shire Hall Communications and the case for Hepatitis B immunization". *British Medical Journal*, Sep 28; 313: 825. Available from <http://www.bmj.bmjjournals.com/cgi/content/full/313/7060/825>

20 Hilleman, M.R. 1981. "Merck's profit plan for Hepatitis B vaccine". *Chemical Weekly*, Nov 25; pp. 12 and 14.

21 NVAC. 1997. "United States vaccine research: a delicate fabric of public and private collaboration". *Pediatrics*, Dec; 100(6): 1015–20. PMID: 9411380.

49 An Encouragement for Those Who Get Lost

Just as Auckland Hospital and the Domain are alongside each other, the same is true of Greenlane Hospital and Cornwall Park. Stark contrasts between those who are fit and well enjoying the beauty and peace of these green oases, and those who, because of some health problem, are contained within the multi-storey, hugely expensive buildings, standing cold and stark.

Across the road from Greenlane Hospital is the Auckland Showgrounds, and some years ago, Hilary and I attended a craft exhibition occupying one of the large halls making up this complex.

Included in this exhibition were some of Hilary's Japanese embroideries. Apart from these works of art which I had watched being completed at home over many months, I was not sure what else I would see displayed as we entered the exhibition hall.

There were plenty of people with plenty of oohs and aahs. All around for as far as the eye could see were the exhibits grouped in little islands, hung from the "ceiling" or walls; on tables; in enclosures; stand-alones: an amazing array of beautiful and exquisite work from very skilled people.

Where do you start?

How do you do justice to what appeared to be totally disorganized confusion?

I felt overwhelmed.

A mere male out of his depth.

Fortunately I had Hilary with me to guide me through the maze.

Naturally enough we homed in first of all to the small section devoted to Japanese embroidery.

And there they were. Those two beautifully crafted cranes (who still look down haughtily at me every morning at home.) Their plumage glowing gloriously under carefully placed spotlights.

Nearby were some quilted bed covers standing tall in their allotted space.

I began to try to take it all in. A little bit at a time. The creators of all these displays could talk at great length on a whole range of technical matters. Many admirers could nod their heads in understanding – it made perfect sense to them.

But me? I was a "layman" not accustomed to, or knowledgeable in, the finer points.

In a sense, I was lost.

I moved step by step from one place to the next trying to piece together the progressions, the sequences, the interwoven threads that were essential to understanding the unique "stories" they were telling.

But I still felt lost and was getting more and more out of my depth.

Suddenly I realized that I had also lost Hilary. Where was she in all this crowd? In this seemingly complicated maze?

What should I do? Find a reference point. That's what.

Find something that was familiar. Begin again from there. Surely I would find Hilary. She wouldn't be far away.

So I started looking for those horrible haughty herons. You can see what a scrambled state my mind was in!

Yes I found them. Quite easily in fact. They weren't far away at all.

And I found Hilary too. Just on the other side of an obstacle really.

Together we explored the exhibition. From different points of view, mind you!

I came away from that experience having learnt an awful lot. No, certainly not everything. I could never fully see everything through Hilary's eyes but I reckon I could see things clearly that maybe Hilary couldn't see.

As you read this book, you may be like me.

You get lost.

You feel confused.

You can't follow the "threads".

Well, find a reference point. Go back to what you do understand and keep going.

The "picture" will take shape.

The story will make sense.

Hilary is still there in spite of any obstacles that get in the way.

And you will see things that will be just right ***for you****.*

Those who really seek ***will*** *find.*

50 "No One is Listening": A Mother's Story

I was about five weeks pregnant with our second child, Candace, when the doctors diagnosed Giardia, and gave me one large bolus dose of antibiotics to "kill" it. At about six weeks I started spotting and getting stomach pains as I had with my first pregnancy, and again at about eleven weeks.

As the doctors had with my first pregnancy, they gave me the anti-D jab as I am "O" negative and my partner is "O" positive.

For two months before Candace was born I was given antibiotics for a bad cough, which didn't clear up, and lasted another month after Candace was born. In retrospect, it could well have been whooping cough, but I was never tested for it.

About four years before Candace was born I had a rubella vaccination and got sick afterwards. My doctor thought the symptoms were due to a thyroid problem but all the tests came back OK, but looking back, I now believe it was a vaccine reaction. My partner also had a reaction to the MMR vaccine when he was a baby – which we only found out about after Candace's reaction.

Candace was born five weeks prematurely, weighing 6lb 1oz. She was grunting when she breathed, so they took her and put her in an incubator and gave her, and me, antibiotics, because they weren't sure why she was so early and they thought there was a risk of infection.

The nurses had been told she was to be breast-fed and I had expressed colostrum for her. I waited in the ward, as advised, for them to call me to feed her. They didn't. Finally I went down to find out why. I found them giving her formula. What's worse, they had already given her two previous feeds of formula. I felt totally betrayed by them – knowing she was premature with a history of asthma on her father's side, there was a more than normal reason for being breast-fed. I was terrified she would not take to the breast after this. As soon as they would let Candace leave, we went back to our local small country maternity unit for a few days, to allow me time to get used to our tiny baby.

Candace was slightly jaundiced so they had me feeding her three-hourly to help clear it.

When I came home, the midwives were happy with Candace's weight gain, and the jaundice had cleared up, so they put her up to four-hourly feeds. She was a model baby. She ate, slept and poohed like clockwork every four hours. She hardly ever cried. We sometimes wondered whether we had a baby in the house. She had perfect skin and everyone said she looked like a little doll.

Breast-feeding was easy. Candace was a natural and knew what to do straight away, and I had no problems. She started sleeping longer between feeds and at night up to about eight to ten hours. She had also started to coo and make noises and turn over and hold things in her hand.

She used to suck her fingers sometimes, but she never needed a dummy. She went to sleep on her own, and was a model, totally contented, placid baby – so totally different to her older sister, who was chronically constipated and colicky.

Vaccine day

9.00 am – Because she was born five weeks premature, we waited an extra five weeks before giving her six-week shots, so she was about eleven weeks old. The nurse rubbed arnica cream on the jab immediately. After the initial screaming she had a breast-feed and we waited for 10 minutes for any immediate reaction.

When we got home I gave her pamol as instructed by the nurse and she slept for about 45 minutes, then woke up screaming, and nothing would comfort her. It was a gut-wrenching inconsolable scream; she arched her back with her fists tightly clenched, and her face bright red and puffy, and this went on for about three hours.

I wondered if it was colic but that didn't seem logical. This was too intense for such a normally placid baby, and more than I could remember from colic. (My mum later said that when I had the vaccines as a baby, I screamed for hours as well and had a fever and my leg came up all red and swollen.) Candace went straight off her feeds . . . she would have a couple of sucks and then start screaming again.

This was really upsetting for me because normally a breast-feed would settle any upset or fright. Now not even this sacred bonding act would work.

It also seemed as though, when she did sleep, her little body was twitching now and then as if she were having a bad dream – normally she sleeps so soundly you had to go and touch her to see if she was still breathing.

She finally went to sleep again for about another ¾ of an hour, and again woke up with the same gut-wrenching inconsolable scream, arching back with fists tightly clenched and her face bright red and puffy.

She was hot, but never really had a high fever.

Her right leg came up red and swollen at the site of the jab. I phoned the nurse and told her Candace's symptoms and how much she was screaming. She said, "Just keep giving her pamol, some babies get unsettled like that."

She had also done a really smelly bright orange pooh almost like stewed apricots, which smelled terrible. Candace wasn't on solids – and I knew it wasn't from the breast milk.

The nurse phoned the next day to see how Candace was, and I told her she was a bit better, but still very unsettled and grizzly which was most unlike her. She said she would probably be a bit unsettled for a few days.

Nearly two weeks later I wrote:

> ***Candace is constantly grizzly for no apparent reason. She has started banging her hands against the side of her body. It's like an involuntary act and she isn't able to control it. It's as if she is trying to get something out of her and can't, and is getting frustrated because she can't communicate it. It's a very aggressive act for such a placid baby.***

Something is wrong with my baby and no one is listening to me.

Six weeks after Candace's first shots, my diary entries continued to record the story of her constant screaming and lack of sleep; of her swollen legs and convulsive movements; of rashes and disrupted breathing and unusual bowel movements.

The doctor I consulted wanted to give Candace an oral steroid for the swelling, and was horrified when I questioned vaccines. The nightmare of screaming and of fever continued, as did the nightmare of the medical profession's denying it was a reaction to vaccine. They had no explanation when Candace had seizures in hospital, and her left eye started looking into the centre. Diagnoses like *colic* and *viral infection* and *eczema* were offered, though a discharge notice stated "Serum sickness". So it continued throughout the month of January, by the end of which I knew that I would never let Candace have any more shots. I changed GP and used homoeopathy and Vitamin C, and slowly she got better, but has never returned to normality.

Every time she gets sick now, she gets a cough and it seems to go straight to her chest, and her rash also gets worse. Candace has had just about every bug that has been going around. It's as if there is something wrong with her immune system. We have kept her off dairy products and we try to keep wheat and gluten out of her diet as much as possible which seems to help.

The Sodium Ascorbate (Vit C), the Homoeopathic and the Osteopathic treatments seem to have been a big help and at least gave us more answers and solutions than the medical profession have been able to give us.

One thing that upset me was that every time we saw the doctors it seemed that the only important thing to them was that we give her more vaccines under supervision. The three months we had gone through just didn't matter. They wanted us to take her to hospital and have more done there. As one of the doctors said, "Then we can revive her if anything happens".

Many of my questions to them remain unanswered: "Can you guarantee that the next time won't cause permanent damage?" "How can you reverse brain damage?" "What have the vaccines done to her immune system?" And, "Why would I want to put my baby through something like that again?"

I would rather risk her getting the illness than knowingly inject another vaccine into her that could make things so much worse. I am now starting to wonder whether my first child's glue ear problems may have been as a result of a reaction to her vaccines.

We went to the doctor with Candace in July – our doctor was away and the locum just happened to be the doctor who saw Candace when she had her reaction in December. I told him what had happened since then and all the problems Candace had been having, and the answers the doctors have been giving me and that I was pretty sure no one had reported the reaction. It was a relief to finally talk to someone who had been there at the time and knew what had happened – who didn't automatically assume that I was imagining her symptoms.

He was amazed at the lack of action by any of the doctors. He said he thought the hospital would have reported it, but he would report it for me now, and wrote down the general details I told him and though I asked him if he wanted a copy of the notes I had been keeping on Candace, he said he didn't need them. I phoned a day or two later to get a copy of his report and the nurses said they didn't keep one on her file because everything went to CARM.

Several weeks after I saw the locum, I was back at the doctor and happened to see a letter in our file from CARM. I had not been told about it and was very upset to read they were asking for more details and that CARM suggested it could have been a reaction to the Hepatitis B jab. I immediately asked for a copy of the letter, and got no answer as to why I hadn't been told about the letter.

The explanation in the letter didn't make sense to me, so I typed up my diary entries and sent them down to CARM to provide them with more information as requested.

To me, a major problem seems to be that some of the medical profession just aren't interested in reporting vaccine reactions if they can help it. The medical profession can't prove to me it was or wasn't the shots but there are some who still want me to continue giving her them anyway. I ***now*** know I could have reported the reaction myself, which would probably have got this settled a lot earlier and been a lot less hassle.

I feel that if vaccine reactions were recognized and reported properly they might be able to find out why some children react and not others, and I hope that describing my baby's suffering and my feelings may help other mothers I know whose stories haven't been told, to stand up for themselves, and to feel less alone.

Candace's mother sent me a copy of a letter sent her by CARM[1] 18 months after the vaccines were given, which seemed to be making sense until I saw this part:

> "*. . . it is unfortunate that in the case of Candace there was a more profound and visible immune response to immunizations. Whilst these reactions are unpleasant they are an indication that the body is mounting an immune response to the foreign antigen in the anticipated manner.*"

What mother would honestly consider a combination of urticaria (hives) mild broncho-oedema, seizures, and encephalitis-type irritation, with repeat systemic reactions following the second injections, an anticipated immune response to foreign antigens?

1 Centre for Adverse Reactions Monitoring.

51 Benefits from Chicken Pox

Towards the end of January one year, I administered some attainment and diagnostic tests to quite a large group of homeschoolers in Pukekohe. Among them were our children.

During the first weekend of February there was a national homeschoolers' conference to be held in Palmerston North and I had been invited to be one of the speakers. We travelled down the Island as a family in our house bus, stopping overnight at several places, one of which was the camping ground at Whakapapa on the slopes of Mount Ruapehu. While we were there, the children began to feel unwell and it looked like chickenpox. We did some quick calculations and the penny dropped. One of the families who had been at the testing days in Pukekohe had had chicken pox, but because they were over the worst of the disease, had not wanted to miss the tests (spread over three days) and so had been mixing with all the others during that time.

Now we were headed to a much larger gathering of homeschoolers in Palmerston North. We would be living in the bus in the parking area of the conference venue.

But would our Ian and David be welcome?!

We explained the situation to the organizers who although very understanding did not feel it would be politic for them to take part in the Conference activities.

We resisted the temptation to hang a little notice saying, "Unclean, unclean" on our bus door!

Apart from some evidence of the chickenpox on exposed parts of their bodies, the boys behaved very much like normal.

Well, you can't keep kids away from kids, but while I was fulfilling my commitments, Hilary took the boys on numerous walks to the children's playground at Ongley Park, and when I could I did the same. We walked many miles in the process.

During the few days we were there it was interesting to note the different reactions of the parents attending the gathering, towards the "threat" of their children being exposed to this illness.

However, David and Ian got their natural immunity and enjoyed all the rich experiences which our few days of travelling here and there gave them. Apart from the usual itching that accompanies chickenpox, they were their usual selves.

Although conference participation was "restricted", Hilary did have the opportunity to spend time in the city with a couple of families who had problems arising from vaccinations and with whom she had been working. There were also opportunities during the conference, and on the journey home, to share with other families the practical outworking of an all-embracing lifestyle – including chickenpox.

52 Dr Archie Kalokerinos

In 1992, and 1995 the Immunization Awareness Society organised two conferences, where international speakers came to talk about vaccines.

The issue of why babies react to vaccine was still very high on my list of priorities, because the 1991 MMR vaccine campaign had produced the usual spate of parents with sick babies and sick children.

During the first conference, I sat down with Archie Kalokerinos, a tremendous admirer of the work of Dr Reisinger, who explained how he used the endotoxaemia information to eliminate SIDS in his practice. He said that it was when Dr Reisinger explained the whole of the *E-coli* link to vaccines that his eyes were opened clinically to what was happening right under his nose.

Archie has been in medicine a long time. When he first started he noticed that Aborigine children were susceptible to high levels of infection, and were also very susceptible to what looked like shock after vaccines, and to begin with, in his practice, they just died, with the deaths always being labelled as SIDS.

He scoured the literature to see what could be done with shock and what might cause it. He felt that the primary cause was their diet which had plenty of flour, jam, meat and alcohol, a drug that Aborigines have no tolerance for, and that their general emotional and physical condition was the cause of their ill health.

Their infant mortality rate of about 100 in 1000 horrified him. Often these children would be brought in, maybe with mild diarrhoea, to have a vaccine, then without warning they would become shocked, fail to respond to measures like cortisone and intravenous fluid, and just die. Or they would come into hospital sick with pneumonia, languish and then after a few days would die.

He did autopsies and found abnormalities which made no sense and had no readily understood explanation. He also saw similar things in the European babies in these areas, so decided to keep records of everything to present the problems to senior colleagues. They thought that worry was making him a little strange.

Dr Kalokerinos decided that the next time he had another pneumonia case languishing he would take the child to a specialist and chose Dr Douglas Harbison, 220 miles from his practice. Dr Harbison diagnosed scurvy, and immediately injected the baby with an injection of Vitamin C with such dramatic results that Archie almost didn't believe what he had seen. Since the specialist diagnosed scurvy, the child was treated for scurvy.

The problem Archie had with the diagnosis was that the baby did not exhibit even one sign of classical infantile scurvy, except perhaps irritability. He concluded that maybe the child might have got better anyway, that he had just selected the wrong specialist to look at the child, put the case away in his head, and carried on as before. But the baby deaths mounted, to the point where he became despondent with his inability to stem the deaths, packed up his medical bags, and went opal mining.

At the opal mines he mostly kept the fact he was a doctor quiet, except from his mining partner, who would tease him and say, "Are you sorry now that you gave away medicine Doc?" He would say, "No", but deep inside, thought of the eyes of the little dead dark faces and wondered.

For three years he dug opals, photographed them all, later becoming one of the world's most renowned published ex-opal miners. During that time, he noticed a lot of the aborigine children at the mine had infections, weepy eyes and ears discharging pus. He tried to get the mothers to let him look at them, but they didn't trust this white man.

Then one day, a miner arrived with an injured dog. Archie decided the dog couldn't be left untreated with a compound fracture of the hind leg, so operated on her using an improvised truck tray as a table. The whole village watched, including the Aborigines who were fascinated, as he injected the anaesthetic into the leg vein, repaired the damaged muscles, sewed up the skin, applied a plaster cast, gave antibiotics, etc, and they all waited until the dog came around. She was able to stand gingerly, but painlessly, on her plaster-cast leg.

Next morning, an Aborigine mother arrived with her boy covered in pus, maggots and flies. The distrust had gone. She pushed the boy gently towards him as if saying, "If you can do it to a dog, can you do it to my boy?"

He cleaned away the pus, washed the eyes, ears and nose, and instilled antibiotic drops. Nature did the rest. That day, he decided he would return to medicine because he wanted to find the answers to questions to help the Aborigine people in whatever way he could.

Going back to Collarenebri after three years was like returning to another world. Nothing had altered except his attitude. His patients noticed it, particularly the Aborigines. Foremost in his mind was the case of scurvy he had dismissed all those years before. He decided that since nothing else had worked beforehand, if he had any more cases like it he would take a punt and just do what Dr Harbison had done and give them Vitamin C injections.

To him, it was a logical, simple, cheap treatment, with no side-effects. He quickly found it worked, and death rates in his practice plummeted. He didn't realize that otherwise sensible people were about to start frothing at the mouth when word got around that there were no more babies dropping dead in Collarenebri, and that Vitamin C injections were about to become a huge sore point with the Australian medical authorities.

He researched the literature and found it was crammed with references proving beyond doubt that during infections there was an increased utilization of Vitamin C, and that many references illustrated the need for far more than 30 mg of Vitamin C under a wide variety of conditions. In the conditions in which Aborigines and some Europeans lived, very large doses were required. And in many situations, repeated injections were necessary.

Archie also discovered that along with Vitamin C deficiencies, these children were often showing Vitamin B deficiencies as well. Acute Vitamin B deficiencies could also cause shock. Usually this happened when glucose was given intravenously to counter dehydration. The glucose needs Vitamin B to metabolize and if there is a deficiency that is marginal, it too can result in shock and death.

He started to see these patterns, but also to realize that orally-administered antibiotics could make things worse. There was a parasite problem often seen in Aborigine children, so initially he put most of it down to that.

He discussed these problems with doctors who then considered him barking mad. A letter published in the *Medical Journal of Australia* brought the roof down on his head. A specialist said that there was no such thing as scurvy in Aborigines.

So Archie turned to his other speciality: photography. Within a few months he had amassed stacks of photographs clearly showing all the clinical signs of scurvy, but met nothing but continual stubborn resistance and derision from his colleagues.

In the late 1970s he met Dr Reisinger, who spent some time explaining the role of endotoxin to him, which put the central part of the complex jigsaw puzzle in place, and gave an explanation for why Vitamin C worked so well. He realized that the X-factor wasn't parasites, but endotoxic shock from the gut from die-off after oral antibiotics were given. He also saw that endotoxin shock from the gut didn't just happen after vaccines, but that it also happened in connection with other diseases, including viral infections.

What he also found interesting was ignored medical literature which showed that many other diseases and medical conditions have an endotoxin content, including animal diseases which can be dependent upon endotoxin. For instance, parvovirus in dogs, which is like measles in humans, has no affect on the dog at all, if there isn't endotoxin in the dog's gut.

The medical literature showed gut endotoxin to have a huge impact on simple things in humans like surgery, even in ***"graft versus host"*** disease. There are now people looking at marathon runners who suddenly die, supposedly of heart failure. Some blood tests are showing up curlin in their system. It seems that some of them, like babies, absorb an overwhelming dose of gut endotoxin or curlin, the end-point of which is bradycardia and heart failure.

Ebola, though a virus, is another disease which has a huge endotoxin content, which results in blood pouring out the body from everywhere. Yet even now, with all the available evidence on the use of Vitamin C with sepsis involving DIC[1] (and there is a mass of it), doctors won't

1 DIC = disseminated intravascular coagulation.

try intravenous Vitamin C for Ebola victims. What is there to lose?

Archie was finding out that what is to *lose* is professional standing and reputation. To put something so simple to such efficient use, appeared to threaten not only his peers' ideas about useful drugs, but also their mindsets as to the value of "just a vitamin", and the whole basic understanding of disease processes.

I sat down with Archie to discuss two problems with him.

The first was one of my own. The arthritis from the Rubella injection was getting to the hair-tearing stage. Archie explained to me that one of the things found in people who had high rubella titres after a vaccine, but also had vaccine reactions like arthritis, was an antigen/antibody complex.[2] If there was something about my immune system that wasn't working right, my immune system wouldn't deal with the virus.

He explained that Vitamin C was a very effective anti-viral, how it worked, and that if the arthritis was caused by the rubella virus, then Vitamin C might break the cycle. I didn't see that I had much to lose trying it, so we worked out a management plan based on the fact that when tissue saturation of Vitamin C is reached, the unneeded extra is pushed out via urine, which showed up as a change in colour on the C-stix which was a bit like litmus paper.

I was horrified on the first day when I did not get urinary spillover, or diarrhoea, until after 60 grams had been given. Gradually, it was possible to decrease the amount until by the end of the third month, I was getting urinary spillover after 8 grams. Best of all, the arthritis I had had for so many years had gone.

A year later, I would get urinary spillover after about 4 grams on a good day, and after perhaps 20 grams on a day with lots of stress. Now, I can't get the C-stix any more, so just go by diarrhoea.

The second thing I wanted to talk to him about was his use of Vitamin C for vaccine reactions. We talked around the subject thoroughly and I decided that, as he had done in the past, that I would suggest the use of Vitamin C after vaccine reactions.

Why? Because a medical profession that denies the existence of vaccine reactions has nothing to offer. In the unlikely event that they do recognize them anyway, they still have nothing to offer that works. Again, what is there to lose?

---

2 Coyle, P.K. 1982. "Rubella-specific immune complexes after congenital infection and vaccination". *Infection and Immunity*, May; 32(2): 498–503. PMID: 7085069.

It would work, or not, but either way, it couldn't do any more harm than doing nothing. The biggest problem was to get mothers to give enough. The RDA[3] rule that *"60 mg a day is enough"* has been so ingrained that the idea of giving much larger doses sends some parents into fits of hysteria. I found, though, that the more severe the reaction, the less advice doctors had offered, and the more desperate the parent, the more likely they were just to use it.

Sometimes the parents just wouldn't believe me, or wouldn't give any Vitamin C. They were scared. So I'd give them Archie's telephone number so they could ring him. After all, he was a doctor, I wasn't. Then they would give it. And . . . it worked. Children would literally *"come alive"*. Parents started to see some of the things that Archie described in his book called *Every Second Child*.[4]

BUT . . . there was a problem. They would then be so delighted that they wanted to go and tell their doctors what they should have done. I'd say, "Don't do that. For a start they will consider you are mad. Secondly they won't believe you. Third, you'll have to change doctors. It's better to say nothing."

Some parents didn't believe me. Sure enough, some found themselves confronted by enraged frothing-at-the-mouth doctors who considered that these parents had just become a danger to their children.

Even though I was wising up to some aspects of some doctors' intolerance to certain ideas, one thing I didn't wise up to was that I soon wasn't going to be able to talk to some doctors and immunologists whose doors had previously been open. Looking back, the first IAS conference was where professional suppression started to come to the fore.

After the discussions with Dr Lloyd Cairns at Auckland medical school, I had discussed with Professor Murdoch the possibility of applying to do another trial comparing vaccinated with never-vaccinated children. He was keen on the idea, and put forward a proposal which was stubbornly resisted, and he copped flack in the process. I guess there is only so much flack anyone can cope with.

I knew there was even more tension between myself and Professor Murdoch when he had withdrawn as a speaker from the first conference.

---

3 RDA = recommended daily allowance

4 Kalokerinos, A. 1974. *Every Second Child*. 1974. Australia: Thomas Nelson. ISBN 17 001987 X (has been reprinted since).

Professor Murdoch had been interviewed for a *Metro* article in December the year before. The journalist who had done the article had asked to use the Immunization Awareness Society's Library. The IAS saw no reason why not, basically opening the door and saying, "Go for it". In the article appeared a verbatim quote from Professor Murdoch from a video tape of the Christchurch seminar where he took the blood sample from me. All speakers had given permission to be filmed, and for the videos to be part of a freely available public record. I couldn't be bothered looking after my copies of talks or seminars so had dumped them at the time, with all my other videos, into the IAS library.

Professor Murdoch was livid. He reamed me and the journalist out. He hadn't been asked if he wanted that comment to go into the article but when the journalist asked him if the comment he made was incorrect, and he said it wasn't, but that he wouldn't have wanted it reported.

Shortly after the conference, on 25 July 1992, I was invited by a Hamilton doctor to give a talk to the Waikato Postgraduate Medical Society. Another speaker from the international symposium was also going, and picked me up on the way. Stepping into the car was like stepping into a refrigerator, but I didn't understand why.

At the seminar, a doctor prominent in the provaccine scene, and I came to verbal blows. I had mentioned in my talk, that New Zealand was using the Urabe mumps strain which was withdrawn overseas, because it had unacceptable side-effects. This doctor said, as an aside directed at me, that New Zealand didn't use the Urabe strain at all. I stood straight up and said, "I'm sorry, but we do. It's called Pluserix." Again, the doctor refused to admit that Pluserix contained the Urabe strain.

I sat down, silenced, livid at myself, because I was stupid enough to have left the manufacturer's brochure at home, so I couldn't prove I was correct. At lunchtime, I mentioned it in somewhat annoyed whispering to the speaker who had been at the IAS conference. I was stonily ignored, and suddenly, it dawned on me that the heat might have been put on; an ultimatum given. Perhaps that was the reason for the sudden coldness, the distance. I had plenty to think about on the way home.

Sure enough, not long afterwards I heard from a third party that an ultimatum had been given along the lines of "shut your mouth or lose your job". Was this academic freedom, and encouraging intellectual honesty? Not long after that, Professor Murdoch left New Zealand and later medical articles showed he is still out of the country.

In September of that year, amidst big fanfare, New Zealand withdrew the offending Pluserix MMR vaccine, because it contained the mumps Urabe strain.

Looking back now, the most significant signpost I see is that the very people who, way back then, publicly, vehemently opposed everything I said still hold the jobs they had then, to this day.

Other medical people who were prepared to openly discuss issues, not just with me, but with parents of vaccine-damaged children, and actively look at the problems raised, or those who even considered serious study proposals suggested, were no longer in the posts they held.

If there is one thing I deeply regret about doing this work, it is the thought that I might have been part of the reason these sincere and honest people appear to no longer be able to discuss any issues related to vaccination. It would have been better to have kept them all at more than arms' length. But then, had I done that, imagine what might have been said. What the authorities might have implied that that conveyed. You can't win, either way.

Thinking back, on the way home from the Waikato talk, I started to get a sense of when I should have been alerted to this new divide; that is, at the first International Conference.

A previously friendly speaker there, on the second day, was very ill at ease, whereas previously this had not been the case. The Health Department and ACC were at this conference in force, and bailed some of the speakers up in corners at lunch times. I was busy at the time, but others had commented that the body language was very negative, and it looked like the Health Department was applying heat. It's fair to say that the Conference was tense in many respects, and with vaccination and the immune system being openly talked about the Health Department people weren't going to like it. But I never thought they'd take the opportunity to hit on speakers.

The dismissive attitude towards vaccine-damaged children came through loud and clear from a high-up member of the medical audience as he resumed his seat with his colleagues, to hear from Hiria Potae's father about their walk through vaccine reaction denial, and the minefield of attempting to prove a case. He said in mocking falsetto tones to his peers, "Take out your hankies everyone, here comes the emotional blackmail".

53 House Bus #2

We had to wait just over six years before we were able to buy our second bus.

On 12 December 1991, we purchased a 1957 AEC, ex-Wellington City Transport vehicle from Commercial Buses in New Lynn. In configuration it was completely different to the Ford. It had a type of pre-select gearbox and fluid flywheel, with a mid-mounted 466 Bedford diesel. As there was no clutch to operate, my left foot had to learn that it was superfluous when driving the bus, but that it **was** required when driving our trusty 1975 Hillman Hunter station wagon!

With this bus, we started fitting it out from scratch. Five months after purchase it was comfortable enough to be usable. During the eleven years we had this house bus we kept on refining the fitting out until it became uniquely us.

It had to have a name of course, and what better than "Beyond Conformity". The following poem attempts to put in verse something of the lifestyle we had embraced.

BEYOND CONFORMITY

Yes, there's a story
Behind the writing on our bus.

One day in Glory
'Twill be more fully told by us.

Daily we learn more;
We can but share a little now
'Bout the time we saw
What right decisions would allow.

Why be different?
To swim against the "normal" flow?
Surely it is meant
For types others don't want to know?

What is the reason
For rolling wheels and moving on?
Whate'er the season
Freedom can be won.

Not to be conformed
To all the many things that bind,
But to be transformed
By the renewing of the mind.

There's a price to pay
For a lifestyle without clutter,
Cutting adrift may
Cause the bravest heart to flutter.

When there's conviction
That the way you've chosen is so right,
There'll be lots of fun
To fill the hours of day and night.

So for all to see
The message is declared in name –

"BEYOND CONFORMITY".

Hi there, to those who think the same.

During the years we had this house bus we did manage to get away for a week or two at a time, as well as numbers of shorter spells. These trips took us from Kaikohe in the north to Palmerston North in the south as well as up the west side of the North Island.

But the reality was that whether we liked it or not, our lifestyle was increasingly having to deal with "clutter". Clutter both literal and metaphorical. The ties that tended to keep us in and around our backyard were becoming more difficult to sever. The children's extra-curricular activities and sports, for instance.

Hilary's involvements were now extending into time-consuming ACC claims that often took years to settle, and requests for help from overseas as well.

"Beyond Conformity" could not go unnoticed in our backyard! It was a constant reminder of a lifestyle we had chosen. We were having to make adjustments, but I was determined that we were not going to be squeezed into the moulds of systems and structures which were attempting to tell us what to think and how we should act. We still had the right to make informed choices, even though this right might come with a price tag.

However, the time came when we down sized from the 10-metre mobile home to a smaller 6-metre bus. But it is still "BEYOND CONFORMITY" by name.

54 Measles 1985–1998

"Yesterday forenoon the Tarawera arrived from Sydney and it was found that an adult and a child were suffering from measles . . . were all placed in quarantine . . . until the authorities from Wellington were communicated with, could hold a meeting and direct the health officer how he was to drive his buggy through the regulations.

It is quite a screaming farce.

Only a week or two ago, measles were in almost every house in the city and nobody thought anything of it. It was proposed a few weeks ago, that the Government should have such an alteration of the law made as would take measles from the category of diseases which have to be specially dealt with."[1]

When our children were born, measles was not a notifiable disease, presumably because it wasn't considered serious enough to be on the list. The only figures kept, appear to have been hospitalization cases, and deaths.

On 10 January 1985, our two children had been diagnosed as having classical measles. That's behind me now, I thought.

The Auckland measles vaccination campaign in November 1985

1 1883. *New Zealand Herald,* 18 September, 1883. (printed 1993 p. 9, "100 years ago").

which was kicked off with a dramatic headline,[2] set the foundation for the measles campaigns to come later:

Big Drive to Beat Measles Epidemic

". . . to try and control the worst measles epidemic in Auckland for 20 years . . . The measles outbreak has killed two children and put more than 200 in hospital . . ."

An initial investigation showed that most were under two years, and the majority were Maori and Pacific Island children. Cases were scattered but concentrated in Mangere and Otara . . . which had an immunization rate of 64.6%.[3]

Dr Diana Lennon wanted a *"Measles Monday"*[4] on 18 November, because hospitalized *"problem cases" were just "the tip of the iceberg."* "The cause of this *'outbreak',"* she said, "was children not being immunized." She stated that Maori or Pacific Island children were ten times more likely to be admitted to hospital. Dr Ip[5] estimated 8000 Auckland children were unprotected, with about 800 children having never received a measles immunization. There was much talk of how dangerous the disease could be. It could maim and kill.

By December 1985 we were told: *"Measles Monday has worked"*.

Apparently, 500 Auckland children[6] had been vaccinated. Interestingly, letters started appearing in papers[7] like this one in the Courier:

Sir – Our family had three weeks of measles so far. All our children were vaccinated as recommended, but still caught the disease. As a caring parent it annoys me that a minority who cannot be bothered getting their children immunized causing other children and families to suffer. Despite what the human rights lobby may say, it is time to penalize such people – for example by withholding family benefit payments.
Time for Action (Glenfield)

2 1985. "Big drive to beat measles epidemic". *New Zealand Herald*, 18 November.
3 Mitchell, E.A. et al. 1985. "Measles immunization in South Auckland". Nov 27; 98(791):1016–7. PMID: 3866190.
4 Levy, F. 1985. "Monday – measles day". *New Zealand Woman's Weekly*, 19 November.
5 Ip, S. 1985. "Measles war first for health officer". *Auckland Star*, 15 November.
6 1985. "Measles Monday has worked". *Manukau Courier*, 26 December: [PAGE?].
7 Letter to the Editor "Time for Action". 1985. "Spot of bother". *New Zealand Herald*, 7 December.

How extraordinary that unvaccinated people should be presumed to be the cause? Wasn't the vaccine supposed to work in their children? Did TfA miss the point that their vaccinated children with measles were also generously donating their measles infection to others, along with a whole raft of other vaccinated children?

Details[8] were published about the two children who died in 1985. One was a six-year-old with non-Hodgkins lymphoma, on chemotherapy, who had previously been immunized at 10 months, and the other was an unimmunized six-year-old girl with I-cell disease (a mucolipidosis).

In 1987, we spent Christmas day with a Warkworth family, whose children had been vaccinated in the 1985 Measles Monday campaign. We entertained their very spotty youngest daughter, who had previously had two measles shots, and was now spending Christmas Day in bed.

Because I had believed measles could only be had once, I initially missed the diagnosis, but by 4 January, 1988, both the children had measles[9] again.

The first warning that there was another outbreak came in June 1991[10] when we were told that Pacific Island children were bearing the brunt of a measles epidemic that had been raging for a fortnight. In July when it was reported that two babies under one had died in Wellington[11] that 1312 notified cases had occurred[12] and by the end of the month[13] that there had been 2200 cases nationwide. Then immunized children in Western Auckland came down with measles which was blamed on inadequate storage and handling procedures by doctors.[14] Shortly after, we were told that at least 15,000 people might have had measles. The Health Department based these figures on school absences,[15] maintaining parents didn't take their children to the doctor, so this was the only way to estimate the numbers.

From July onwards, Headlines like: ***"Parent's 'panicking' . . . Measles cases tagged 'huge' . . . 'Jab rush over killer measles***

8 Hardy, R.B. et al. 1987. "Measles epidemic in Auckland 1984–85". *New Zealand Medical Journal*, May 13; 100(823): 273–5. PMID: 3455494.
9 See "The battle begins".
10 NZPA. 1991. "Islanders fall to measles". *Auckland Star*, 28 June (Midnight extra): 8.
11 NZPA. 1991. "Babies die of measles". *Auckland Star*, 1 July.
12 NZPA. 1991. "Measles experts jab plea for kids". *Auckland Star*, 16 July.
13 1991. "Measles cases". *New Zealand Herald*, 30 July.
14 1991. "Reimmunization call after vaccine failure". *Western Leader*, 17 September.
15 NZPA. 1991. "15,000 may have had measles". *New Zealand Herald*, 10 October: Quoting from "Health".

. . . Auckland parents are rushing to get children vaccinated against measles as the epidemic creeps nearer. . .'"[16]

The Health Department said:

> *"Of all reported hospital admissions, 36 per cent were Pacific Islanders (Pacific Islanders make up around seven per cent of the population in Wellington)".*

The immediate response of Wellington's Department of Health Chief Medical Officer, Dr Gillian Durham, was to launch a[17] *"vaccinate all school children regardless"* campaign. Television had a field day.

In 1993, we were told the reason we had to have the 1991 vaccination campaign was because a 1991 immunization survey[18] had shown that:

> *"a 60% vaccination rate is not enough to protect children against a disease like measles . . ."*

In 1985, newspapers constantly warned about low South Auckland vaccination rates being the worst in the country and Otara and Mangere were reported to have the worst immunization rates in the Auckland District with only 11% of the 35.4% of MMR unvaccinated responding to requests to do so.[19] You have to ask the question why, after a nationwide MMR vaccination campaign in 1991, this new nationwide figure of 60% immunization is less than that publicized in Otara and Mangere in 1985.

Ironically, across the country more than 50% of the 10 year olds who contracted measles in 1991 had been immunized,[20] some more than once. In Waikato, Dr Dell Hood (the then medical officer of health) said[21]

> *About 60 per cent of the reported cases of measles in teenagers in her district had been previously immunized.*

---

16 Bilby, L. 1991. "Jab rush over killer measles". *Auckland Star*, 2 July.
17 Neville, P. 1991. "Measles Shock". *New Zealand Woman's Weeky*, 2 September: 46.
18 Sarney, E. 1993. "Measles scare!" Reporting Dr Michael Baker an epidemiologist at the Communicable Disease Centre quoting a 1991 survey. *New Zealand Woman's Weekly*, 8 February: 52–53.
19 Mitchell, E.A. et al. 1985. "Measles immunization in South Auckland". Nov 27; 98(791):1016–7. PMID: 3866190.
20 Ashton, J. 1991. "Measles – fighting the epidemic". *Health*, Spring: 40(17): 6.
21 Legat, N. 1991. "Measles on Elm Street". *Metro*, December.

However, a GP who attended a Waikato Health Department meeting the following year, reported back that the insider figure for vaccinated cases was 68%.[22] Other doctors at the same meeting also verified that figure. The Health Department refused to reply to letters asking for written confirmation of the true vaccination rates for cases, or the numbers of shots the children concerned had received.

Why were all these fully vaccinated kids getting measles in 1991? Were fridges too warm? Was there incorrect handling? Or maybe the vaccine simply wasn't working?

Then we were told, *"Two shots are necessary"*.[23] Yet the view put was that the second shot was only to pick up those who didn't have it the first time. A few parents asked for blood tests to see if their children had antibodies to measles, but were told that two needles (one for the blood test, and maybe one vaccine if the child wasn't immune) was cruel for children, and since the vaccine was said to be so safe, why check for immunity? It's just easier to jab them again, because the second would work.

Yet in reality, even with a lowish vaccination rate before 1991, with the amount of measles cases and vaccinations there had been since 1991, you couldn't say only 60% of children were immune.

In terms of hospitalized measles, case numbers hadn't reduced significantly since the monovalent measles vaccine was introduced decades before, so plenty of vaccinated kids would have had exposure to wild measles as well as the vaccine.

According to vaccine manufacturer information for 95% of children vaccinated with ONE MMR, a second shot should not have been necessary.

Age of immunization was again extended downwards to all babies over 6 months, because the three deaths reported previously in the media, were all in the under ones . . .

What interested me about reports at the time was the new introduction of the words *"at least"* and *"probably"*[24]. ('At least 15,000 may have had measles'.) Probably the case numbers were closer to 15,000 cases in 1991, according to the latest *Health* Magazine.[25]

22 Personal communication.
23 Ashton, J. 1991. "Measles fighting the epidemic". *Health*, Spring: 40(17): 6. "Last year the Communicable Disease Conrol Advisory Commitee . . . recommended that all children be given a second dose of MMR vaccine . . ."
24 NZPA. 1991. "15,000 may have had measles". *New Zealand Herald*, 10 October:.
25 Ashton, J. 1991. "Measles fighting the epidemic". *Health*, Spring: 40(17): 4.

Suddenly, after a review of school absences, the Health Department upgraded the figure to 30,000 cases, because school absences were three times higher than doctors' notifications, so they concluded that measles numbers must have been higher as well. And probably, we were told by the same *Health* magazine, some hospital admissions and possibly, some deaths may have gone unreported. Wouldn't a death like that have shown up at autopsy and been reported? There was speculation as before, that parents who hadn't immunized their children could have been too ashamed and not taken their measled children to the doctor.

The Immunization Awareness society presented the contradictory data to the Holmes Show, and suggested that he run it all in front of epidemiologists and experts in number crunching to try to get to the bottom of these ever-changing numbers.

Holmes thought it sufficiently interesting to schedule a show for 2 July 1991. The plan was that Wendy Lydall, myself and two people from the medical profession would discuss these issues. Things started to look shaky, when the day before, the producer said that when the idea had been mooted, the Health Department while agreeing, had been most irate and protested to the research people that:

> ***"these 'anti' people are always shouting their heads off and confusing people."***

However, everything was still all go, as far as they knew.

Taxi time drew near with just two hours to go when the phone rang with the official call to tell me that the producer had decided that I ***"was too provocative, controversial and would confuse people."*** A second behind-the-scenes call told me that the Health Department had pulled out, putting the acid on the producers.

I have to admit that my immediate reaction was to express annoyance, for which I apologized quickly. The programme went ahead in a Clayton's format, leaving Wendy Lydall to hold the fort. She's a brick of a girl, with excellent brains and a focused mind, but was in my view given no leeway, while Holmes solemnly lectured viewers on the terribly destructive and lethal nature of measles.

I felt like ringing back, and apologizing for apologizing.

Other sympathetic journalists told IAS that a Health Department directive had gone out (whether verbal or written, we never found out) that during the rest of the 1991 vaccination campaign, debate was officially off limits.

When asked by Metro why the medical people pulled out Paul Stephenson, Auckland area Health Board media manager offered this explanation:[26]

> ***"We didn't want to get into another debate on immunization and anti-immunization theories at that point. Having people making the sorts of allegations that the anti-immunization people often make could have scared a lot of people away from having their children immunized when it was vital that they did. It wasn't helpful to what was a serious campaign to prevent lots of young people getting a painful and nasty disease – spending many days feeling sick and, at the end of the day, possibly dying."***

In 1992 doctors were told[27] there had been 9239 reported cases of measles and 230 patients requiring hospitalization in 1991. 43% of patients were over 10 years old, and 6% were 20 years or older, and in 1996 doctors were told[28] there had been four deaths.

Just before the 1997 epidemic, measles became a notifiable disease.

In January 1997, doctors[29] had put a new and different spin on the 1991 epidemic. Gone was the word ***"probably"*** for a start.

> ***Page 1 "The 1991 measles epidemic was the largest ever recorded . . . approximately 640 children hospitalized . . . six deaths . . . 30,000 or more cases . . . cost estimated at $5–8 million".***

Dr Charles Essex made a suggestion that New Zealand should look at doing what the United Kingdom did in 1994[30], by repeating the 1991 mass-MMR school campaign, because, he said, the UK MR campaign had eradicated measles and rubella in the United Kingdom.

---

26 Legat, N. 1991. "Measles on elm street". *Metro*, December: 95.

27 Raymond, N.J. et al. 1992. "Adult measles in Auckland Hospital, 1991". *New Zealand Medical Journal*, Sep 9; 105(941): 359–60. PMID: 1436831.

28 Essex, C. 1996. "Elimination of measles and rubella in New Zealand a possibility". *New Zealand Medical Journal*, Aug 9; 109(1027): 303. PMID: 8773678.

29 Tobias, M. 1997. "Predicting the next measles epidemic". *New Zealand Public Health Report*, January: Vol 14, No. 1: p. 1.

30 Essex, C. 1996. "Elimination of measles and rubella in New Zealand a possibility". *New Zealand Medical Journal*, Aug 9; 109(1027): 303. PMID: 8773678. "UK used the MR vaccine, not the MMR."

By August 1998, doctors were now being told[31] that in 1991, there had been *30–60,000* cases, 629 hospitalizations and 7 deaths.

In January 1997, Martin Tobias and Dr Osman Mansoor stated that *"mathematical modelling suggests that New Zealand would experience a measles epidemic in 1997 or 1998."*

So it was no surprise when the first 1997 headline I saw was:[32]

GP's warned of killer measles

We were told that the 1997 epidemic would be larger than 1991.[33] Again the blame was laid on inadequate vaccine coverage. The article said that the 80.2% vaccination rate only applied to the baby dose. Had anyone been keeping stats for the Form 1 dose, which had been going for 7 years? It appears not. A review of previous vaccination coverage (with catch-up shots at 5 years) stated:

- the 1979 survey found a 77% baby vaccination coverage, with 30% of unimmunized children vaccinated at 5 yrs of age
- 1980–1992 = 82% baby coverage and 20% of unimmunized at 5 years.
- 1993–1996, 84% baby coverage plus 10% of unimmunized at 5 years.[34]
- Catch-up shots at 5 years was discontinued in 1991 with the introduction of 1st Form 2nd MMR.
- (and) since 1992 70% of previously *unimmunized* children had a first dose. 90% of previously immunized had second dose.[35]

If you have a baby coverage of 84% as above, and add to that figure the 70% of the previously unvaccinated 16% as above, the total

31 Jones, N. et al. 1998. "1997 measles epidemic in Auckland". *The New Zealand Public Health Report*, August: Vol 5, No. 8: pp. 57–60.

32 Young, A. 1997. "GPs warned of killer measles". *New Zealand Herald*, 14 January: A3.

33 Tobias, M. et al. 1997. "Predicting the next measles epidemic". *New Zealand Public Health Report*, January: Vol 4, No. 4: 1.

34 McNicholas, Q. et al. 1996. "Immunization coverage in New Zealand 1995". *New Zealand Public Health Report*, Vol 3: 83–4.

35 Tobias, M. et al. 1997. "Predicting the next measles epidemic". *New Zealand Public Health Report*, Vol 4, No. 4: 2. "Since 1992, at age 11 years, 70% of previously unimmunsed children receive a first dose of vaccine while 90% of previously immunized children receive a second dose".

receiving one MMR vaccine equals 95% and 80% of children would have received two MMR vaccine. To estimate community immunity you have to add into that figure immunity gained by children who caught measles in the community over that time, as well.

That community immunity was way above the 60% figure touted by the Health Department is confirmed by a Department of Health serological survey in 1996 which showed that over all ages, community immunity[36] to measles was 94.7%. Measles immunity was 85.5% between one and 19 years of age and ***"Individuals aged 20 and above have been found to have adequate immunity against measles."***

In April, the Herald said: ***Measle jabs for half a million***[37] (*New Zealand Herald*'s spelling!)

> ***The Ministry of Health estimates that the disease could kill up to 10 people and put 900 in hospital. . . . It regards 95% coverage as necessary to stop the epidemic . . . Health officials are racing against time . . . the disease is already well established in Auckland and expected to spread rapidly when children go back to school next week . . . In the past three weeks 23 cases of measles have been recorded, compared with none for the whole of last year . . .***

This graph shows the estimated proportion of susceptibles to a predicted epidemic in 1998.[38] The article reads: ***"The threshold for the triggering of an epidemic, of around 140,000 susceptible children aged 1–10 years. Two thirds of the susceptibles aged 2–10-years are unimmunized and one third are vaccine failures."***

Therefore the math works out as 93,400 unvaccinated + 46,700 vaccine failures = 140,000 susceptibles to trigger the proposed epidemic.

This report[39] recommended that ***"all children aged 2–10 years who had never received measles immunization should be offered MMR."***

---

36 Department of Health. 1997. "Special vaccination campaign for measles in 1997". Special Edition: *Public Health & Epidemiology Bulletin*, August.

37 Laxton, A. 1997. "Measle jab for half a million". *New Zealand Herald*, 24 April: A3.

38 Tobias, M. et al. 1997. Predicting the next measles epidemic". *New Zealand Public Health Report*, January: 4(1):2 (Figure 2).

39 Tobias, M. et al. 1997. "Predicting the next measles epidemic". *New Zealand Public Health Report*, January: 4(1):2 (Figure 2).

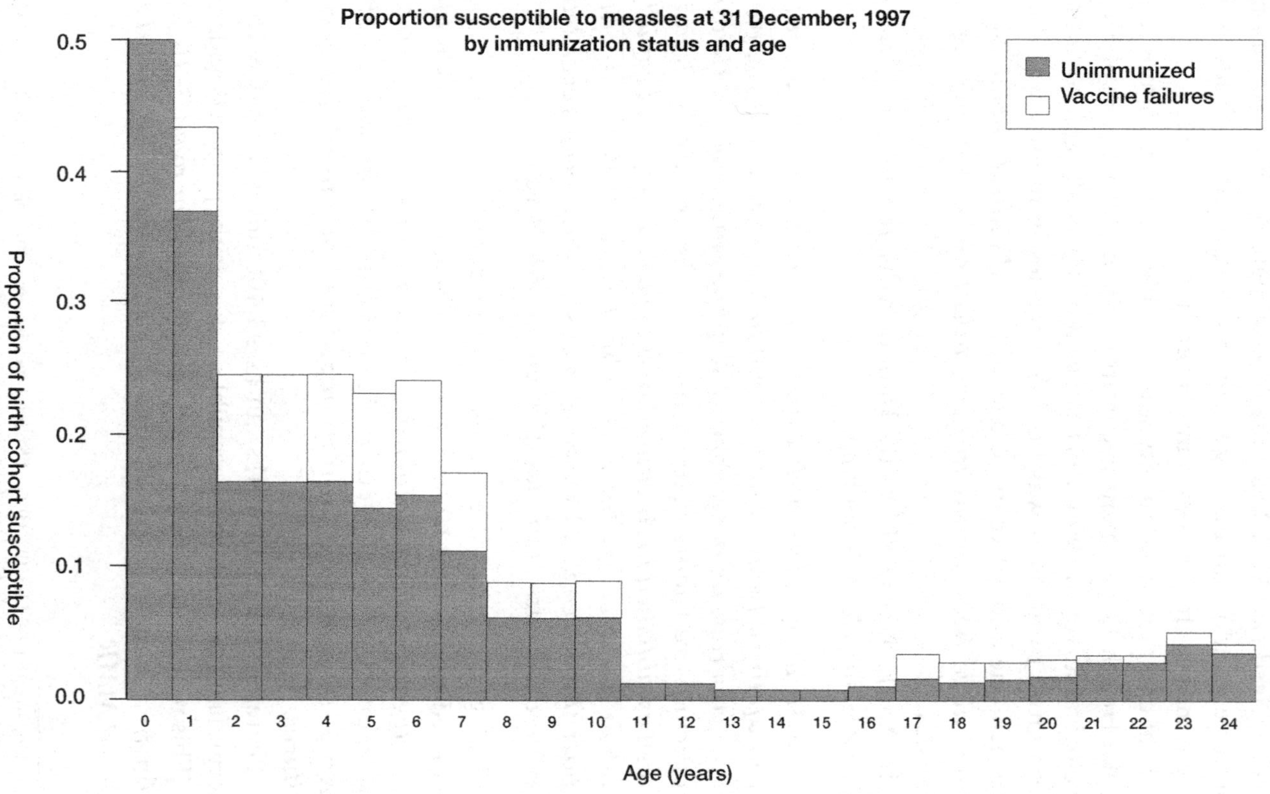

Source: Tobias, M. et al. 1997. "Predicting the next measles epidemic". New Zealand Public Health Report, Jan: 4(1); 2 (Figure 2).

This being too complicated, the KISS principle was invoked again, and letters send out by Health Authorities instructed that all 2–10-year-olds should be jabbed regardless of their immunization status, and all babies between 6–11-months should be vaccinated.

Supplies were slow coming and in May, the vaccine ran out. Masses of articles with *"Killer measles"* headlines tumbled off the presses and out onto the TV screen.

In this nation with a 94.7% community immunity rate the year before, the talkback callers were suddenly reduced to hysterical rubble, so a national hotline was set up, which only caused even more confusion, by giving conflicting advice.

Interestingly a special report[40] showed that of the cases in the first six months of 1997 by which time there had been 927 cases,[41] 50% had been immunized. ***"This was a significant sign of waning immunity or vaccine failure."***

Vaccination got underway properly in June in Auckland, and didn't finish until late November in the South Island.

By December 1997 when the epidemic was over, the 1991 figures were changed yet again, but the Ministry was still predicting an epidemic in 1998:

"Using the Ministry's figures of some 60–70,000 cases, 629 hospitalizations and 7 deaths in the 1991 epidemics . . . [42] the prediction was that ***"the size and age structure of an epidemic occurring in 1998 is estimated to be roughly similar to the 1991 epidemic. Approximately 45,000 cases would be expected with 600–900 hospitalization and 6–9 deaths".***

Why were they using the size of the 1991 epidemic as a projection for 1998, when they alleged in 1991, that immunization levels were 60% and a 1996 serological survey showed the community immunity rate was actually 94.7%? Should that not have changed the mathematics?

When the vaccination statistics for the nationwide campaign in 1997 were added up, the vaccine acceptance rate[43] was 60% of European

---

40 Department of Health. 1997. "Special vaccination campaign for measles in 1997". *Public Health and Epidemiology Bulletin,* Special Edition, August: 1.

41 Eyles, R. et al. June 1997. "Measles monthly report". Downloaded from the Ministry of Health on 8 July, 1997 at 10.55 am.

42 Cullen, R. 1997. "Should New Zealand eliminate measles." *New Zealand Medical Journal,* Dec 12; 110(1057): 470. PMID: 9451416.

43 ACCEPTANCE RATE is where parents signed the consent for to allow their child to

children, 43% of Polynesian children, 40% of Maori children, and 53% other ethnicities. Coverage for children 6–11-months-old was estimated at about 57%.[44]

The measles epidemic went from April 1997, to December 1997 (1964 cases[45]) 1225 cases (62%) occurred in the Auckland region. Totals from January 1997, to February 1998 (to mop up odd cases either side) were 2095 cases[46] (16.1% were in babies under 12 months of age), 216 hospitalization and no deaths. Of the hospitalized cases, 20% were under 1's, 19% under 2's, 30% in the 15–30 year old group. The ethnic strike rates were 199.3 per 100,000 for Pacific Islanders, 54.1 per 100,000 for Maori and 30.3 per 100,000 for Europeans, 120.4 per 100,000 other.[47]

In terms of the vaccination campaign, 56% of 6–10-year-old were estimated to have been revaccinated, including those previously fully vaccinated.[48]

The low uptake rate didn't stop Dr Nikki Turner from writing a follow-up article[49] which she illustrated with a fancy graph, saying ***"Last year we had a measles epidemic. When it hit the news there was a tremendous uptake in the vaccine which dramatically stopped the spread of measles and prevented 90–95% of the cases. A great response from parents and the result was only 2000 cases, 313 hospital admissions and no deaths."***

She also said this: ***"New Zealand rates for MMR vaccination are around 80–85%. Another 5–10% of our children being vaccinated and we have a realistic chance of never seeing these diseases again."***

Let's focus on these figures for a moment. Community immunity was 94.7% before the vaccination campaign started. The prediction was 140,000 susceptibles aged 6-months–10-years-old, leading to a predicted epidemic of 45,000 cases in susceptibles. 45,000 cases

---

be vaccinated.

44 Compiled from the Weekly and Monthly reports off the Ministry of Health's website at the time.

45 Jones, N. et al. 1998. "1997 measles epidemic in Auckland". *The New Zealand Public Health Report*, August: Vol 5, No. 8: pp. 57–60.

46 Kieft, C., and Short, J. 1998. *Measles Monthly Report*, February: Downloaded 20 April, 1998.

47 Kieft, C., and Short, J. 1998. *Measles Monthly Report*, February: Downloaded 20 April, 1998.

48 Jones, N. et al. 1998. "1997 measles epidemic in Auckland". *The New Zealand Public Health Report*, August: Vol 5, No. 8: pp. 57–60.

49 Turner, N. 1998. "Be wise, immunize – and minimize disease. *Healthwise*, August–September: p. 17.

among 140,000, comes to 32%. The vaccination campaign records show that:

57% of those 140,000 were vaccinated	=	79,800 people.
43% of 140,000 were not vaccinated	=	60,200 people.

Out of the 2095 cases in 1997, half of the cases occurred before vaccination really got under way in June, and of the year's total, 1055 were not in the susceptible group upon which projections were based. On the basis of a calculation that 32% of ALL 140,000 susceptibles would get measles, then there should have been around 20,000 cases during the whole epidemic among the 60,200 subsequently non-vaccinated susceptibles nationwide (or at least 10,000 before the vaccination programme started), assuming viral circulation in that group – which was the basis of their estimates.

Dr Turner assumes that the top of the epidemic graph spike in June would have been the beginning of the epidemic, yet in comparison with previous epidemic graphs, the pattern is identical. Furthermore, if you look at the susceptibles proportions graph compared with the age groups in which the cases actually occurred, the premise of the estimated ages in which cases would occur which she says were prevented by vaccination, were faulty.

To then claim the vaccination campaign of 79,800 children throughout New Zealand, many of whom were fully vaccinated anyway, prevented 40,000 cases of measles in susceptible New Zealand children is very strange.

Their estimation of 32% of any group catching measles in an epidemic is also false. Epidemiological studies[50] in the most severe epidemic prior to the use of vaccine had found infection rates were normally 15%.

Summary: In my opinion, the Ministry of Health gradually over time, turned generalized data into inflated assertions, hence the notified 9239 cases in 1991[51] and two acknowledged deaths was quickly suggested to have been 15,000 who might have had measles, then exploded into 60–70,000 cases, with 629 hospitalizations and 7 deaths by December 1997. Furthermore claims of low vaccination

50 Sencer, D.J. et al. "Epidemiologic basis for eradication of measles in 1967". *USA Public Health Reports*, March: 82(3): 255.

51 Raymond, N.J. 1992. "Adult measles in Auckland Hospital, 1991". *New Zealand Medical Journal*, Sep 9; 105(941): 359–60. PMID: 1436831.

rates of 60% didn't stack up with published medical literature, showing a 95% vaccination rate for 1 MMR, an 85.5% vaccination rate for two, alongside a 1996 measles serological survey showing a 94.7% measles immunity rate.

Therefore their predictions of a huge epidemic were grossly exaggerated, and subsequent claims that the vaccination campaign prevented an epidemic of the scale they predicted are logically unsustainable.

55 Today

4.20 am.

Another two hours to go. Give or take a few minutes.

Will I go back to sleep?

I don't know.

So I lie there in bed and . . .

Think!

You know, the mind is a funny thing. My mind is anyway.

I try and concentrate on something – to think it through – and all sorts of other thoughts invade that "space".

And somewhere in this exercising of the grey matter I think a bit of dozing takes place too!

But I keep refocusing on what I want to think about, which is . . . the new day about to unfold over the next eighteen hours or so.

I do this each day in some way. When we are both awake, Hilary and I do it together. It's almost a morning ritual.

Why is it so important?

Because like it or not, we can only live one day at a time.

Actually, we live by the hour, or the minutes or sometimes, the seconds.

None of us know for sure what the future holds.

Yes, we can make plans, and if all goes well everything may turn out exactly to the letter.

The more structured arrangements are, the less flexibility there is.

Our unique lifestyles will be determined by convictions, goals, objectives, people and all sorts of other variables. Things can become very complicated.

***Simply** though, each day is lived according to the realities of the present. The issues we have to face* TODAY.

5.30 *am*.

What are the realities today for me and Hilary?

Well, I don't have any sinking feeling in my stomach – no dread or apprehension or anguish,

no pain,

no despair or sorrow carried over from yesterday.

Hope, joy, contentedness? Yes, nothing disturbing those things.

Concerns?

Yes, some I guess.

So I mentally examine them.

6.05 *am*.

I still keep coming back to thinking about today.

It's all so personal; so hidden; so tentative; so vulnerable to unbidden, intruding thoughts – usually from the past – yesterday, maybe, or way, way back. An intricate web of thought associations.

Dreams? About the future?

Yes, they can be mixed up with everything else which will include what other people's day will turn out to be and the impact of that on us.

6.30 *am*.

Time I got up for a while. Get some fresh air and enjoy the sunrise.

I'll come back shortly when Hilary's awake and we'll talk things over and work out what could happen today.

What has lying in bed thinking, got to do with this book? Surely it's irrelevant? Just disjointed rambling!

Whether or not you do it when you're getting ready for the new day, doesn't really matter. The point is that at the beginning of each new day it has to be thought about. If it isn't, it could become an aimless, drifting, twiddle-my-thumbs, waste of time. Or will we allow other people to decide it for us?

I believe each day needs to be lived to the full, according to broad pre-determined **priorities**. These will be like a framework, at the start of the day, on which the fleshing out will take place, and reviewed as the day progresses. Consideration for the needs and feelings of others must not be overlooked.

As far as is possible the agenda set should be achievable for all concerned, and should include time to relax and wind down.

There will, of course, be times when the unexpected and emergency-type situations can throw everything into what seems to be total disarray.

At a time like this, lifestyle priorities should kick into action, automatically, because they form the basis for **each new day**. They should have been well rehearsed and practised on a daily basis.

I can almost hear readers muttering all sorts of deprecations under their breath. Others may be more vociferous and tell me to "get real"!

Thanks. But I am being real – for me at least.

I am not telling anyone how to run their lives, nor have I provided sets of priorities to be used as check lists.

I am just suggesting that today – right now – there are opportunities to be recognized and used to the full. I may not be around tomorrow. And you mightn't be either.

This book identifies some issues which could be placed in the broad category of "health". But it also goes much further for anyone who wants to read between the lines, thinking things through; personalizing it.

After a long life of many and varied experiences resulting from interacting with lots of parents and children – unique families – I just long that each **day** we live – me and mine, you and yours – will be determined by well-thought-about choices that will enable you and me to say, "I know this is right for me (or for us)".

Are the foundations being strengthened day by day by day?

I heard a true story the other day. A lady went to visit her chiropractor, who passed on to her some information on non-vaccination. At her next visit the lady expressed indignation at being given something to read which was different to the Health Department's blurb. "I don't want any more of that stuff thank you. I HAVE TO THINK! It's much easier to do what the vaccination campaign brochure says."

Another typical example comes to mind.

A proud father called around to see us and lovingly showed us their recently born baby. In the course of conversation the question arose:

"Are you going to have your baby immunized?"

"I don't know," he replied. "I'd rather he wasn't. He's probably due for his first jab. I don't think my wife's had him done yet."

Talking about each new day **is** important.

Life-changing decisions may be involved.

A question asked hundreds of years ago still needs to be confronted today:

"Can two walk together, unless they be agreed?"

56 Which Groups are Most at Risk of Measles?

One choice criterion when it comes to vaccination is to answer the question, "Is it necessary?" Parents have to balance risks and benefits, and to do that they need an accurate risk assessment of what the chances of their child getting that disease are. They also need to know, if their children get a disease, how likely they are to get really ill, or die?

Sir MacFarlane Burnet[1] was one of the great and really knowledgeable virologists/bacteriologists of the time when measles was supposedly a major killer. He wrote:

> ***"Most parents and doctors feel that if a healthy young school child is exposed to measles, there is nothing to be gained by trying to prevent infection. Provided a doctor is on hand to watch for and deal with any complications like middle-ear infection, the disease presents no danger to a healthy child."***

Also, Sir MacFarlane Burnett's prognosis for immuno-compromised children was that they normally get through measles quite well if their nutrition is okay. Immuno-compromised children without antibodies do just fine, and have a normal progression of measles. But children

1 MacFarlane, B. (Sir). 1953. *Viruses and Man.* London and Baltimore: Penguin Books. p. 57.

treated with chemotherapy, or immunosuppressive drugs, even if they are immunized, will succumb to measles, because the medical treatment is what train-wrecks the rest of their immune systems which would otherwise deal with the virus reasonably well.

An infectious disease doctor wrote this in 1989:

> *"Measles used to be a common cause of severe illness although the outlook was always good."*[2]

In 1990 the *Herald*[3] reported an interesting medical study showing that:

> *"High doses of Vitamin A considerably reduced the duration of measles and cut the death rate by more than half . . . an American study has found . . . the authors of the new study recommended that ill children with severe measles should be given vitamin A supplements regardless of whether or not they were deficient in vitamin A."*

In 1997, the strike rates for measles in Northland and Auckland were as follows:[4] Polynesians: 230 per 100,000, Maori: 67 per 100,000, European: 53 per 100,000. Nationwide they were 199.3 per 100,000 for Pacific Islanders; 54.1 per 100,000 for Maori; 30.3 per 100,000 for Europeans, and 120.4 per 100,000 for other groups.

We also know that acute rheumatic fever in Maori in the early 1980s[5] was 125 per 100,000 and for Pacific Island children the corresponding figure was 114 per 100,000.

In a fax to TVNZ, Ossi Mansoor[6] said this:

> *"Measles, like most diseases, predominantly affects Maori, Pacific Island people and the socioeconomically disadvantaged. In the case of measles this is aggravated by*

2 Family Doctor by Iatros. 1998. *New Zealand Herald*, 24 January: Section 2: 2. (Written by a prominent New Zealand Infectious Disease expert of the time.)

3 1990. Medical Frontiers. "PMT drug questioned". *New Zealand Herald*, 24 July.

4 Jones, N. et al. 1998. "1997 measles epidemic in Auckland". *New Zealand Public Health Report*, Vol. 5(8): 58.

5 Martin, D.R. et al. 1994. "Acute rheumatic fever in Auckland, New Zealand: spectrum of association Group A streptococci different from expected". *Pediatr Infect Dis J*, 13: 264–9. (The article also found that a much wider spectrum of Group P streptococcal M types caused ARG than those usually listed. Naturally the focus of the article was to direct attention to the needs of any vaccine that might come up in the future.)

6 11/02/97 (G:\PP\OSSI\IMM\MEDIA2.DOC) page 2 of 12. "Response for TV3 on immunization questions." 12 page fax from Dr O. Mansoor – TV3.

> ***the fact that these groups tend to have lower immunization coverage. In the 1991 epidemic, the Maori rate of hospitalization for measles was eight times the non-Maori rate."*** (emphasis mine)

In 1991 and 1997 parents were not told clearly who the risk groups were. They were also not told all the facts about what influences the outcomes of ANY infectious disease even in normal children. There was no discussion on the risks for immunocompromised children. One of the health authorities' arguments was that everyone has to have the vaccine, because immunocompromised children die from measles. Which is not what Sir MacFarlane Burnet says:[7]

> ***"With the recognition of considerable numbers of children with agammaglobulinaemia and their maintenance in fair health by immunoglobulin injections, it was inevitable that some of them would contract measles. To everyone's surprise they showed a normal measles course with a typical rash, which faded at the normal time and was followed by just as substantial immunity against reinfection as would be shown by any other convalescent. Antibody production is therefore not necessary either for recovery from or for the development of immunity to measles."***

So why is antibody level after a vaccine said to be the only way of developing immunity to measles? Doctors though might point to immunoglobulin given by injection, but this doctor doesn't think that's the whole story.

The author then looks at measles in children who have acute leukaemia that is treated with steroids:

> ***"the combination of disease and treatment virtually paralyses the T-system . . . Measles usually kills these children, but in quite abnormal fashion. There is no rash and the children die of what is called 'giant-cell pneumonia' in which the lung is choked with large cells containing many nuclei."*** (Emphasis mine.)

I also wonder if steroid treatment in asthmatic patients increases their

7 Burnet, M. (Sir). 1972. *Natural History of Infectious Disease*, Cambridge. p. 79.

risks of infectious diseases being more severe, for similar reasons.

As parents we also need to consider the likely severity of the disease in normal children. Did it really help us to make an informed choice, when we read in 1997:[8]

> *"Starship general manager Grant Close said measles was the most virulent disease known to man . . ."*

Do you really think measles has been the most virulent disease known to man and worse than ebola, smallpox, HIV, or the plague?

History has interesting lessons to teach. In 1932, on page 7 of the Appendices to the New Zealand Parliamentary Journals, the then Director General of Health wrote:

> *"We still experience epidemics of scarlet fever, diphtheria, measles and whooping-cough, but these epidemics give an annual death rate very much lower than that experienced in former epidemics, while in the intervening non-epidemic years, the sporadic cases have assumed a milder type and give a reduced death rate . . .*
>
> *These reductions are so great and so sustained that one is forced to the conclusion that good environment (to use a comprehensive term which includes measures taken to improve diet and hygiene) is steadily removing these diseases . . . The thought then arises, despite the prophesies of certain epidemiologists who, on historical grounds, predict a recurrence of high infectious disease virulence and mortality and perhaps undervalue the influence of improved environment, and those of immunologists who regard the subject as essentially one of acquired immunity, whether or not New Zealand and even closely populated England can by the maintenance or even the improvement of a good environment, retain the natural resistance of their peoples to these diseases."* (Emphasis in the report itself.)

In 1982,[9] Dr A.J. Tyrell wrote about the importance of the host:

> *"It has been pointed out repeatedly that the decline of*

8 NZPA. 1997. "Measles campaign begins". *The Press*, 9 May.
9 Tyrell, A.J. 1982. "The importance of the host". Nuffields Provincial Hospital Trusts publication: p. 23. (ISBN 090 0574 39 9).

> *infectious diseases in Britain since the mid-nineteenth century may have had little to do with specifically anti-infectious measures . . . it is likely that other less well-defined changes, probably in housing and diet, reduced the mortality of diseases such as whooping-cough, measles and tuberculosis; certainly they were declining before measures such as vaccination or antibiotic treatment had any effect."*

Dr Tyrell then diverges onto a personal impression that Florence Nightingale's influence had more effect than realized in the decrease in death rates from infectious diseases. She had become a role model, with parents taking note of her methods, and therefore resting sick children, giving more fluid, and proper nourishment. Given that Florence Nightingale was such a heroine of the day to parents, perhaps there's something in that. Dr Tyrell talks about economic improvements and medical care changes but doubts that they can explain the changes. Epigeneticists should have a field day with this:

> *"A converse phenomenon has been seen, namely that after personal stress, individuals are prone to infection – there is a real truth in the cliché that 'war and famine' are followed by 'pestilence'. Refugees from Uganda had been mostly well fed and housed and then came to Britain in the early 1970s. They showed a greatly increased incidence of tuberculosis, though the strains they were infected with were acquired in Britain . . . some . . . failed to show signs of an immune response by either skin test or lymphocyte response and this is presumably why the disease was progressing.*
>
> *Sometimes after treatment for a while, the immune response seemed to develop quite suddenly and they felt worse, because of the inflammation in infected tissue and the fever. However, we used to regard that as a good sign indicating that a satisfactory host response had returned."* (Emphasis mine.)

He also talks about how an accident can change the types of bacteria in the pharynx, and then discusses a study in which it was found that introverted *"volunteers"* shed more virus than those with extroverted personalities, but the study had no idea of the connections between the two . . .

What is important is that both previous quotations are from doctors, one writing in Parliamentary Journals in 1932, and another writing in 1982. Both recognize a paradigm of their time that immunologists and epidemiologists do not consider relevant in infectious diseases today, namely that nutrition, host factors, or life's circumstances can undermine the immune system. These factors continue to be ignored in 2006.

Even in 1981 these authors[10] discuss a statement with which they do not totally agree, but cannot totally dismiss either:

"Children who die from measles are typically those with malnutrition or some other severe intercurrent condition who would soon die from some other cause if not from measles."

Then they say:

"To what extent should the issue of who dies from measles decide whether or not to promote measles vaccination? This was examined in the United Kingdom during early discussions over the advisability of a national measles vaccination programme. Half of the 132 deaths attributed to measles in the first six months of 1961 were in children with serious chronic disease or disability. The fact that many of the children who died of measles had at best a short expectation of life, did not cancel the overall benefits to be gained from the programme."

Another interesting old article makes a relevant comparison where the author discusses his experience in Africa and the UK, and compares the severity of measles in industrial and developing countries. He discusses and acknowledges that the severity of the disease and the death rate as a result of measles radically declined before the medical people could do anything about it. He then discusses the very real clinical differences in the severity of measles in African children, between those who are reasonably well fed, and those who are not:

"The nutritional state of the child before and during

10 Editorial. 1981. "Rationalising Measles Vaccination". *The Lancet*, August: 2(8240): 236–7. PMID: 6114288.

> ***the attack from measles may be the dominant factor in producing the severe form of the disease described above.***"[11]

He compares the symptoms described in two UK studies (Glasgow, and Drinkwater), where impoverished families had high death rates, with the symptoms he saw in Africa. He noted and compared the "*dark rashes*" in UK studies, with the dark rashes he saw in the very impoverished African children, and stated very clearly that the most severe measles as seen in all countries was where malnutrition is the worst.

In 1997, I provided for all media outlets several articles on Vitamin A, including an article[12] showing:

> ***"Vitamin A deficiency is associated with increased mortality (deaths) and morbidity (severity) from infectious diseases. Vitamin A enhances immunity in humans . . . Vitamin A supplementation reduces severe illness and deaths from infectious diseases in children.' (p. 490) 'Even sub-clinical Vitamin A deficiency is associated with more severe disease in children.' (p.491) The impact of Vitamin A supplementation on death and severity in measles is striking. High-dose Vitamin A supplementation has reduced severity and deaths even among children with no clinical signs of vitamin A deficiency." (p. 493)***

All the articles made it clear that Vitamin A deficiency is common in socio-economically deprived children of *any* country, and a Vitamin-A-deficient child with measles will also have other nutrient deficiencies as well. The articles also showed that all infectious diseases have a worse outcome if vitamin A isn't at optimal levels. Everyone who wanted this information was given it, and a lot who didn't want it were given it too.

The *Herald* had an attack of editorial amnesia, and forgot it had published something along these lines in 1990, and like other newspapers started reporting medical personnel saying that the only relevant prevention was vaccination. In the official rebuttal sheets,

11 Morley, D.C. 1967. "Measles in pre-industrial countries". *Modern Trends in Medical Virology*, Vol 1(6): 141–161.

12 Semba, R.D. 1994. "Vitamin A, Immunity, and Infection". *Clin Infect Dis*. September: 19(3): 489–99. PMID: 7811869.

the Health Department emphasised that Vitamin A was of no use, and that only vaccination would do. No one challenged the medical profession using their own literature.

The Honorable Neil Kirton, on 30 June 1997, even graced my desk with three pages of admonitions including the statement that Vitamin A had only been shown to be effective in treating measles in developing countries. I felt that I was being told to shut up.

However, suddenly in 2005[13] there was the *Herald* article which said that:

> ***"One in every 10 Auckland infants is growing up with Third World-type vitamin deficiencies.***

Dr Cameron Grant had discovered that a four-year study found 12% of Auckland babies 6 months to 2 years of age were vitamin A deficient, 24% were iron deficient (similar to USA 30 years ago) and 10% vitamin D deficiency. He said that this implied that there would be other micronutrient deficiencies as well, which might undermine these children's health. He commented that while vitamin A deficiency wasn't common in countries like New Zealand, because New Zealand infectious disease patterns were similar to third world countries they had decided to study some vitamins.

He commented that childhood pneumonia here was 5–10 times higher than in USA, and while that was partly due to over crowding, it also stemmed from poor nutrition. He said:

> ***"If a child is admitted to hospital with measles, we give them a treatment of Vitamin A."***

Did this mean that everything said about appalling diet in measles cases and the need to use Vitamin A, which authorities had publicly dismissed in 1991 and 1997, was now a fact, but only because Dr Grant had done a study? Vitamin A has been known as the anti-infective vitamin since 1930. What about selenium and zinc, two other crucial micronutrients intimately involved in the immune system?

The medical profession will claim for ever and a day that the cases of measles and the deaths that occurred in 1987, 1991, and 1997 could have been prevented *IF* the children had been vaccinated. Maybe

---

13 Collins, S. 2005. "Vitamin lacking in 1 of 10 toddlers". *New Zealand Herald*, [Internet] Available from <http://www.nzherald.co.nz/index.cfm?c_id=1&ObjectID=9006061 10> Accessed on 18 September, 2005.

most of the hospital complications and some of the deaths COULD have been prevented if the medical profession had told parents about decades' worth of information on the use of Vitamin A and other nutrients, and given Vitamin A to all those children in their care whether at a doctor's office or in hospital.

Dr Ossi Mansoor hit the nail on the head when he said that most measles cases (and that also applies to most other infectious diseases) occur among Polynesian and Maori children. You have to wonder why it is that it took so long for a medical person to work it out. Perhaps it is, as a recent *NZMJ* editorial said[14], that they mostly live in the rarefied intellectual atmosphere of their offices.

Nutrition and lifestyle dramatically change the equation of personal risk versus benefit for every individual and society as a whole. Certain sectors of society are much more at risk in every area of health because of poor nutrition, smoking, toxicity levels, damp housing, stress and other environmental issues. Therefore, instead of just pushing vaccines, shouldn't medical people be seriously asking, "How can we really help people to effectively reduce the risks across the spectrum of all the diseases they are more at risk for?"

I put this to infectious disease experts on BMJ rapid responses.[15] Like Dr Mansoor, they considered it ***"too hard"***. Even more interesting, when the question was put to them, whether even in a utopian society they would still want to use vaccines, the inference was ***"yes"***, because as one doctor pointed out, vaccines were cheap, easy and expedient.

So, even if we could prove that unvaccinated properly fed children could get through all these diseases relatively problem free, it wouldn't make any difference. The mindsets are so fixed that vaccination as the right (and only) concept has become enshrined, no matter what.

---

14 Kearns, R. et al. 2005. "Widening the lens on child health". *New Zealand Medical Journal*, Dec 16; 118(1227): U1785. PMID: 16372034. "Experience can be accessed through encountering others and observing their environments in situ. With their retreat from home visiting, members of the medical profession increasingly encounter people only within clinical and institutional settings . . . While processes and places of everyday life most accurately reveal exposure to the distal determinants of health, the synergies between diverse domains of human experience have only recently been considered in policy."

15 Retrieved on 18 September, 2005 from <http://bmj.bmjjournals.com/cgi/eletters/330/7483/112-d>.

57 Just Another Call

It was just after 8.30 in the evening.

The telephone rang.

I was washing the dinner dishes.

Flicking the water from my hands I picked up the receiver.

"Hello", I said.

"I don't know whether I've got the right number or not, but I was wanting some information about immunizing my daughter."

"You've got the right number. Just a moment, and I'll hand you over to my wife."

Back to the dishes.

Skim through the newspaper.

Do my daily crossword puzzle.

Maybe time for a game of Patience.

10 o'clock and the yawns are getting more persistent.

Hilary's still on the phone.

I wrap my arms around her as I bend down to give her a kiss. I nibble her unoccupied ear.

"Good night my lovely. God bless you. See you sometime," I whisper.

58 On the Matter of the 1991 Deaths

In May 1997, when the medical profession kept emphasizing the seven deaths from measles, I tried to find out what the real figures were, but was told the information was "confidential".

Then, one night, I got an interesting phone call. It was a doctor not previously known to me, who had heard me on the radio, and thought I would be interested to know that a meeting had been held for GPs. At that meeting it was stated that of the six cases, there was no data for two of them, but of the other four, three were immunocompromised and one might have been immunocrompromised.

Interesting. I sat back and thought about it. I didn't know this doctor and felt unsure, wondering if this could be a plant, as in "let's throw something out there and watch someone fire off without checking, and therefore make a fool of herself".

But then I had two more calls, both from doctors I did know, who confirmed the comments of the first doctor. I wrote a letter to the person responsible for the meeting repeating back what three doctors had now confirmed, and asking for clarification. No reply. I also wrote to Dr Gillian Durham and relayed the exact information and got no response. On the second reminder, Dr Durham wrote back that the doctor could only comment on one patient treated, and that patient was immunocompromised.

Eventually, the data was found. The Morbidity and Demographic Data 1991 for Measles deaths was incomplete:

Page 21 – Males:	1	(0–1)	+	1	(10–15)
Page 31 – Females:	1	(1–2)	+	1	(5–10)

A letter[1] stated:

"Four of the six deaths recorded in 1991 were children. Their ages were 12 years, 8 years, 1 year and 9 months. So far as is known, none had any underlying illness and none were immunized . . . One death has been recorded from 1992 to the present – an adult, aged 44 years, in 1994."

By July 1997, I had found the following data on the deaths: three males, aged 9 months, 2 years and 12 years. Four females, aged 13 months, 8 years, 18 years, and 80 years. One was a Pacific Islander, one was Maori, and five were other. The 44-year-old had disappeared somehow.

To this day, I am unsatisfied with Dr Durham's explanation about what was said in the GPs' meeting. I believe that what the three doctors reported to me was what was said at that meeting.

1 Dr John Eastwood, in a letter dated 13 May 1997.

59 Collateral Damage

The official line on serious MMR vaccine reactions in 1997 is that there were none.

Parents in this country didn't hear about the many personal tragedies. I did. Some stories were only partially told, like the case of the 11-year-old vaccinated boy on life support in a regional hospital that TV1 tried to investigate. They got the constant fob-off and in the end, the paediatrician would only say to the reporter, "We may never know".

But there were many times I picked up the phone and listened to stories of personal nightmares. There was, for example, the single father, with custody of his child, whose son was vaccinated, and started seizuring. He took the child to a doctor who found nothing wrong. When they got home, the child had another fit, and the doctor advised them to go to the hospital. At the hospital, every test under the sun showed nothing. The man persisted, refused to go, and got so upset that staff got two doctors' signatures and had him taken to a psychiatric unit. Shortly after he had been forcibly removed from the hospital, the child had a seizure in front of the staff. Yet, even in spite of that, it took the man's doctor and lawyer considerable time and expense to have the man released from the psychiatric unit. The man was far too scared to complain. He didn't want to make trouble in case he lost custody of his child.

If all the stories were told, they would all relate tales of dismissal, denial and distraught parents.

I heard about some cases from people in the system. In 1997, there was a child who was transferred from Starship to Christchurch hospital, and subsequently quarantined with measles. All Christchurch registrars were given the MMR vaccine. Unfortunately, a registrar who dealt with immunocompromised patients got measles. The virus was PCR-typed by the laboratory and the result came back as vaccine virus, not wild virus.

The public never heard about that. I checked the papers and in Christchurch, people had been told in November[1] that:

Jabs beat measles epidemic

Then[2] an oops article appeared:

Local measles epidemic reverses national trend

According to Dr Briesman, it was mostly young adults being hit rather than children. No mention of whether or not the adults were amongst the doubly fully vaccinated schoolchildren under 16 year olds from the 1991 campaign, or whether the medical profession checked if the cases were from the vaccine strain, or from a wild virus.

Two parents would like the record set straight, about there being no serious vaccine reactions.

RAYMOND'S STORY[3]

Written by his mother.

We live on a farm, out the back of Taupo. Raymond was a tough, stubborn, strong-willed seven-and-a-half year old, with an older and a younger brother, who was popular with his mates, very gregarious and just loved his soccer.

I was worried about the up-coming MMR school campaign, but didn't know why, so rang the local public health nurse. I was sent the

1 Newman, A. 1997. "Jabs beats measles epidemic". *Christchurch Mail*, 3 November.
2 1997. "Local measles epidemic reverses national trend". *Christchurch Star*, 3 December.
3 Names have been changed for legal reasons.

official *Immunization Choices* booklet, and the measles pamphlet.

I signed the consent form, with a heavy heart, because it didn't sit totally right with me, but I didn't want my child to get encephalitis or die; what mother would?

The day of the shot was Friday, 20 June 1997.

Raymond got off the bus, crying. I asked him, "What's the matter?" He said, "I feel all hot, and I've got a horrible headache." I wanted to know, "When did it start?"

"After the injection," he replied.

The next morning, he seemed no better, but wanted to play soccer. His team depended on him, and he felt he would let them down if he didn't. So, even though he wasn't well, he went and played. He scored all the goals that day, but was exhausted when he came off the field, and slept for most of the remainder of the day.

I just made sure he had plenty to drink, gave him some Panadol, and sponged him down to control his fever. He had a headache, no energy and no appetite.

On Monday morning he seemed to look a bit better, but when he opened his mouth, he started asking stupid questions. "Where's Dad, I need to find Dad," but his father was there. He couldn't find his way around a house that had been his home for the previous two years. I even had to show him where the toilet was. We became very frightened and worried by his condition and decided to make an appointment with the family doctor as soon as it was opening time.

At the doctor's visit, I made the doctor aware that Raymond had just been vaccinated. The doctor said reactions were possible, but felt the headaches were more likely to be connected to the fact that I get headaches myself. He felt the deliriousness was the brain's reaction to high temperatures and to check that it wasn't something more serious, he would refer Raymond to a paediatrician. Unfortunately, there was a huge waiting list and it was going to take some time to get an appointment.

I took him home, watched him closely and nursed him as though he had a bad dose of the flu.

By Friday that week, Raymond was physically better, with no fever, but not right mentally. He didn't seem to be connecting things as he normally did. It was hard for me to put a finger on what the symptoms I was seeing, meant. I rang and explained Raymond's situation to his teacher and she suggested I send him to school and she would ring me if he wasn't coping and I'd go and get him. He lasted the day but came home exhausted.

Over July, Raymond's health was up and down, so I took him back to the doctor and asked him to test for everything and the rest besides. The only thing that showed was anaemia and he started taking Fergon. A welcome phone call was received in mid-July from the Paediatrician's nurse. There had been a cancellation the next day and could I come? Absolutely – I was looking forward to getting some answers, but as Raymond's high temperatures had settled and the deliriousness was pretty much gone, the paediatrician wasn't concerned about Raymond's vague unwellness and lethargy. He booked him in for a CT scan, but the appointment never came up before he died.

Over the next month Raymond suffered general unwellness, and was hoping he'd be well enough to go to his older brother's birthday party where they were going to play mini-golf. Anything to do with sport had Raymond's competitive nature keen to go. The day before the party, 13 August, Raymond started vomiting and had fevers and headaches again, so he missed the mini-golf. His brother brought him some lollies and cake, but he never got to eat them.

On Saturday the 16th of August, there was a soccer game. It was an important match for the team and he felt he had to go. I knew he couldn't play, but he was so unhappy with my decision, I told him I'd take him so he could watch and cheer his team-mates on. Just to get to and from the game was exhausting and when we got back home, he flaked out on the couch and went straight to sleep. When he woke, his temperature was back up, he had another headache and started vomiting all over the place.

By Tuesday Raymond was showing no signs of improving and when his Dad arrived home from work that evening we decided that we needed a doctor to see him. He was very ill – fever, occasionally vomiting and was delirious again. He was very wobbly on his feet and needed help walking.

However, the Doctor decided Raymond had the flu and home we went. I was very worried and kept thinking, "This has all happened since he was immunized," but obviously I was the only one who felt that way – none of the doctors we had seen and talked to about it, felt there was a link.

Raymond's bed was a top bunk but I didn't want him further off the floor than a mattress so we both slept in the lounge on mattresses. The night was very disturbed with Raymond vomiting and unsettled. Around 6.30 I woke and saw Raymond peaceful and still in his bed. He obviously had got to sleep. I got up and had a shower, then Raymond was going back to the doctor, and I wasn't being sent home again!

Halfway through my shower, I heard my husband yelling for me. I rushed out and found him holding Raymond who was fitting. I held him while my husband rang for an ambulance. Because we lived ten minutes out of town, he told the ambulance we'd drive in to meet it. With him driving and me and Raymond in the back, I realized Raymond wasn't breathing. I started mouth-to-mouth and continued for what seemed ages until we met the ambulance. What a relief! Someone else could take over the responsibility. As they took over, Raymond fitted again. They gave him oxygen and we raced to the small local hospital Accident and Emergency department. He was put on a ventilator and continued to fit until the medication he was given stopped the fits.

The hospital rang the retrieval team from the main hospital who flew down in the Westpac helicopter with a doctor and nurse and the equipment to keep him alive. I flew in the chopper with him while my husband drove home to organize the other children, grab us some bits and pieces, and then drive to the hospital.

Raymond was admitted to the Intensive Care Unit where the specialist asked lots of questions. Every time we tried to ask him about the vaccine, he kept saying, "It can't be the vaccine, because we've never seen anything like this from the vaccine before." They just wouldn't listen.

He was tested for a whole lot of things including blood tests, a lumbar puncture and a CT scan. All the important tests gave negative results, and they couldn't tell us what was causing the coma. They couldn't give us a time frame, but they expected him to come out of it. We stayed close to him, looking for any sign of change. Then in the early hours of the next morning we noticed a nurse flash her torch light onto Raymond's eyes – she redid it – then went to get a colleague to do the same. His eyes were big, black and very scary! The specialist organized for Raymond to have another CT scan – this time they found something – there was some swelling to the brain. He was put on a cold mattress to try to reduce swelling and obviously received medication – but I wasn't aware of what he was being treated for specifically – it was all a blur.

During the day various family members and friends arrived to share our distress and support us. Nothing changed and the seriousness of the situation was devastating and terribly frightening. By Thursday afternoon the doctors were concerned about the blood flow to Raymond's brain and did another CT scan. The worst news came back. His brain had swelled so much that the blood supply was cut off and although he was being kept alive by machines, his brain was dead.

We were now able to do what we had wanted to do over the two previous days which was to take him off the bed and hold him in our arms and cuddle him tight. Only this was for the last time. We had decided to turn the ventilator off and let him join his Nana and two Poppas in Heaven. Fifteen minutes later we could feel his body going really cold and knew he had slipped away from this life on 21 August, two months and one day after receiving the MMR vaccine.

We discussed with the specialists the possibility of using Raymond's organs to help someone else, but they refused, saying that because they didn't know what he died of, they couldn't do that.

The subject of an autopsy came up, to find a cause, but they said we needed to be the ones to decide whether to have an autopsy or not – what an awful decision to make when your child has just died. We didn't want an autopsy right then, but looking back we wish the doctors had done one. After all, they didn't know what had caused all this. We both felt that the MMR vaccine was the start of all the trouble, and maybe, had there been a proper autopsy, and proper blood work done, something might have been found that would have given us something other than no answer.

(Addendum: one blood test showed positive to Coxsackie virus.)

Raymond wasn't the only child to land up in ICU in hospital. There was a child in Hawke's Bay Hospital, another in Christchurch Hospital, another who lived in Marton, another in Auckland. Later I heard a child died in Palmerston North Hospital after being given the MMR vaccine. From around the country, I heard from eight parents (other than Raymond's) whose children had been in hospital. I heard from parents about a few very sick children who had not been admitted to hospital. But all the children had had similar, though not so dramatic, unwanted direct effects from the MMR.

I wonder how many MORE children reacted to the MMR, whose parents weren't listened to either, who didn't know about the Immunization Awareness Society, and had no one to talk to about what they were seeing?

It will be interesting in future to see if we continue to be told that there were no reactions to the MMR vaccine in 1997, because . . . no one had ever seen it before in this country, or any other, so it doesn't exist.

The remark that sticks in my mind most of all when one mother first told me her story, was of when she left the hospital. A nurse who had been there and seen it all, stopped them as they were going out. She had heard what was said, and knew the parents considered the vaccine to be the cause. She said to the mother very quietly, before she left, "Don't think that your child is the only one who's been in here after the MMR. He's not." And walked off.

60 The Secret

"I want to let you in on a secret!"

Has anyone ever said that to you?

Have you ever said it?

Then something else is added, in a very serious and confidential way.

"Promise you won't tell anyone."

Of course, as everyone knows, that's the quickest way to make sure everyone does know!!

Well, I ***want*** *to let you in on a "secret".*

And I ***want*** *you to tell anyone and everyone.*

You may already know it, but for some people in high places, it is very hush-hush.

Did you know that in most, if not all systems, those in authority presume a superiority, an expertise, about how to live, raise children, become or stay healthy, how to know what is right or wrong, and what the "truth" is. They try to control the details of our every thought, act and decision. They want to do this so we will yield to their opinions – to be conformed and compliant.

My reaction to this "state secret" is indignation. "What makes anyone presume that they know better than I do? Do they think they know everything and I know nothing?"

Bluster, fume, rant and rave!

At last I calm down sufficiently to ask another question:

"What happens when they're proved wrong; when faced with failure; when statistics don't show the right figures?"

Well, the answer is usually that they increase doing what they're doing now. They do more of the things that have already failed. This may include more control and more money spent. Lying by omission is also a favourite ploy.

Do you want to share my "secret" with others?

Or for your own peace of mind, stop thinking? Keep it hush-hush and become a clone!

Knowing the truth can hurt.

Knowing the truth is costly.

Knowing the truth can be dangerous.

It's not easy, is it, but then no-one ever said it would be.

61 Pita James Highland

My son was born on 2 July 1996. I have a history of being allergic to penicillin and sulpha drugs and have a sibling family history of asthma and allergies. Pita's father is partly deaf and has migraines sometimes.

Right up until six weeks, the Plunket nurse was really pleased with Pita's development, so he had his first DPTH, first HepB, and first oral polio vaccines. At eight weeks he developed intermittent vomiting, which continued for a long time. Later I was told the name for this is Gastro-oesophageal reflux and that he would grow out of it. I asked the Plunket nurse what the rash on the top of his chest, under his chin, was. She didn't know, but thought it might be fungal and wrote that in his book. It gradually turned into eczema, and then spread onto his tummy, his wrists, his knees and stayed there for years.

Ten days after his three-month shots he developed a cold, and a few days later, ear infections and so he was put on antibiotics. Because his weight was below 50% on the graph, he was put onto SMA, and his weight quickly climbed up to the 75% mark.

On his nine month assessment, everything was perfect. Then at ten months, on 12 May 1997, just before lunch I took him to the doctor because he had had a cold for four days, was coughing, bunged up and had green mucus coming out of his nose. The doctor gave him Amoxil, and then vaccinated him with MMR.

He cried at lot that afternoon, and was very tired and whingy.

He wouldn't play with my brother when he came home, which was unusual, and was generally grumpy. Two days later, he broke out in a rash on his body. His cold got worse and I thought maybe it was a flu.

After that, he only ate little bits of food, and generally moped around, and often appeared sleepy. Then I noticed he was not moving smoothly any more. Sometimes it was jerky, like when he was a little baby. Then he started to have awful smelly poos. Not diarrhoea, but just horrible smelling. These have continued ever since, when Pita gets stressed by anything.

Also one eye was looking inwards, so I rang the doctor and made an appointment. A few days later (4 June 1997) the doctor, who said he had a "right squint" referred him to hospital for the squint and also because he had started vomiting every day, several times.

Then, on the morning of 10 June, he was really strange for quite a long time. He went stiff, floppy and then went to sleep, so I took him straight around to the doctor. The doctor didn't seem concerned and thought he was okay, but wrote in the notes that he was not eating and just wanted to sleep and had been floppy.

Over the next few days I noticed little things but not enough to really get upset about, but gradually Pita stopped vocalizing, and also stopped crawling and trying to sit, so I made another appointment with the doctor on the 15th. His eczema was getting worse as well.

The squint was worse, and the doctor decided to refer him back to hospital again, as he also now had *alternating strabismus* which means that both eyes looked inwards sometimes.

We got in to hospital on 23 June. The only thing apart from the squint that they noticed was that he didn't have much body tone. They wrote "hypotonia" in his file, but weakness on his right side. They felt his head was a bit small as well, and wrote "global developmental delay". I tried to describe what I was worried about, but they didn't seem to think it was important.

They thought maybe, because there had been some dips on his foetal heart monitor in my labour, that it was lack of oxygen in labour.

But in August things got really bad. On the 10th, he started having lots of seizures. By this time, I knew what they were, whereas in the beginning we didn't know if he was staring, or what he was doing. He had three seizures within 90 minutes so I took him to hospital. They weren't sure what to make of my descriptions and I thought they didn't believe me, but then he had one in front of them, so they were able to see for themselves, and they wrote their own description.

I took him to the doctor again on the 21st, because the seizures were happening a lot, and the doctor gave us an urgent referral to the hospital.

On the 25th, he had a big seizure lasting 20 minutes. We finally got to hospital on the urgent referral on the 27th and they sent him for a Cat scan, and we went home. The next day he had more seizures.

On 4 September we were back in because he'd had more seizures, and was very flushed, out of it, and had a rash over his body. He didn't have a temperature or anything.

Another interesting thing is that the hospital records show that every time he went in to hospital, they always gave him paracetamol. Even after this visit, if we landed up in ED, the first thing they did was give him paracetamol. They did a spinal tap and lots of tests. They put him on Cisapride, but that made it worse, so they stopped that.

They noted ***"used to wave, now doesn't; used to crawl around furniture, now doesn't. Falls to Left side a lot more . . . skull shape abnormal . . ."*** Under impression: ***"developmental regression – neuro-developmental . . . degenerative condition/metabolic."*** We went home on the 8th September. The discharge letter said ***"Gastro-oesophageal reflux, delayed development and seizure disorder"***, and they wanted him to have an EEG. He was referred for hearing tests and to an ophthalmologist for the strabismus.

On 26 September we went for the EEG and Pita had a seizure in the middle of it, and again at the end.

The hearing tests came back normal, the CT scan was normal, and the ophthalmologist didn't see the squint that day, so he said Pita was normal.

On 2 November, he had seizures all day. On 30 November, the hospital faxed the EEG results to our doctor. They said it was abnormal with "erratic epileptiform disturbances multi-focal in origin" and affecting both sides of the brain.

For those interested, amongst the tests, the Cerebrospinal fluid tests and other bug tests came back normal. Abnormal results showed that the Alk Phos was very high, Chloride was low, the Neutrophils and monocytes were below normal, and his PCO2 and ACT Bicarb were also low.

On 5 March 1998, we saw the paediatrician because Pita had a rotavirus, and he had had more seizures. They reassessed everything, and said the problem was microcephaly. They explained this by saying that his head had stopped growing and it was genetic, and that it was defective "karotypes genes" in us. Or something. We wanted tests done. The doctor said they weren't necessary, but we had them done anyway, and they came back clear. They decided to order an MRI. We stayed there three days. Every day they gave him paracetamol every four hours . . .

The MRI was done on the 18th, and on 26th the results came back normal.

We were very unhappy about the diagnosis. It seemed silly. To us, we couldn't get passed the fact that he was fine before the MMR.

Also, Pita had started banging his head on the wall. Really hard, and he didn't cry. He would do it about three times a day. It was as if there was something annoying him.

He started pinching people and playing differently, repetitively and was starting to get very rough, and frustrated.

His hurt reflexes were strange too, and still are. If he jammed his fingers he would wait about five seconds, then maybe cry, or maybe not. I started to have to watch him around fires and the oven, because he didn't seem to register heat for a while, like the jamming of the fingers. He was leaning to the left a lot. When he drank something he drank to the left, looked to the left, and used his left arm more than his right. Everything on his right side just didn't work properly.

Not long after that my mother saw an article by Hilary Butler, in *Healthy Options*, so we rang her, and we both had a long talk to her.

She didn't agree with the Microcephaly diagnosis and felt it was a fob-off. She said she had heard of other children diagnosed like that, but after they had had cranial osteopathy their heads grew again. The closest person to us who she knew of was a naturopath, Paul Hume, so we went to see him. We decided not to tell Paul what the problem was but just ask him to look at Pita and tell us how he saw him. He checked him all over and when he got to the head, he said the head plates were locked together. Then we told him about the vaccine, and the diagnosis. He treated Pita for it twice. Not long after that, at another Plunket session the medical staff were very surprised, because his head had started to grow again.

Hilary also suggested we see Dr Mike Godfrey. He gave us some remedies to help detoxify the system. Pita's eczema went away completely straight after that and the seizures stopped, so I took him off his medication. He never had another seizure again. We noticed a big difference within weeks.

But there were still some things that were worrying me. Pita was still not talking. He was walking better, but with his feet wider apart. There were no more seizures though, and his head kept growing.

We went back to the specialists in July, who were also surprised to see his head growing again, and that his seizures had stopped, so they referred us to a Neurologist. On the first visit on 15 January 1999, the neurologist wasn't sure what was wrong, but didn't think it was microcephaly. Pita was okay, except his eyes, and the doctor called the condition esotropia. But his head shape and size were fine.

She thought it was encephalopathy, and that it could be from the MMR, but first she wanted to do more tests to see if there was a *"mitochondrial"* cause for the encephalopathy, and wanted more tests to rule out *"underlying metabolic predisposing"* conditions. It was the first time anyone had mentioned *"encephalopathy"* to us. Up until then, it had been blamed on my labour, or microcephaly.

After the tests came back, Pita was evaluated by another professor who agreed, and we applied for ACC for encephalopathy following the MMR vaccination. On 19 October 1999, we got a letter saying it had been approved. ACC then sent us for more evaluations and assessments by another Professor, and a serious injury scoping report, which found that Pita was now displaying autistic features as well.

Pita is now at a special school for disabled children. We haven't been back to hospital for sickness since early 1999, and he doesn't have seizures at all. Pita has a new paediatrician now, who doesn't believe it was the vaccine. He told us that vaccines don't do those sorts of things. As far as we are concerned, we know what we know, and he isn't going to convince us otherwise.

When we first took Pita to the special needs school, the principal told us there were a few children at the school funded by ACC. There is another boy Pita's age who had exactly the same things happen, except he's on medication. But he has the same problems as well. His parents think his was from vaccinations, but they never pushed the doctors for a proper explanation like we did, and didn't go for compensation from the vaccine.

Ever since we saw Mike Godfrey, Pita's never been sick or had a seizure, all his eczema went, and has never returned. But he still gets these horrible smelly poos all the time if his routine is changed or he gets stressed. So we are going to go back to Mike Godfrey soon, because we think there must be something else we can do to help Pita. I've looked at all sorts of treatments, including supplements, but Pita is like other autistic children. Getting him to take tablets or eat different food to normal is almost impossible.

While he has *"autistic spectrum"* behaviours, we think he's more *"Asperger's"* than *"autistic"*, because he's too intelligent for the class he's in, and too intelligent for the next class up. The occupational therapist has told us that she also thinks he's more Asperger's than autistic, and we'd like to mainstream him to see if that will help. But the nearest school with a satellite class isn't fenced. He has to be in a fenced area, or else he will wander off.

We are sure he can read, because every now and again, he sees words and tries to say them. But he can't express himself verbally well enough, because he will only say 30 words, and his ability to say sounds, gets jumbled. He can understand ordinary sign language, but won't use it. He will only use the sign language he makes up for himself.

We know he understands everything we say perfectly. He responds to anything we ask him to do. We think that he is thinking normally, but he can't say what he needs to say, and we can't work out his thinking, or what his frustrations are, and that is the hardest thing to live with. We don't know how to assess his intelligence, or how to progress it so that he can learn better, we can understand him better, and encourage him to try harder. Perhaps he's too lazy, because everyone assumes "he can't" at the special school. And maybe we do too, but it's very hard to assess what he can say and what he can't. Being clever, he may be having us on a lot of the time.

We want to do more for Pita, but vitamin and mineral supplements are very expensive, and alternative medicine is too. ACC hasn't offered to pay for any of that so we are limited in what we feel we can do.

The biggest problem within family life, is that Pita still doesn't feel pain, and doesn't understand consequences. He's gone through stages of setting things on fire, sucking water from the toilet into the vacuum cleaner, putting water in the drier and the TV remote in the microwave and switching the microwave on, which caused a fire. He pulled a jug over onto himself and scalded himself and after we sorted that out, he went straight back to do it again. So I had to buy a different jug to stop him doing that.

Sometimes, dangerous situations just make him laugh hysterically when it involves himself. When he set his mattress on fire he thought it was funny. But if he sees someone else frightened or upset, because of something he has done, then he won't do it again.

He's really on to it in many ways. He can manipulate situations, and get out of doing something he doesn't want to do. The problem with that is he also picks up other people's bad habits as well. The other children at his school are more autistic than he is and do things I don't want Pita to do. He sometimes copies them just to see if there is a pay-off for doing that. He sees them get what they want when they do that. But we try not to let him get away with that.

Physically, he's still weak on the left side, and sometimes we wonder if perhaps it wasn't so much encephalopathy, but maybe that he had a stroke.

Pita is certainly autistic in one sense. He has supersonic hearing and he loves wind chimes. He buys them at the market, and carries them around with him, sleeps with them and plays with them until they are broken. The sound fascinates him, and he has a huge collection of useless wind chimes. If he hears one, houses away, he has to go and find it. When the Harcourt's "houses for sale" magazine comes, he will look through it to find all the wind chimes in the pictures.

Pita is nearly ten. But he's the size of a 14-year-old. A lot of the children who have the same problems as he has are also large for their age.

Every second weekend he goes to a community house around the corner on Saturday morning until Sunday night. Living with a child like Pita is so stressful that I need time out just to unwind, and give his younger brother, Dre, the time he needs.

Dre is not vaccinated, and never will be. He has never had eczema, or any health problems at all. He's three, talking well, and was toilet trained at two, whereas Pita is still in night nappies. In so many ways, we can see in Dre what Pita could have been. When you live with a child like Pita, you can't plan anything. He doesn't like routines being broken, or doing new things. We live day by day, and it's very hard.

People often come and ask me about vaccines, but I won't talk about them. I tell people to go and research it and make up their own minds. To talk about them just brings back all the hurts, and I remember all the times when I kept saying to the doctors it was the vaccine, and they always said that it couldn't be. "Vaccines don't do that. We've not seen it before."

Well, that's strange, because I know a lot of people now, who think that their damaged children were damaged by vaccines but their doctors say the same things to them too.

I wonder how many Pitas there are out there, whose mothers have been ignored as well.

They didn't have a supportive mother like I did. I'd like to thank my mother here, in this book. Without her support and her coming with me to all the appointments, and pushing me to carry on trying to find out what was wrong, I might have given up like most other people do. It was my mother who pushed and pushed. It was her anger at the constant denial of the paediatricians that kept me focused through the despair and hurt that I felt.

There are other people I'd thank too, but I'd rather not accidentally miss one out. You know who you are, and all I can say is thank you.

I also want to talk about what I regret. After the vaccine when things started to go wrong, people would say, "Oh, that's normal" but it wasn't. I wish I'd taken Pita to the doctor earlier. But looking back, perhaps there was no point. Apart from tests, and drugs and fobbing me off, hospital doctors didn't have anything to offer Pita to help him get better, apart from loads of paracetamol. My GP was very sympathetic and very persistent trying to get the specialists to see Pita, but he didn't know how to help either. The first person to recognize what the problem actually was, was the neurologist, for which we are very thankful, because the funding from ACC is the only thing that enables us to get some help. Without that, I don't know what we would do.

I wish I'd asked a lot more questions about a lot of things. Looking back, I trusted people too much and didn't ask enough questions, or push enough at the beginning.

62 The Day the Nurse Jabbed Herself

Mary Smith stretched and sighed as she thought about the new day before her. Twenty new-entrant five-year-olds occupied so much of her time and energies. She had all sorts of activities planned for her class today. First up there would be a visit from . . .

The phone rang. Mary groped for the receiver somewhere near her pillow.

"Hello".

"Hello Mary. It's Leigh White here. Sorry to ring so early, but I won't be able to do that health talk with your class this morning. I'm having a day or two off. I don't feel too good at all."

"Nothing serious, I hope," said Mary, already trying to rearrange her day.

"No, I don't think so. I don't know whether there's any connection but I was giving a baby another injection the other day. The little rascal must have recognized me and started to struggle and scream. To cut a long story short, I jabbed myself in my thumb. It's never happened before. But I think I'd better err on the side of caution. I'll call in and make another time for that talk. I've got a few catch-up jabs to do at the school. See you."

"O.K. Bye for now," said Mary as she rolled out of bed.

Sometime later Mary Smith sat on her little chair surrounded by her class of children. The settling-down routines had been completed and fertile minds were waiting for Miss Smith to speak.

"Well children, Miss White the Health Nurse was going to visit us this morning, but unfortunately she can't come. Let's just have our usual morning talks time, but instead of you giving me all your news, I'd like us to talk about the work Miss White does. Hands up those of you who have met Miss White before you started school?"

A few hands went up somewhat tentatively.

"Can anyone tell me what her work is?" prompted Miss Smith.

"She comes to see sick people," called out Terry.

"She gives people injections," said Rangi, "and they're not nice."

Rangi's comment seemed to awaken memories and soon a number of children were clamouring to be heard.

"One at a time please. What do you want to say, Jamie?"

"Yeah. They hurt. She told me that it was just a little prick and I wouldn't feel it. But I did and my arm was sore for a . . ."

"But I like the sweets and stickers she gives . . ." interrupted Rachel.

"She stuck a needle into our little baby's bottom and he screamed awful loud," added Beth.

"Miss Smiff, my Mum says that when I was a wee baby I got some jabs and I did the same thing. She said I was unconsellable because I cried so much."

Miss Smith smiled at the last speaker. "Jackie, I'm sure your Mummy said that you were inconsolable."

"No she didn't," insisted Jackie. "She said she wouldn't even have been able to give me away. I carried on for hours. I was unsellable, my Mum said!"

In an attempt to change the subject, Miss Smith asked, "Who doesn't cry when they get immunized?"

Quite a lot of hands went up.

"You're a fibber Robert," accused Helen. "I saw you crying at Kindy and your Mum had to help you blow your nose."

"That's not true," said Robert. "I had a cold and a runny nose. Anyway, what about you? You can't talk!"

"Maybe we should think about what you should do next time, seeing that you are all getting to be big people now. Perhaps we should all learn how to grin and pretend it doesn't hurt. We can practise what we could call our "vaccination smiles" every time we look in a mirror. Don't you think that would be a good idea? After all we need to get used to having these little pricks."

"I don't want any more," declared Billy. "My Mum and Dad are going to write a notice on my arms if there are any more injections at school so that the nurse can see them, and I won't get jabbed."

"You don't have to have them," said Gaylene quietly. "I heard Mum talking to Dad about it. That's why I haven't had any. That's right, isn't it Miss Smith?"

Mary Smith thought it was about time she moved on to something more comfortable and unrelated, like Numeracy. "We'll get Nurse White to talk about that when she comes next time."

As Mary started to collect the maths equipment, she couldn't help musing to herself, "Phew! Who'd be a health nurse? Trying to get kids to like you by sticking needles into them. I'm glad no one asked me what I do when that happens to me! Poor little Jackie! Unconsellable! What a price to pay!"

63 Diphtheria? Check-Mated

One of the hats I wore years ago was that of a gymnastics coach. I had decided to throw this hat in the ring again, because our eldest needed a couple of years' gymnastics to improve his timing and flexibility. To save money, I agreed to teach again. As I loved being with the kids and seeing them achieve, it was no hardship.

Officially in 1992, there were ***zero*** cases of diphtheria. But that isn't actually the whole story.

It was June. A fellow coach had a daughter at the club, one of a group of elite gymnasts who regularly travelled over to the North Shore, in order to take advantage of the skills of a newly immigrated Russian coach. He occasionally came over to the club as well, as we had some promising gymnasts in the club.

That week, a fellow coach arrived in a real sweat, none too happy about her daughter who wasn't well. By Friday lunchtime, the girl was seriously ill, and the doctor called an ambulance, to take her to a large hospital where she was put on life support, stabilized and flown to a more suitable hospital. This mother's aunt had been a nurse in the 1940s. She arrived at the hospital to visit ICU, looked the child over, smelled mouse and sagely nodded her head. "Diphtheria," she said.

On Monday morning, a doctor queried the test results because it was positive only for diphtheria, and the notes said the child was immunized. The mother confirmed that was so. The doctor replied that they had better do some more tests then, since it couldn't possibly be diphtheria in an immunized child. The new tests came back positive again for diphtheria, but with the addition of haemophilus as well.

The discharge letter said that the tests had shown diphtheria and haemophilus but that the clinical disease was compatible with neither.

Then a friend told me that another child from the club, with identical symptoms, was taken to hospital. This had to remain hearsay, because, my friend told me, the parents didn't want to talk to me. But a week later she told me that they hadn't been given a clear diagnosis either. They'd been told something about "infected asthma" and a strange word which made no sense to me, unless it was epiglottitis and they had heard it wrong.

I shrugged my shoulders. The only thing different at the club since the beginning of June had been a strange sort of cough everyone had, but in winter you expect the odd cough.

The girl came back to gymnastics. She was worked quietly to one side of my group one day, not doing that much, but I wasn't chuffed with either her timing, or her colour. As any coach can tell you, there comes a level where timing is crucial in gymnastics. It's an unforgiving sport, and the potential for serious injury looms if your timing is off. I went over to this girl, and took her heart rate. For someone doing not much, a heart rate over 200 a minute was a big deal. It only came down to 160. When her mother arrived, I sat down with her and told her I was worried.

"Why?" she asked.

"Well, have they resolved the issue of what she had yet?"

"No," she said. "Why?"

"I think you need to. Her heart rate is high, and I don't like her colour or her timing. If it was diphtheria then she should not be here. Clinical diphtheria is serious, and can stress the heart, and she is just not well enough to be doing this. If it was diphtheria, then you should know. Then you know what you are dealing with, and what she might be able to cope with."

"Well, what can we do now? It's all over!"

"No it's not," I replied. "You can have the hospital sample tested for diphtheria antibodies, and have another one drawn and retested. Even a third if you want. You need to look for a four-fold increase in diphtheria antibodies. Find that out, and then you will have your answer. Ask them to check for diphtheria, haemophilus or both, but ask them not to leave you hanging like this."

She asked her doctor, who didn't know and asked the hospital. They said it wasn't necessary. The mother started to push and probably would have made enough fuss to make them do it, except that her daughter had had enough needles stuck into her, and refused to do it.

Fair enough. I could relate to that. My eight months in bed at the age of 16 had been one long monotonous bi-weekly vampire session, so why push something?

Then something happened to make me somewhat annoyed. I heard from a friend that there was a bit or gossip amongst a few parents who knew I tended to challenge convention with regard to vaccines. A huge spread in *Metro* six months before had possibly fuelled the talk. One day, a comment reached my ears that someone was suggesting that just maybe, my unvaccinated kids might have brought something into the club and caused all the trouble.

That made me very angry. After all, even if my children had brought diphtheria into the club, shouldn't the vaccine have worked in others? And how come my kids weren't in hospital on life support?

The social implications of this hit like a brick. Just imagine what would happen if MY CHILD landed up in hospital, on life support, with these symptoms, these test results and a blank vaccination chart!

You can hear it now. Papers and TV stations, hounding us daily. A newsreader intoning

"Nation brought to knees by non-vaccinating monster mother . . ." Well, probably not the "monster" bit, but it would be insinuated.

I would have been media mincemeat, which made me want to get to the bottom of what the problem with these two children was. I asked around locally, and found that other children in the schools where gym club children came from, had this cough as well. Maybe it wasn't just a cough, because the two kids in hospital just started with a cough.

An edgy comment here, an odd angry look at me there, made me realize how easy it would be for most people to follow the majority and cave in to pressure. One of the few positives of being a vaccinating parent is that you can't be treated like lepers of old, or modern pariahs, and doctors can't irrationally accuse you of starting a diphtheria epidemic amongst vaccinated kids.

Of course, in the event of a vaccinated child being proven to be the first case, they would have said to that mother, "Never mind, you did the right thing."

Under these circumstances it isn't easy being a non-vaccinating parent, so I decided to take the bull by the horns. I went to see a doctor I knew who was tolerant of my position, and explained the whole situation to him. He asked me what I wanted to do about it.

In my frustration I said, "Well, you know, if the Health Department was to actually take this seriously instead of seemingly covering it up, they should come out here and swab the whole gym club, the schools these kids go to, and find out what this is. They know FULL WELL that there is an epidemic in Russia and . . . (a light dawned . . .) you know what? Some of these kids have been working with Russian coaches . . . there is a newish Russian émigré community over North Shore . . . do you think that . . .? What do you think? I wonder what would happen if they typed her diphtheria sample, and typed it back to the Russian strains going around?"

He hadn't known about that. I knew, because there was a huge fuss at the time, when parents in Russia refused to have their kids and themselves jabbed yet again. A friend of mine from Alaska had sent me articles about it. The authorities were refusing to use single-use syringes, and the fact that the children had already had so many diphtheria jabs previously was making many Russian mothers rebel. The Russian media was also full of it, and reporting dissent readily.

I had also spoken to some Russian doctors who weren't happy, because while the American CDC doctors were saying that Russians weren't vaccinating enough babies, these doctors pointed out to me that by the time many Russian adults got to their mid-twenties, they had actually had eight (8) diphtheria shots, and if they were in the medical field, the police or the military they would have had ten shots, and that most of the cases they saw, were more than fully vaccinated by Western standards.

"I think," this doctor said, "I'll have a quiet word on the side, with a friend of mine in Wellington."

A few nights later, he rang me at home. Surprisingly he said that people in Wellington not only knew about the two cases, but also knew

I was a gymnastics coach at the club. I wondered with whom they had been talking. What business of theirs was that? As to the Russia issue, apparently that hadn't crossed their minds, and the person spoken to, thought my reasoning rather funny. Seemingly they were more interested in what I might do . . .

"What do you mean?" I said, not understanding. After all, if I believed the story that these girls had been on life-support for nothing in particular, there would be nothing I would do.

"Well," he said, "As you know the two 'disputed isolates' came from vaccinated children. If for example, you decide to insist that further testing be done, or if you had your two boys tested and they came back diphtheria positive, they would come here. But the Public Health Act entitles them to not only test who they want, but vaccinate anyone, whether they consent or not."

"Righty then," I said, incredulous. "So I have two choices. Keep my mouth shut, and do nothing, or open my mouth and possibly my kids pay."

"That might about sum it up," he said.

I left the issue alone.

Are you thinking . . . *Cowardice*?

I decided to keep my mouth shut for other reasons as well. The main reason was that, as I said, it's hard to be a non-vaccinating parent with flot like that going around. I was learning what it is like to live in a whispering society where a tiny minority talk behind your back.

Had I pressed the issue just to shut up a tiny clique of people, not only would my kids have been at the rough end of the deal, but so would I.

Can you imagine what the parents of all the kids the Health Department might have lined up, to test, then maybe decide to treat, would have THEN said about me, and to my face?

The whole issue would have been opened up to broad gossip, not just a few discontents. I, the "unvaccinating" parent, "was now requiring all stones to be turned . . ." What for? Maybe to protect my unvaccinated children? Was I now running scared? Hiding behind all their vaccinated kids? The possible flow-on implications to me as a person, and my children from their children were very clear, if I made it an issue.

What if the Health Department did find diphtheria? What then? Would it be prophylactic antibiotics en masse, and public vaccination clinics? Would I get the blame for that too, and become a public pariah?

I certainly wasn't scared of diphtheria. I knew enough about the disease to know what I would do if push came to shove with regard to a clinical diphtheria infection. I discussed that and all the ramifications of Health Department involvement with the doctor, and decided that it was discreet to walk away from it. I knew that diphtheria isn't nearly as infectious, or as scary as the medical profession would have us believe, and that in a society like ours today, it is highly unlikely to produce membranes or the more serious manifestations in the majority of people. That has been borne out since, by just who in Russia succumbed to serious disease. Contrary to publicity, the highest rates of deaths occurred in predominantly well-vaccinated people who became susceptible, not through lack of vaccines, but because of war, social dislocation, food shortages. The group who had the highest death rates were the vaccinated homeless alcoholics. Go on to Ukraine's TV channel[1] and you will see that TB levels are epidemic. So are typhoid, measles and the flu. None of that is to do with lack of vaccines. It's due to the appalling socio-economic situation exemplified by an item from the military bemoaning the lack of recruits because of the unhealthy state of the young.

I thought that would be the end of the story, and wrote it all up, pretty much as it is here, except with the title of "Politically incorrect disease" and filed it under "useless information", where it remained until August 1998.

---

1 Ukraine TV available from <http://5tv.com.ua/>

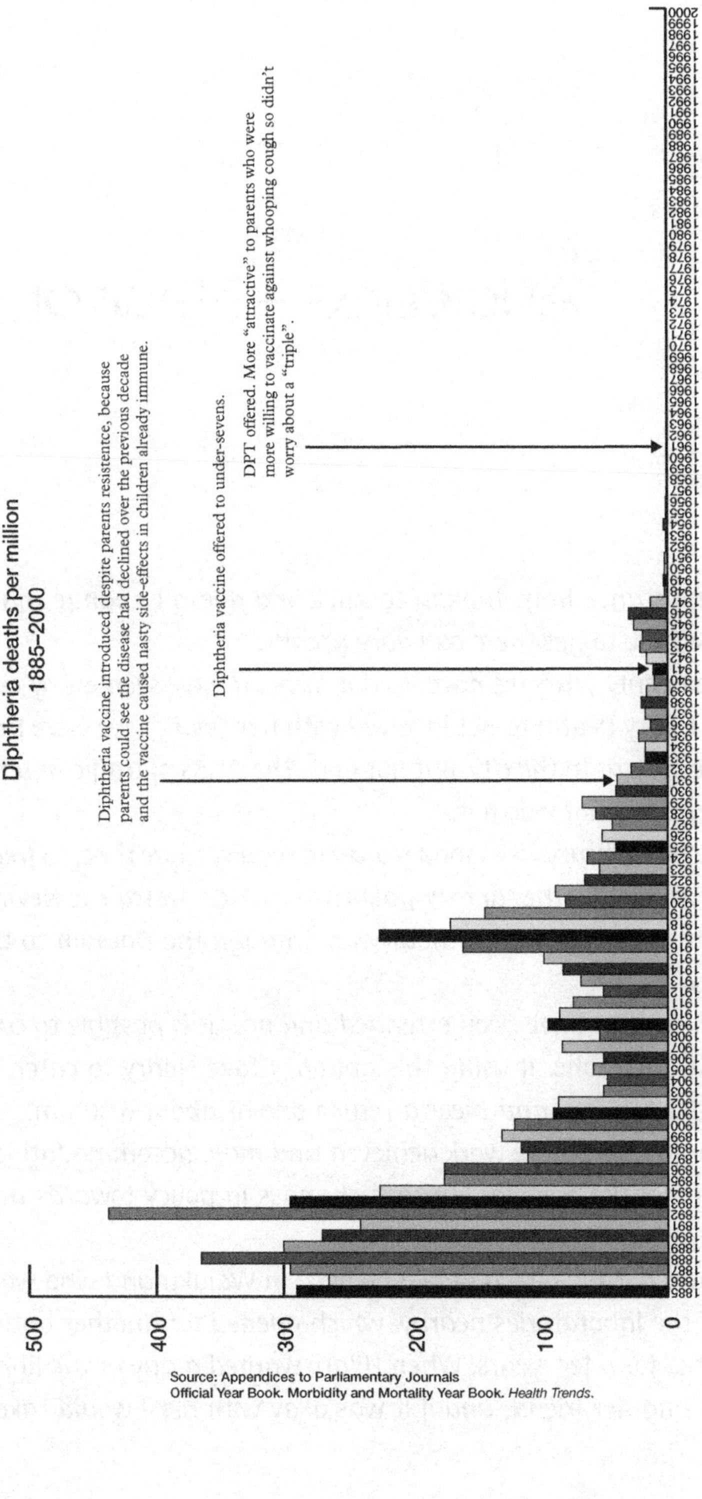

Source: Appendices to Parliamentary Journals
Official Year Book. Morbidity and Mortality Year Book. *Health Trends*.

64 Auckland – Near or Far

The distance from Tuakau to Auckland doesn't change much, but the time to get there can vary greatly.

The twenty years we have lived in Tuakau have seen many changes. When Hilary began to get involved with her "work", we were prepared to take our car to the city. But not now. The stress of traffic and parking problems are not worth it.

The Med Library visits soon began to require more time, so frequently Hilary would take the car to Papakura and catch the train to Newmarket. From there it is a quarter-hour walk through the Domain to the Med Library.

Rail services have been extended and now it is possible to catch the train at Pukekohe. If using this option, I take Hilary to catch a train at about 7.15 am and meet a return one at about 6.30 pm. A longer day for her, but more work achieved and more accommodating of the vagaries of the medical library's changes in policy towards members of the general public.

Hilary got to know a lady who lived in Waiuku and who worked at one of the laboratories nearby, which opened up another option that was used for a few years. When Hilary wanted a day at the library she would ring her friend, and if it was okay with her I would take Hilary to a meeting place where the Waiuku and Pukekohe roads merge, and they would go together in her friend's car. I'd pick her up again in the afternoon.

These types of arrangement could also be used if Hilary had a day-meeting in Auckland. However, if a radio or TV station wanted Hilary for an interview or talkback at night or early in the morning, then they had no option but to arrange taxis, or no Hilary!

As the children grew older it became more difficult to combine Hilary's "work" requirements with other family activities. There were too many conflicts of interest to fit together the times available to do things, within the restrictions of transport time-tables.

It is pleasant to live well away from the rat-race of the City, but if you have to spend a day breathing the traffic fumes and trying to cope with the rush and bustle then you pay for it in more ways than one!

65 The Making of a Pariah

I watched in dismay as the TV cameras and written media started ramping up a story about a wee boy, who had contracted the "killer" disease diphtheria, which was now threatening Auckland, and the nation, and, while we are at it, all unimmunized children should be banned . . . And their parents . . . well, you'd think we lived in the middle ages.

Who needs "burning at the stake" when you see what the medical profession can do in the media?

All those thoughts and feelings that had coursed through our family discussions in 1992 came to the fore. The media were shown on TV, camping outside the family's house. The family were trapped in their own home. I decided that whatever the situation, I would be there for them, because I was pretty sure they would be hung out to dry.

Over the next few days, at every opportunity, I asked questions on the radio, rang reporters, asked if they had seen the test results. Nothing. Then . . . I had an anonymous call from someone in the system to let me know that the tests were equivocal. Yes, there was a diphtheria isolate, but there was also a Strep A pyogenes isolate as well. And there were no clinical symptoms compatible with diphtheria.

I was due to go in to the TV studio two days later, to appear with Nikki Turner and presenter Susan Woods. I walked in, to find the intellectual temperatures were freezing, and if looks could have killed, the camera-operators would have also been dead. Nikki Turner however, was very chirpily seated next to Susan, who leaned forward in what appeared to me to be a very buddy way, and informed her that she had just had a diphtheria booster.

Not a good start. As the programme progressed I could see it was getting nowhere and felt that Susan Woods was making sure that I got little traction, or none at all. I didn't agree with anything Nikki Turner (the doctor who headed the pro-vaccine organization called the Immunization Advisory Centre (IMAC) was saying, but hardly got a chance to challenge it. Suddenly it was all over and I was unceremoniously ushered to the corridor. Wondering how all that had happened, I regathered my wits, while Nikki Turner bounced out of the studio, looking to me as if she had eaten two months' worth of Irish cream.

At the end of that week, the parents snuck out of hiding to come and see me, after they had heard some of my interviews on the radio, and seen me on TV. The father told me they had requested privacy and for their names not to be released to the media for the sake of the children, but their request was denied.

The inference made in the papers, on TV and talkback radio was that they were horrible people who had brought diphtheria into the community because they didn't vaccinate their son. The constant hammering by the medical profession with this innuendo was starting to impact on their relationships with the community and their friends, and the hysteria and nastiness on talkback programmes after Nikki Turner's appearance on Susan Woods' show, was just about the last straw for them.

The first thing I suggested, was to get a full set of the hospital files. What a drama that turned out to be.

EVENTUALLY they managed to get them. The files were very interesting. The parents then went to the news media wanting their side of the story told, but a late story is a dead story, so they got flicked off.

It would mean showing that an unvaccinated child was used mercilessly at huge cost to a family, as a medical political football. Just as I might have been, in 1992, had things been rather different for us.

So what exactly did happen?

Here is the story from the medical files, and the family. It is the story they were never allowed to tell. I hope it makes up for the years of pain that were to follow:

On 30 June 1998, the boy's grandparents arrived at his house to take care of him while his parents and brother went to Indonesia for a holiday. Because their oldest son had had a severe reaction to the DPT vaccine, the parents had decided not to vaccinate the younger son. He was in the care of his grandparents because they felt travel was an unnecessary disruption for a 2½-year-old. They returned to New Zealand on 13 July.

Eleven days after returning from Indonesia, a graze on the father's chin became infected. The infection had spread to his nose by 28 July when the doctor started treatment with antibiotics. An ESR doctor, in a published report on the boy, considered this important because there were no swabs taken from his father's chin – the unproven insinuation being that the infected chin would have been diphtheria, which then infected the child.

Three days before A[1] got tonsillitis, there had been a big rainstorm on the North Shore. The stormwater drains overflowed into the sewage system and large amounts of raw sewage spilled onto the property next door – something too interesting for a 2½-year-old to leave unexplored.

It was also something too uninteresting for the Public Health people to investigate when it was brought to their attention later, even though New Zealand has had historical precedents of diphtheria following raw sewage flowing onto land.[2] And even more relevant, this was the area in which many of the Russian émigrés settled – a group who go regularly between here and their homeland. At this time, many were in direct contact with areas of Russia experiencing a huge epidemic of diphtheria.

When the tonsillitis became obvious, A's mother took him to the doctor who did not think he was particularly unwell, but took swabs, which showed normal flora, and prescribed the antibiotic, amoxycillin.

On 30 July, A's mother became concerned that there was no improvement. A had become quite hoarse, wasn't interested in food or drink, and was coughing. So in the late afternoon, the mother's sister took them back to the doctor, who decided to refer him to Starship. The doctor saw a yellow green exudate on the tonsils, and swollen

1 A is not his real name.
2 Maclean, F.S. 1964. *Challenge for Health*. Govt Printer. Chapter 15. pp. 349–52.

glands. He wondered about diphtheria, purely because the parents had been overseas, the child was unvaccinated, and the antibiotics weren't working. He rang ahead to Starship. His admission letter to the hospital gave name and address, and stated:

"Problem:

1) Severe tonsillopharyngitis with confluent yellow green exudate.

2) Cervical nodes in swelling.

3) Unvaccinated child.

Many thanks for seeing this young boy. I have swabs off at Diagnostic for CTS and Diptheria [as spelt by doctor]. Many thanks, with regards . . ."

The parents arrived, their doctor having primed them to expect masks, white gowns and immediate isolation. Instead, they were put into a six-bed room with other children, two of whom had immunodeficiencies. A nurse and student GP interviewed the parents who on both occasions gave the full story. During this time, their son played happily with the other children. A was finally seen by a doctor at 7.24 pm. The first question was, "Why haven't you immunized A?" A's mother said that right now, they wanted A looked at, not their choices questioned. The first line this doctor wrote in the file was:

"Referral from GP? Diphtheria."

"Previous history" written into the files included: "cough and fever, four days . . . 2½-year-old boy unimmunized (underlined twice) . . . no others in family unwell . . . Alert and happy playing, Temp 37, . . . throat pus on tonsils – exudate green, no grey. Confined to tonsillar bed, no pharynx . . . diagnosis, tonsillitis in well unimmunized 2-year-old – low likelihood of C. diphtheria . . . explained above to parents." The history was thorough with a lot of lists, no this, no that, no the other; clearly ruling out clinical diphtheria.

His parents were told that it was probably some virus, or tonsillitis, that the doctor could see no evidence of any form of diphtheria, to continue using the amoxycillin, that no follow-up necessary, and that A could return to play centre.

They asked what the hospital could do if it was diphtheria, and he mentioned an ECG, but that he didn't think it was necessary. The parents refused to leave until A had one. They also discussed anti-toxin, and the doctor said he didn't know much about it, if there was any in the country or where to get it from, but he considered it academic, since he didn't think A had diphtheria. Just before they left, he said in an offhand manner – almost as an after-thought – "Oh, I had better give A a swab".

A discharge letter reads:

Under *"Reason for attendance (Primary diagnosis)"* was written *"tonsillitis"*. Under *"Medications"* was written *"Amoxycillin"*. Under *"Disposition from the Emergency Department and Follow up"* was written, *"Discharge, No Follow-up"*. Under *"Other comments": "Concern re ? Corynebacterium diphtheriae in unimmunized child. Well in CED. No "mousy" breath, Exudate confined to tonsils. ECG normal."*

On 7 August at around 10.00 am., the doctor received notification that the swab taken on 30 July had grown a heavy growth of Streptococcus group A (pyogenes), a common cause of tonsillitis and sensitive to amoxycillin, and a heavy growth of Corynebacterium diphtheria (usually treated with Erythromycin). The doctor wrote and faxed the mother the test results with an urgent letter for readmission to Starship for review, which states on the last line:

> *"It may be appropriate to notify staff who saw the patient whilst last in Starship."*

On arrival the family were again asked to wait with other people, even after the father pointed out that their son had had a positive test result for diphtheria. Meanwhile, A was having great fun playing in the playhouse with other children. The hospital was treating this as a normal, everyday event, which surprised the parents. A nurse from Public Health came and asked them whom they had seen, and where they had been. The father again pointed out that diphtheria was supposed to be serious, and asked why they were still in a public area, and whether all staff and families in the same ward as they had been in over a week ago, should be notified?

Starship staff were unconcerned, as A was playing enthusiastically, and on viewing the files, noted that the admitting doctor hadn't see any signs of disease.

Someone went off and referred to the infectious diseases protocol and finally decided to put A into isolation. There he was seen by people in NASA-type suits who could find nothing other than a perfectly healthy, fit child. The notes from that day show nothing of any sort of infection, so the staff wrote "***parental perception of illness***"*: "1/52 throat infection, drinking down and fever. ? Diphtheria"*

Staff then dropped the "NASA" suits in a wheelchair next to reception, gave A his second ECG, said he was fine and sent them home at 5.40 pm.

However, one doctor who ***did not*** see A the first day, wrote in the file on 7 August 1998 at 1700:

> ***"Presented 7–10 days ago with clinical naso-pharyngeal diphtheria – green membrane on tonsils Rx Amoxyl . . . Now back to self."*** (Underlining mine.)

This is the key file entry, because according to all other records, the doctor the week before, could find absolutely nothing related to clinical symptoms of diphtheria whatsoever.

The family was returning home when their brother-in-law, who had gone to the doctor's to check on them, phoned to see how the family was doing, and was told nothing was happening. The doctor then phoned them, and asked them to come back to the surgery instead of going straight home. Just as they got into his room, the doctor was called away. The husband asked for a drink of water, which he was drinking when the doctor came in. The door banged the father who spilled the water down his front, which was the last straw after a long day. The children were tired, fed up, thirsty and hungry, having not been offered anything at all during the time in hospital, and having had had enough of being pushed from pillar to post with no one seeming to know what to do next, the parents went home. After all, A had been declared just fine, so what was the problem?

The dates show that the next thing that happened was that the Minister of Health was being interviewed on TV intoning with the utmost gravity that the Ministry of Health had taken over, as this was now a national emergency, and so it went on, with the media continuing to camp at the front as well as rear of the family's house.

The next day the family decided that the management of A had been so atrocious that if anyone wanted to do anything further they could come to their house and run the media gauntlet, since the family had done everything asked of them. The father repeatedly rang the head of Starship hospital to discuss the matter, but he would not return the call. However, the supervisor at the hospital did ring back twice; the first time was to say that they didn't have any antitoxin in the country; the second time was to say that it was on a plane from CSL laboratories in Australia[3], and could they please bring A to Starship the next day to be re-evaluated by infectious disease specialists.

The Public Health people went to their home, took swabs from everyone and wanted to give them all diphtheria boosters.

At midday next day, A was seen at Starship for specialist review. The written purpose of the visit was:

- Clinical Review.
- Throat swabs.
- ECG.

The notes, written by two doctors, state that: *"Dr XXXX and I explained the rarity of this disease and that throat swabs are not usually cultured in such a way as to detect it."* . . . a comment which raises the interesting question as to how many incidental diphtheroid isolates are routinely missed, because the normal culture medium is not able to grow diphtheria. The records show:

> *"As strep A pyogenes was also cultured as a much more common cause of tonsillitis which fitted the clinical picture, the C. diphth could (emphasis in file) have been carried, not causing disease, but having been found, illness and contacts have to be managed as such."* (Underlining mine.)

Note the words *"having been found, illness . . ."* If throat isolates were routinely cultured on media sensitive to diphtheria, and if bacteria were regularly found, would each isolate become a national crisis? After all, in 2003 there were 9 isolates. Did we hear about them?

The parents had it explained to them that to use anti-toxin with no

3 The health department subsequently denied this conversation took place, saying that anti-toxin was in the country all the time, and shipped up from Wellington. I asked the father if he was sure he was told CSL Australia, and he said yes. On checking, CSL is the manufacturer of the NZ antitoxin. I find it highly unlikely that a father who up till then knew nothing about diphtheria would have made that up.

sign of infection could be dangerous and cause quite nasty, side-effects which you wouldn't want in a healthy child. The records read:

> ***"However, there are no clear guidelines for its use so far into illness (resolved) and antibiotics and in mild disease which this must qualify as, as the exudate had gone by Friday. The antitoxin is only effective prior to absorption by cells so is unlikely to affect outcome now."***

By now, the parents were somewhat confused . . . a viral infection, just tonsillitis, go back to playcentre, no follow up required, and now ***"Mild disease which this must qualify as . . ."***?

When did a staff member, at any point see any clinical illness compatible with diphtheria? In a later letter[4] to the Health and Disability Commissioner, the mother complained that at no point was blood taken to look for antibody rises to prove whether or not he had diphtheria, something she had wanted done.

It's easy enough to do. Two blood samples, four weeks apart with the second showing a four-fold rise in antibodies would have proved that A had had subclinical diphtheria.

On Sunday night the family went home with a perfectly healthy child who infectious disease experts had refused to treat any further, because they couldn't find anything to treat.

The next day was the interview by Susan Woods on the Breakfast show, with Dr Nikki Turner. The tape of this interview is extraordinary. Nikki Turner is saying A was a seriously sick child, being treated in hospital, that you had to get in fast with anti-toxin, and that the play centre where he had been was being tested, treated and basically under lock-down to prevent the spread of an epidemic to the rest of the country. It's hard to believe she hadn't been kept informed.

The next few weeks was like watching a soap opera, minus the orchestra, but with all the hysteria. The story was milked nationwide, by the medical profession and editors who all moralized on parents and expounded the merits of banning unimmunized children from education or day-care facilities. The mental instability attributed to such parents who could dare to put such stress on the country was analysed to the enth degree, in papers and on talk-back. The venom of some of the judgementalism heard on the radio was such that it's small

4 9 January 1999, mother to Robin Stent.

wonder the family felt under siege. The newspaper articles have to be seen to be believed, particularly when laid alongside the hospital files.

It's even worse when you know that even before the first article was printed in the media the hospital, the admitting doctor and all the other doctors who later wrote articles in papers must have known that this child was perfectly well and never had clinical diphtheria.

But I wasn't surprised to see the medical profession decide to make the incident into a momentous occasion in their own literature. It could so easily have happened to us.

Worse was to come as far as the family was concerned. Up until September A was classified officially as an "isolate". The Public Health Report accurately stated:[5]

> *"A toxigenic strain was isolated from the throat of a 32-month old Auckland boy."*

But then the article stated: *"A greenish exudate on tonsils and pharynx"*. (Underlining mine.) No pharynx exudate was involved. But they did say he was treated with antibiotics, did not require antitoxin and was not admitted to hospital.

But by October, the same publication[6] said:

> *"The first notified case of respiratory diphtheria in New Zealand for 19 years occurred in Auckland in August 1998. The case was an unimmunized 32-month-old European male who presented with pharyngitis from which toxigenic Corynebacterium diphtheriae was isolated."*

The author, defined respiratory diphtheria as:

> *"In the respiratory tract, infection causes patches of thick, adherent greyish membrane."*

The author, who never saw A, classified pharyngotonsillar diphtheria this way: *"May result in a sore throat, enlarged cervical nodes, and swelling of the neck in severe cases."*

"Laryngeal and tracheobronchial diphtheria may cause dyspnoea, stridor, and progressive respiratory obstruction, particularly in young children and infants."

---

5 1998. "The New Zealand Public Report". Sep; 5(9): 68.

6 Baker, M. et al. 1998. "A case of diphtheria in Auckland – implications for disease control". *New Zealand Public Health Report*, October: 5(10): 73–6.

Did the admitting doctor leave his glasses at home? He did seem to know exactly what to look for, and what should be done.

A's radiology report in the hospital files, taken on the first visit to hospital as a precaution, stated:

> ***". . . the mild bronchial wall thickening with hyperinflation . . . was consistent with bronchiolitis."***

The article author does state:

> ***"Membranous pharyngitis is, however, also associated with infection by other organisms, such as Streptococci, Epstein Barr virus, Adenovirus and Corynebacterium pseudodiphtheriticum . . . Patients with suspected respiratory diphtheria should be isolated and treated on the basis of their clinical presentation . . . Antitoxin should be administered promptly with the dose based on the site and size of the diphtheritic membrane, the degree of toxicity, and the duration of illness."*** (Underlining mine.)

Wasn't A treated on the basis of his clinical presentation? No membrane, no mousy breath, no bull neck, and no symptoms of diphtheria. Just tonsillitis. You can be sure, that had there been anything to indicate clinical diphtheria, it would have been found.

The article author then says:

> ***"Based on the extent of the tonsillopharyngeal membrane and resolution within a week, this case would be classified as mild."*** (Underlining mine.)

The *extent* of what membrane . . . exactly?

It seemed to the family as if it was a case of "don't let the facts get in the way of a useful cautionary tale of respiratory diphtheria."

The first medical person to refer to A was Dr Diana Lennon in the *Herald* on 18 August:

> ***"When a disease such as diphtheria, which we believe we have conquered, reappears . . ."***

Why didn't she talk about the other positive diphtheria tests in 1996, 1995; 1994; 1993; the mysteriously blank year of 1992 when I had to chew cud on the issue; in 1991; 1990 etc? Why was there no mention that diphtheria was routinely tested for until the early 80's then discontinued, which no doubt contributed to the large drop in isolate numbers. Theoretically, I and my son should make it into those books in 1981, since we both returned positive diphtheria tests while in Middlemore hospital. But neither of us had any infection.

Then came the editorials about how it was time to act against parents who wouldn't vaccinate; let's make vaccination compulsory; social obligations must override individual rights; take them to court, make non-vaccinators pay the price!

Suddenly, amazing statistics started flying around the country. The editor in a Napier paper came up with the ultimate in inflated statistics by saying that diphtheria was a disease ***"that killed almost 800 New Zealanders a year, earlier this century."***[7] This figure, it turned out had been stated by a Health Department doctor on radio.[8] Nothing could have been further from the truth. The only year that records show 800 deaths is 1874. Dr F. S. Maclean[9] reports the highest death rate for the 20's as 88 in 1921, and the New Zealand Health trends[10] which only goes from 1922, states 93 deaths in 1929.

One journalist from the *New Zealand Herald*, who later read the full hospital files, started getting suspicious, and asked tricky questions and was given contradictory answers. One area of concern was that if this was so serious, why had the child not been isolated in hospital from the start? The other was the lack of clinical symptoms. Another journalist knew some of the people who had serious reactions to unnecessary antibiotics given. After the hospital files were circulated, a few journalists realized the ethical implications of propaganda hype, and some started to have some sympathy for the toll this was taking on the family. It seemed their editors disagreed.

When they finally wanted to talk to the family, the family had had enough and went underground leaving all their records and information with me for me to try to say what I could on their behalf. I also provided the reporters with an affidavit of the people and events in 1992[11] which I was told was shown to Nikki Turner and the Health

7 Editorial. 1998. "Time for action over immunization". *Daily Telegraph*, 12 August.
8 Mansoor, O. 1998. *Radio Pacific*, August 13. "The figures we have are that in the 1920s there were 800 deaths every year."
9 "Challenge for Health" Govt Printer 1964.
10 Page 13 (no date, I only photocopied the page).
11 The affidavit had correct day and month, but incorrect year (1993), but that didn't matter because in a letter to me Dr Turner indicated she knew the "cases" and had spoken to the specialists.

Department. Given that I know someone in Wellington knew, they should have been able to figure out who the cases were.

Not long after, a doctor from Wellington Health Department headquarters rang me, wanting to know more about the two cases in the affidavit, that I had subsequently mentioned on the radio, asking if I wanted them investigated fully. I said that I didn't, since I doubted there would be anything so inconvenient to find. But that if he thought it worth his own while, then to go right ahead. I never heard any more on that issue.

One Press Association journalist, concerned at the plethora of pre-prepared press-releases available on every minute facet of the issue, tackled the head of the hospital on why the hospital took such a lax attitude to the isolation procedures. After all, if it had been Ebola in the making, what would have happened then? Several papers reported that:

> ***". . . a senior registrar found the child showed no signs of diphtheria on July 30. The accompanying referral note from the child's general practitioner showed a diagnosis earlier that day of a sore throat."***[12]

So, why then did the hospital so carefully turn it into a media circus when the parents requested anonymity? While the hospital was now trying to play down diagnostic issues, Nikki Turner, was trying to play it up. The *Waikato Times*[13] was only one of many papers to report these comments:

> ***"New Zealand is open to huge risks of infectious diseases due to selfish parents protecting their individual rights not to immunize their children, a health specialist says. 'The health of the nation is in real danger when rare diseases such as diphtheria are again a threat . . .' Nikki Turner said."***
>
> ***Dr Turner . . . said the unvaccinated Auckland toddler at the centre of a diphtheria scare this week was likely to have got the acute infection from his parents after they holidayed last month in Indonesia. 'If the parents can bring***

12 NZPA. 1998. "Boy's diphtheria not detected for 8 days". *Otago Daily Times*, 12 August.

13 NZPA. 1998. "Selfish parents exposing nation to diseases: specialist". *Waikato Times*, 13 August: 2.

diphtheria back and give it to their child, they can easily give it to their neighbours . . .'"

If A's supposedly acute infection of diphtheria was so easy to give to their neighbours, relatives and family, then why didn't it happen? The reality was that some of the doctors involved long after the admitting doctor, appeared not to know what to do. Dr Lennon[14] admitted as much saying, "The rarity of the disease meant doctors had to return to their textbooks and consult older physicians about the best way to treat the boy." Perhaps they should have brought in an older doctor to have a proper look as well.

When I asked a Professor of General Practice what they taught medical students about diphtheria I was told that they only taught them that they didn't need to teach them anything since a vaccine had eliminated it. Ignorance about the disease, wasn't the only problem.

Dr Jones[15] said: ***"Diphtheria bacteria is carried around by a small proportion of the population, but immunization fights off the toxins that the bacteria produces."***

Had Dr Jones been taught the work of the world's most renowned writer on the subject[16] he might have known that:

> ***"When diphtheria was prevalent in a city before immunization it was usual to find 2–5 per cent of apparently healthy children with bacilli in their throats at any one time. Since each individual could be demonstrated to carry the organism for no more than a few weeks it can be calculated that most of them must have been reinfected on numerous occasions throughout childhood. Yet even in those days not more than 5–10 per cent of children ever suffered from clinical diphtheria so that we can feel sure that on most occasions the presence of diphtheria bacilli in the throat did not produce the disease."***

Burnet could have taught them too, that the current mantra that disease doesn't give immunity, only the vaccine does, was wrong:

---

14 *One Network News*, Tue Aug 11. 16:00 1998. Available from <http://tvone.co.nz/news/general/11Aug1557.html> (inactive URL).

15 1998. "Doctors urge immunization in wake of diphtheria case". *Daily News*, (New Plymouth) 12 August:

16 Sir Macfarlane Burnet Natural history of disease Ch 14, *Diphtheria*, page 195.

> ***"For at least two centuries both Streptococcus pyogenes and Corynebacterium diphtheriae persisted as very common endemic infections of the human throat, producing repeated subclinical infections in childhood with resultant immunity to the effects of the toxin."***[17]

So why is it that the people who worked with diphtheria when it was epidemic realized that its actual infection rate was incredibly low, yet doctors in 1998 made it into a media issue of larger proportions than the plague?

Mind you, their lack of knowledge paled in significance to that of one doctor who wrote a column in which he said that before antitoxin the fatality rate for laryngeal involvement was 35–90 per cent; serotherapy reduced this to below 10%. Strange that New Zealand's death rate has rarely ever hit 4%, and antitoxin and antibiotics made no difference.

Ironically the few people nationwide with the logic to pick up the irony of various suggestions that the vaccinated crèche children were threatened, and a nation of primarily vaccinated people would be in real danger from one unvaccinated child, were primarily writers of letters to the editor.

The parents[18] of the vaccinated crèche children were ***"furious the infected boy . . . had exposed their children to a killer disease"*** and beside themselves with worry. Exactly why were their children vaccinated? So they could sweat if something happened? Were they travelling in a country with endemic diphtheria and vaccinated themselves, would they even think about how much diphtheria they were daily in contact with?

Angered at the relentless innuendo against them, by crèche parents, the community, the papers, and seemingly the country, the parents tried to find out where the isolate did come from. Everything they had read in the medical literature showed genetic typing to the geographical region of source to be standard procedure in all clinical cases, so they requested the results, only to find that the laboratory at ESR (Environmental Science and Research) had not had them done.

The parents asked that they do it. ESR sent samples to Australia,

17 Sir Macfarlane Burnet. 1972. "Natural history of infectious disease". Ch 14, *Diphtheria*, page 200.

18 NZPA. 1998. "Boy's diphtheria not detected for 8 days". *Otago Daily Times*, 12 August.

but the reply was that it wasn't any geographical region they had records of. Given that Indonesia is Australia's neighbour, that was a surprise. ESR then said that Paris and London were being consulted, and said they would get back to the parents when they knew.

A year later, 10 August 1999, ESR still couldn't tell the parents, and to this day, reports say that the source was unknown. ESR enclosed its officially published report in their final letter on A, which further infuriated the parents, who politely asked that the ESR report should be amended to show A as an isolate, since at no time had he shown clinical signs of, or been treated for, diphtheria. The ESR[19] report was never changed, and no apology was ever given, and the parents never heard from ESR again. The report showed all 17 diphtheria isolates from 1989 to 1998, all of which were sporadic in nature with no epidemiological links.[20] If ESR could type all the other isolates, why not A's? 1992 was blank, as I knew it would be.

And it's interesting, that a later case of a four year old in 2002, immunized with four diphtheria vaccines who was admitted to hospital with septic arthritis traced to toxigenic bacteria was never reported in the media. Every year there is an isolate, A is mentioned as a clinical case, yet in the case of this child we are told[21] the child had no toxin-related symptoms, and wasn't a case. Somehow, this child who was really sick with not just a sore throat[22], but required two arthrotomies for septic arthritis, with intravenous therapy with flucloxacillin, and then amoxicillin, isn't a diphtheria case, whereas a child who wasn't sick and wasn't even treated, is a case?

A Health Department doctor had been on radio[23] and said that ***"in the 1920s there were more than 700 cases every year"***, and that without vaccines we could return to those bad old days. He also said that had it not been for antibiotics, the death rates would have been much higher.

---

19 Sneyd, E., and Baker, M. 2003. *Infectious Diseases in New Zealand: 2002 Annual Surveillance Summary*, Available from <http://www.surv.esr.cri.nz/PDF_surveillance/AnnSurvRpt/2002AnnualSurvRpt.pdf> Accessed on 18 September, 2005.

20 Letter from P. Short to parent, 10 August 1999.

21 Sneyd, E., and Baker, M. 2003. *Infectious Diseases in New Zealand: 2002 Annual Surveillance Summary*, p. 25. Available from <http://www.surv.esr.cri.nz/PDF_surveillance/AnnSurvRpt/2002AnnualSurvRpt.pdf> Accessed on 18 September, 2005.

22 Shihab, F. et al. 2003. "Septic arthritis due to a toxigenic strain of Corynebacterium diphtheriae gravis". *New Zealand Medical Journal*, April: 116(1172): 404. Available from <http://www.nzma.org/nz/journal/116-1172/404/> (not accessible on Pubmed).

23 *Radio Pacific* (and possibly others) 12 August 1998.

I had all the statistics for diphtheria cases, deaths, and death rates per million from 1872 onwards, and nowhere was there a statistic like that. So through the IAS[24] I requested the reference to the 700 cases per year in the 1920s, and was referred to the Immunization Handbook. The medical article reference was there, so I checked that. It was an article referring back to a 1964 book which I have, so I checked that too, only to find that the figures used in the medical article and then used by the Health Department bore no relationship to those in the book, thereby making the information in the Handbook incorrect.

Peter Mancer, the then chairman of the Immunization Awareness society, advised the Ministry of this, who replied[25] saying that the Health Department would "modify the statistics" in the next edition of the handbook.

Peter Mancer also rechecked my data from 1872 to 1998 using a comparative computer programme, and sent the doctor a graph showing that contrary to his other statement, antibiotics had made absolutely no difference to the death rates from 1872 as he had alleged:

> ***"What this tells me is that over that period, no effective advancement in diphtheria treatment was made."*** The doctor[26] replied, saying:
>
> ***"The editors are preparing an item for the New Zealand Public Health Report on the diphtheria case, for which they did what you did – getting the historical data. They also came to the same interesting conclusion that the case fatality rate had not changed in this era. But then, anti-toxin has been available throughout this era. Still, one would have thought that antibiotics would make a difference."***

What interested me even more, was the ESR graph.[27] It's very puzzling. Having all the data from 1908 for cases and deaths from 1885 it does, perhaps, bear a faint resemblance to the one we sent the Health Department at the time. Anti-toxin only became available from

24 Immunisation Awareness Society.
25 E-mail to Peter Mancer, 25 August 1998, 9:04.
26 E-mail to Peter Mancer, Thursday 24 September 1998. 16:14.
27 Baker, M. et al. *New Zealand Public Health Report*, October: 5(10): 74.

the late 1890s, after the highest peak, and the death rates remained the same at rates of one in 25 cases throughout, regardless of either anti-toxin or antibiotics.

But one issue needs considering. If diphtheria antitoxin had side-effects potentially far too serious[28] to be given to A who was healthy and had no symptoms, what might those same serious side-effects from anti-toxin do to a seriously ill child with diphtheria? Had the New Zealand medical profession treated A's non-existent diphtheria with anti-toxin on day one as the Public Health article advised, and if A had subsequently died from these serious side-effects of anti-toxin, what would the Health Department have attributed his death to? The diphtheria he never had?

Could it be that historically many of the deaths and serious problems seen in people with diphtheria were actually increased unnecessarily because of the biological dangers of the anti-toxin and the dreadful methods of treating diphtheria right up to 1940? This isn't just an academic question. It's interesting to me that the greatest drop in diphtheria deaths came when doctors abandoned the most atrocious of the treatments available (See Chapter 33 on useless treatments). As in the case of so many medical mysteries, the statistics will never give an answer. But there just might be an answer from Russia.

Russia's clinical experience in the 1990s doesn't appear to have reached medical journals read by English-speaking medical people. Doctors there discovered to their cost that the diphtheria toxin anti-toxin was indeed highly dangerous when administered to patients with serious toxic diphtheria. Its use increased complications three-fold, and myocarditis 4.5 fold. At least, that was the drop they saw when they decreased doses down to a quarter of the recommended regime.[29]

---

28 Anti-toxin side effects are serious and include anaphylaxis, serum sickness, and other resulting immune system problems and even death. Information sheets faxed from CSL at the time advised first giving the patient antihistamine parenterally, then 0.25 mg adrenaline subcutaneously as a prophylactic, to have on hand a syringe of 1 ml adrenaline, and full rescuscitation facilities at the ready, and then 15 minutes after all that, to give the antitoxin intramuscularly. All doctors I spoke to who had used it, spoke with trepidation about using it.

29 Bondarenko, A.L. et al. 2000. Kliniko-epidemiologicheskie osobennosti difterii v Kirovskoii oblasti (Clinical-epidemiological features of diphtheria in the Kirov region). *Eipdemiologiia i infektsionnye bolezni* (Epidemiology and infectious diseases), Vol 2, pp. 26–29 "Giving large doses of anti-diphtheria serum did not shorten the period of treatment. On the contrary, it caused complications . . . After abandoning the large-dose serum treatment (through 1993–1997 the dose was decreased from 400,000 to 100,000 ME in toxic diphtheria) the number of specific complications fell 3-fold, while

No explanation of this phenomenon was suggested. It was stated as an established fact, which as of today, only the Russians appear to appreciate or understand. I also wonder if the phenomenon that Russia discovered partly explains the abrupt rise in cases and death rates in UK, Europe and this country during depression and war years shortly after its use became aggressively applied along with other toxic useless treatments from 1895 onwards through to 1917, and judging by medical literature, even up to 1940 in some places.

As of 7 March 2000, A's parents had still not been told what country their son's alleged diphtheria had come from. They felt as I did, that the "upgrading" of A from an "isolate" to a "case" was a move to justify the needless hysteria the doctors created in the media from day one. Their letters to ESR started to go unanswered. Then they gave up, because the unequal struggle had got to them so much that the ultimate collateral fall-out had occurred. The family unit had disintegrated.

It's one more possible price people end up paying, when left feeling disillusioned, distraught, exposed, abandoned and at the mercy of other people's politics, prejudices, and presumptions.

I am sure none of these experiences were the fate of the family of the fully vaccinated 12 year old in Kimberley Australia[30] who was "successfully treated" after developing clinical diphtheria.

---

the number of myocarditis cases fell 4.5-fold . . ."

30 1992. "Diphtheria case a reminder". *GP Weekly*, August 5.

66 Behind the Scenes

Hilary had gone to Auckland for the day – not an uncommon occurrence.

I was at home – very common.

Hilary had the car.

I had shanks' pony and pedal power – quite adequate unless I needed to go any great distance. So as jack-of-all-trades as well as unofficial secretary/receptionist for Hilary in her absence I commenced my daily duties, one of which I could be sure. Answering the telephone.

By the time Hilary got home there could be quite a long list of logged calls. On this particular day, the usual routine was going to be a bit different.

It started when TV1 rang: "Is Hilary Butler available please?"

"No, I'm sorry. She's out for the day," keeping the "cards" close to my chest. "May I give her a message?"

Then followed an explanation as to the reason for the call. They were wanting to know if Hilary could appear on the Paul Holmes Show that evening. On this particular day, Hilary was not at the medical library. She was with a friend whose telephone number I knew, so I suggested that TV1 ring and speak to Hilary direct.

Later, Hilary rang back to say that she had agreed to go on the *programme but that she would require a taxi to pick her up from Tuakau and then return her after the show.*

I then got another call from Hilary to say that because of developments relating to the proposed item in which Hilary was to appear, the earlier arrangements had had to be shelved.

"What time will you be home, Dear?" I asked, knowing that getting tangled up in the end-of-the-day traffic is never a good idea.

"Well, as there's no deadline to meet now," said my much-sought-after-wife. "I'll take it as it comes."

Time ticked by and I ticked off my list of "jobs to be done".

Late afternoon, the phone rang again. "TV1 here. We've decided to go ahead with the programme tonight. We have a news van available for a live transmission, if we can make suitable arrangements with Hilary." We talked about a convenient location and eventually decided on the Bombay Service Centre. This was ideal for transmission as it was situated at the top of the Bombay hills which gave clear unobstructed views of Auckland city about 40 km away.

"Is there a suitable café or something we could use?"

"The Autobahn Café would probably be the best," I said.

"Leave it to us. We'll make the necessary contacts. But can Hilary make it?" said TV1.

A good question and time was crucial.

"I'll see if she has left Auckland yet and get back to you."

Hilary was still at her friend's place. I explained the latest telephone conversation and we worked out that there should be enough time for her return trip plus tidying up and collecting her wits, before I would drive her the 11 km back to Bombay. Not much leeway for traffic hold-ups though.

A call to TV1 to explain the situation.

"It's all OK this end. Can you be at Bombay, Autobahn Café by 6.40 pm at the latest?"

Now it was countdown!

I mentally sorted out what I needed to do and then eyes on the clock . . . waited.

It was tight, and the adrenalin must have been running. We arrived on location by the prescribed time.

Hilary took off to make herself known to the TV1 News crew, and I resigned myself to another instalment of the waiting game.

I was parked next to the TV1 News van which was all set up to do the transmission on cue from the Auckland studios.

It proved to be a fascinating experience even though I got a numb bum.

Here was a highly organized team who must be doing this sort of thing all the time. A tall telescopic aerial, or mast, disappeared into the night sky. Cables stretched across the footpath and snaked into the Café, where a secluded area with table and chairs, screened off by potted plants and suitable greenery, had been prepared for the telecast. Inside the transmitting van were all the gadgetry, glowing lights, wires and cables needed to get Hilary's face to the nation's viewers.

There were plenty of curious bystanders speculating on what must be some newsworthy event.

Maybe, they conjectured, this had been the scene of a robbery earlier in the day?

Maybe some very distinguished entertainer was being interviewed or was about to perform?

Maybe just something local . . . but . . . and their eyes would wander to the cables, and cameras and the mast away up there. And it was all so ***quiet****.*

For those who could get close enough to peep inside, there was just this woman sitting there talking – to herself it seemed.

What was all the fuss about? Most shrugged their shoulders and moved on.

When it was all over, quiet efficiency again.

All packed up in no time at all, it seemed.

And the mast just came down and down to collapse into nothing.

Fascinating.

Off they went. Just another job. All that for just a few minutes "on air".

Off we went too – to unwind? To put our feet up? To catch up on the day's events?

Not for long. The telephone rang.

The "receptionist" answered.

"I saw your wife on TV tonight. She was great . . ."

Once again, I made the appropriate noises.

Yes, I had seen the organizational side of the media at work.

Things; technology; practised efficiency.

But flesh and blood? My own wife? NO.

And unless someone recorded these programmes, I never experienced at first hand what was said and how it came across.

So near and yet so far.

67 In Front of the Scenes, Facing the Media

Just when you want things to be simple, the simplest thing can go wrong. You work out times for punctures, and other diversions, and take off.

But there is one problem. I try to go up to Auckland and come back at non-peak times when traffic is scarce. I know the scenery, and driving is a cruise.

TV1 had asked me to be at Bombay Autobahn Café at a certain time for an interview with their mobile news crew. This was a different matter. It meant travelling at a time I don't normally travel, with a brain rattling through information not normally processed while driving, in traffic I don't normally have to contend with. At best, it's going to be 50 minutes home, and at worst, who knows?

A combination of having to take extra care jammed in amongst cars, and not being 100% on the job pushes me into the wrong lane at a crucial intersection, and I'm grid-locked, and have no choice but go straight on whether I want to or not. Where this road will take me I have no idea. I'm driving under the south-bound motorway which is where I need to be, and I've never taken this route in my life. There is no map in the car, and it's rush hour, so I sit back and resign myself to the fact that I need to go with the flow or else. There is no point in panicking, and so long as I keep the setting sun to my right shoulder and keep moving, that direction has to take me south, closer to home.

The wherever-it-led me snail-paced traffic route ate into the puncture time, café stop, and the pick-up-the-fish detour. Finally I recognized a turn-off to the airport, and knew exactly how to get home. But there were going to be some tricky busy intersections, and my head was starting to feel the pressure.

This is why when it comes to TV interviews I much preferred to have the taxi, and go to the studio from home. That way, you only have to concentrate on what you have to do, not how to get there or getting there in one piece.

Yes, the time was cut fine, because there was evidentiary proof that had to be faxed to the Holmes show before the show went to air. I was told there were questions Holmes wasn't prepared to ask unless he had the proof in front of him.

Two issues were at stake. The fact that the Health Department had provided TV with a graph that didn't quite equate with the words, and also some left-over unresolved business as a result of the diphtheria case that wasn't.

Let's say also, there were some interpretational differences between me, and someone on the staff of IMAC (Immunization Advisory Centre) which had a direct relationship with the diphtheria-"case" that wasn't . . . in a queer sort of way.

The background of that was the talk given by IMAC the previous year at the Auckland's Parents' show.

In the talk itself, an inflammatory remark was made about me, which caused me to go up to the microphone without invitation and correct it, and offer to send the 'proof' to anyone who wished to see it.

Some of the other staff members associated with IMAC weren't at the talk at that time, but were back at their display stand. They drifted over, after the talk, to handle after-talk enquiries. I was standing around, with a friend of mine, listening to what was being said. Obviously the other staff members didn't know my face, or they might have been more circumspect with what they said. Or not, as the case may be.

Some women were standing around, listening to a woman say that there had been absolutely no proven vaccine damage cases in the country. Not long before, a successful vaccine damage case had featured in *New Idea*.

The article had sparked a flood of calls to the mother, and to me. Later, after articles in *Balance* and *Healthy Options* the mother got more calls and more letters. She took names, addresses and dates of vaccination.

I happened to have the years of the batches, as well as a huge computer print-out from the Centre for Adverse Reactions Monitoring (CARM), which had cost the IAS $500 to get. We took all the dates these children were vaccinated, and it came as no surprise to us, that the majority fitted into a specific date frame of one specific batch, which had been what some might call "hot". That particular lot had been a batch which caused so many reports of side-effects that CARM had it retested in Australia. Most of the cases reported to CARM were not very serious, but were worrying enough for parents.

What this mother and I were now hearing was that there were a lot more parents with children with identical problems to those her son had experienced, saying that their doctors actively opposed reporting the problem. Some were insistent that their doctors had talked to CARM and were told that that batch had no problems, and further, that these sorts of reactions were just one in a million. We weren't surprised. The IAS and I hear this all the time, to this day. It's been the one consistent mantra that has never changed since vaccines were invented.

But what the no problems meant, was that on retesting, the batch, while passing the safety standards, had been observed to have a higher pertussis component potency than normal,[1] though the memo also states:

> *"3) This batch of vaccine is safe and efficacious."*[2]

For anyone who might be reading this, who thinks their child might be one of those, to whom vaccine from that batch was given, the Commonwealth Serum Laboratories Triple vaccine used, was batch number 0433 216. It won't matter if your doctor didn't write it in the book, though hopefully they did, because this batch was used in this country for nearly a year, though the majority of serious reactions from that batch came in the first nine months of 1988.

As this woman from IMAC continued to explain how safe vaccines were and how many deaths from whooping cough were prevented in relation to no vaccine reactions, I quietly asked, "What about that case in *New Idea* a little while back . . .?"

1 Health Board memo, dated 13 February 1989, p. 2.
2 Health Board memo, dated 13 February 1989, p. 3.

"Oh," she said, "We looked at the files of that case, and there was absolutely no relationship."

Interesting. "You *do* mean the case of ______ don't you?"

"Oh yes, we got all the details and that wasn't vaccine damage."

"Funny that," I said. "I did all the work on that case through all stages of proceedings, and have all the paper work, as well as the final judgement. The mother will be most interested in your statement, since no one has asked her, or me, for access to the documents required to review the case."

The faces of the people standing around showed that they understood the implications of the interchange.

In March 1998, Nikki Turner and I had been interviewed on Mary Lambie's *Good Morning*. I had provided Mary Lambie with a letter on IMAC letterhead, signed by a staff member there, which had at the bottom the names of the vaccine companies that funded IMAC and the Goodfellow Unit, from which IMAC worked at the time. I asked Mary to ask Nikki on air, if any IMAC funding came in any way, from vaccine manufacturers. Twice, Nikki Turner was asked the question and twice she replied in the negative. So it would be fair to say that IMAC modus operandi wasn't appreciated after the events of the previous 18 months or more.

The point of the Holmes Show for me, was to bring all this and more, together. Arriving home just in time, after my unscheduled detour, I faxed proof from the hospital files that the case had NOT been clinical diphtheria, as well as other material, in order for Paul to allow me to say certain things.

Then came a call from the producer who had received the faxed material, confirming that if certain things happened, he would allow me to state my case. I was surprised actually, because what with Holmes being married to a doctor at the time, I thought that, as had happened with the 1991 show, they would call it off at the last minute, or squash me, like the debacle with Susan Woods.

But sitting there in Autobahn Café, I was given the opportunity and took it, and challenged both the truthfulness of the graph compared with Nikki Turner's statement, her use of the media and the extra funding I'd heard this had resulted in. She denied it. Afterwards the only unsupportive email I received via the IAS chairperson, was from an IMAC staff member taking me to task for being so horrible to Nikki Turner.

There was another spin-off to the Autobahn interview, which, with hindsight, was also predictable.

The ultimate in risk management by the Health Department appeared to have been pulled out. I don't know the exact mechanism, but I know that there was high-level interference, because recently someone in TV1 told me that the result of that interview is that I've never been on TV since that day: 8 June 1999.

To this day, staff at IMAC will tell you, that not one cent of its funding ever comes from vaccine manufacturers. IMAC is, according to IMAC, the ultimate in providing unbiased independent information.

68 The Tip of an Iceberg

One evening, in April 1988, I logged a call into my exercise book from a woman called Lucy who was worried about her baby, John. He had had two lots of shots, and after each had been admitted to hospital.

The first vaccines were given two days after he was admitted to hospital with apnoeas and weight loss. For whatever reason, it was considered a good idea to vaccinate a baby like this, because to the paediatrician, the baby seemed well enough. Within five hours of the vaccine, John had a fever, irritability and his whole knee had swollen up, two inches below the injection site. Bloodwork showed hypersegmented neutrophils. Hypersegmented neutrophils contain a nucleus with six or more lobes. They are commonly found in cases of folate deficiency and chronic infections. But it seems no one thought to look at this baby to see if there might be immune system problems. Instead, the swelling in his knee was considered to be just cellulitis and treated with antibiotics.

The second shots were given three weeks later, and John's breathing went haywire. He had five large apnoea attacks and was going dusky in colour, so Lucy took him straight to hospital, where he was admitted for observation.

After hearing all this, my advice to her was to not let him have any more vaccines because I believed he had reacted adversely to the other vaccines, and I was worried that something more serious might happen if she did allow more to be administered.

John's paediatrician considered any suggestion that it was a vaccine reaction the most ridiculous thing he had ever heard. After the three-month shot, when John landed in hospital again, Lucy had overheard some very derogatory remarks a doctor made to another staff member saying that in his opinion, John's problems were all in John's parents' minds. John's parents requested another doctor, and all treatment after that was sought privately.

Lucy felt trapped, because on top of the feeling in her gut and her head that the vaccines were causing the problems, she was surrounded by people who said that the vaccine wasn't the problem. Like many people before her, Lucy was talked into believing the assurances that everything would be just fine for the next shots.

So, on 8 June 1988, at 10.30 am John's third DPT vaccine was given.

By 11.15, his whole thigh was swollen, and a rash covered it.

At 12.30, John started screaming and arching his back, and wouldn't stop.

By 2.30 pm Lucy had him back at the doctor and no one could do anything, so he was sent to hospital, where he arrived "Screaming, irritable ++". Doctor's notes state *"Severe reaction to vaccination"*. They took one look at him, and sent him to another hospital.

On arrival John was found to be lustily crying, had buttock erythema, high-pitched and unusual crying, was back-arching and was inconsolable. He had a temperature of 39.5° and a red, excoriated injection site. Urine revealed no infection, and blood cultures were negative. He had neutrophil leucocytosis of 16.3 with 0.2 basophils, 0.6 monocytes, 3 lymphocytes, and total white cell count was 20.1 x 10E9/L.

Interestingly, a note on the bloodwork papers says *"Neutrophil toxic changes present"*. Toxic changes in neutrophils are usually seen in severe infections, burns or exposure to toxic agents.

Hospital notes state *"allergic reaction to DPT"*. Lucy was told that the screaming was called cerebral screaming and that the vaccine *"had gone to his brain"* and that was why he was screaming. But that it would *"go away"*.

By the next morning, John had screamed himself to a standstill, and they were discharged home, hoping that that was the end of it.

John's sleeping patterns changed immediately. He was sleeping far more than before, and becoming very jerky and tense in his movements. His basic nature changed, and he never regained the relaxed temperament and fluid movements he had had before the five-month shots.

Repeated respiratory infections, otitis media, and febrile seizures became common. Regularly, on the dot every couple of months, something would require treatment. Usually yet another standard round of antibiotics was administered.

But by the time John was four it was obvious things were not good at all. He would have strange episodes, which Lucy now believes were complex partial seizures. After these episodes he would always go to bed, and sleep for ages.

Assessment by educational specialists confirmed that John had severe processing problems. In addition, there were behavioural issues, and habits that were bordering on autistic in nature. He hand flapped or "stimmed" and excessive noise drove him up the wall. Special hearing tests showed that he had auditory processing disorders as well, and at one point in the test, the noise level provoked what looked to the tester like a seizure.

This was the first time that anyone had said the word "seizure" to Lucy. She had done quite a bit of research by this time, and come to the conclusion that all reactions to his vaccines, but particularly his five-month shots, had a lot to do with his problems.

So Lucy decided to apply for ACC compensation, to help cover expenses. She realized that recognition of the cause was vital, because without this, his future was less than certain. She wanted some surety for John, but she also wished to put the system on notice.

And so it was in 1995 that our paths crossed again. Lucy was having major trouble with her ACC claim. Lucy never ran into the normal problems and obstacles of getting medical files. She applied for, and received, a complete accurate copy of all records, which made working out the case a lot easier. But in September 1996, for the second time, ACC rejected Lucy's claim. She requested the evidence on which they had made their decision.

ACC replied in a letter, saying:

> ***"The Committee has very full reports before it, including extensive notes relating to John's numerous hospital admissions . . ." etc, etc . . .***

What were all these very full reports?

It turned out to be a four-page letter, plus selective enclosures from her original doctor, who had been replaced when John was three months old.

A reader evaluating this letter would have assumed that this doctor had been John's primary physician for many years. Everything in the letter was worded in such a way that implied, subtly, that everything alleged by Lucy was incorrect. Neither were the full records included. The pages that really mattered were left out.

This doctor had not seen John at the time of the five-month shots, yet inferred that he had "team membership", and stated that the five-month reaction was both mild, local and did not affect John's brain. In other words, John had not had encephalopathy. The previous reactions were also explained away in a very deft creative manner.

But by this time, Lucy had had enough. Using the hospital files, we prepared a very clear letter, enclosing copies of all the relevant pages from the hospital files, and comparing them with the doctor's review in parallel columns. We also enclosed a body of other medical research, which covered all the events that happened to John.

Then Lucy took the factual information, and expanded on that in her own way, stating exactly how she felt about the constructed manner in which she was now being done over yet again, by the very doctor who had contributed so badly to the situation they now had to live with, and whom they had sacked when John was three months of age.

On 24 November, the Committee completely reversed its decision, and handed down the decision that, indeed, her son had had encephalopathy, and that his many problems stemmed from the encephalopathy, which was caused by the vaccine.

Previously I had requested a full break-down from CARM of all vaccine reactions. What fascinated both me and Lucy was that the very batch given to John had provoked huge numbers of adverse reactions.

Gobsmacked, I went back to my telephone log for that year. No wonder I had been rung so often at that time! There were literally pages and pages of entries. I went through the lists and started ringing some of the numbers listed. Most were no longer relevant. The parents had shifted. Some were still having ongoing problems, but all had been fobbed off, with excuses which, in retrospect, simply defied logic.

I suggested to Lucy that it was time to go to the media. She had already decided to do that, and had gone to *New Idea*, which wrote a somewhat disappointing article, very much emphasising how wonderful vaccines were, rather than the aspects of informed consent about possible damage, which Lucy wanted to get across. Overall, the article washed over Lucy's concerns, concentrating on sound-bite data to scare parents into vaccinating.

We did not know the readership figures for *New Idea*, but it would be safe to say that not too many people would have read the article. Lucy rang me, very upset to say that over that weekend 85 people had rung her. After another week, she stopped counting how many calls she had had.

Lucy made a list of the children's ages, and where parents knew this information, the date the vaccine that had caused problems had been administered.

Then we went back and checked this data against the dates when the suspect DPT batch was used. More than three-quarters of those children had been given vaccine from the same batch that John had been given, which raises an interesting question.

John is the only child that we know of, right now, who has received ACC compensation as a result of his reaction to that particular batch of vaccine. Given the hundreds of reported reactions, and if more than 80 sets of parents contacted Lucy after publication of the article, reporting that their children had had similar problems to her son, how many other children in this country, during that time, . . . were affected by that batch?

It would be very interesting to go back and do a retrospective study of all the children to whom that batch of vaccine was given, compare them with a control group of those who had received a vaccine batch that had no reported side-effects, and see if the incidence of learning disorders and behavioural dysfunction was higher in that age group. But that will never be done.

How many of the people who did not read Lucy's story had similarly affected children, but had not the skills, energy, determination or ability to obtain compensation for their children?

Lucy's story underlies an ongoing problem in this country. Parents who are determined to fight for justice, are few and far between.

There are many reasons for this. The biggest one is that the ACC system we now have makes it financially difficult to succeed. Worse, parents face an additional emotional roller-coaster ride because usually every obstacle possible is placed in their way. This makes the process additionally soul destroying. They face a system, where often the very people who judge any medical misadventure case, are the people who advocate the procedures judged, and occasionally have been the ones who applied those procedures in the first place.

I know of only two cases where the medical profession admitted, straight up, that vaccines caused the damage seen.

Most parents face a barrage of denial, deflection and excuses. In some cases, the downright lies they have to endure are awful. In others, CYPS can be brought in, with a request for full psychological evaluation of the parents and family, as if the problem is a mental one. Occasionally, files just disappear. Still others are threatened with withdrawal of medical assistance if they proceed.

Even Lucy did not escape without some mental scarring, though it has made her one of the strongest parents I now know. The problem is that mentally, you cannot undo the kind of damage that attitudes like this cause. You never see the medical profession through the same eyes again.

The problem, for me, was that the doctor concerned regularly sat as 'judge and jury' on the ACC review committee of other cases I was involved in.

Lucy's case was the most provable case of them all because we had all the records, and I felt that it would be ideal as a starting point, to open up the door to other cases which had been unjustifiably refused in my opinion.

But understandably it simply couldn't happen. Sometimes, justice means compromise. For the sake of her family, Lucy, having got compensation, wisely decided to leave the other issues well alone.

John was truly the tip of that iceberg.

The point is that there isn't just the one 1988 iceberg. Vaccine reactions continue to this day. Most parents aren't told everything that COULD happen, because the principle of informed consent still doesn't apply in this country. Parents also live in a different world than even ten years ago. Many children are in day-care; most parents' lives are a high-wire balancing act with little time to think, to analyse, or assess issues properly, even if they were to be given all the information. And some parents just don't want to think about it.

If and when something adverse happens after a vaccine, there is always a quick and ready pat answer to explain it all away as something else. Where do you go, if your child is in serious difficulties? To the very people who vaccinated the child in the first place, or who would have recommended it, had you asked for facts? You are reliant on these people to either treat your child, or get justice. Usually, you can't get both.

If this isn't a conflict of interest, then what is? As a result, it's rare to find a doctor willing to report vaccine reactions, and it is this system's failure that keeps alive the myth that vaccines are safe, effective and risk free.

But there is more to this particular story than the issue of the many unreported vaccine reactions. John's case now stands as the medical hallmark and is discussed with medical students. It is recognized. So why only admit to John's case now?

John's case is totally irrelevant to the vaccine used for whooping cough now. That's the beauty of this case, to the medical profession, who can still look responsible by admitting that one case exists in their records, but in the very next breath, discount it by saying, "That can't happen now. We use a better, safer vaccine."

With the number of cases that have been accepted in the past, and the number of decisions I possess, or have seen, it continues to amaze me that medical people seem to think that the only vaccine-damaged child that exists in this country is John. They seem to infer that they have reviewed every case, which is patently not true. They are even proud to talk about John, because he is, to them, proof that they are vigilant, and prepared to be honest. Which is an illusion, because they fought the case tooth and nail, and only came to the party when in disgust Lucy accused the medical committee of medical dyslexia and asked that the case be referred on to appeal, as she had lost confidence in the process.

Unfortunately, most parents have neither the ability, strength or the emotional courage to do what Lucy did. In order to fight a case, the price of dissent, medically, financially and socially, is usually too high. What's more, it takes a special strength to be prepared to tell it in a book like this. Many were given the option. Few had the courage to accept.

69 A Mother's Diary

"I felt as though he 'left' me."

The trials through which parents of vaccinated children are sometimes put were illustrated for me yet again by the diary which one mother kept and shared with me. Against her better judgement she was persuaded to vaccinate her infant son with DPTH, Hep B and Polio shots. The baby was at once reduced to high pitched, animal-like screaming and back-arching. He produced the frothy, bright orange faeces, which stank, and an angry, blotchy red rash which progressively spread over his body, which I'd been told about so often. *"I felt,"* she said, ***"as though he 'left' me."*** The mother's concerns were at first greeted with the suggestion that she try paracetamol, but she knew something was seriously wrong. His eyes had a glazed look and if she passed her hand in front, or flicked her fingers, there was no response.

When he wasn't screaming, and drawing his legs up, the baby was listless, barely vocalizing any more and hardly feeding. A hard lump developed where the Hep B was given and that remains to this day. One doctor at A&E admitted it might be a reaction to vaccines, but this was hotly denied by others. Exhausted by the extra care she had to give to her distraught and seriously ill child, and repeated visits for medical attention, the mother was shocked when asked patronizingly by one woman doctor whether she was really equipped for motherhood. In response to her concerns, she was told that her child might have a urinary infection. He didn't.

With each visit, fragments of the truth were told to her, when a nurse finally said the problem might be the pertussis vaccine. She provided vaccine reaction forms from CARM[1] to her GP, only to have to listen to an irrationally angry refusal when she asked him to fill them in for her.

Much later, another woman doctor recognized the urticaria and screaming, and advised the mother not to risk giving her baby the whooping cough immunization, or Hepatitis B and reported the reactions for her.

In all this, the mother was appalled that so many in the medical profession had failed to recognize in her baby the classic symptoms of collapse, screaming, or of urticaria, which are listed even in the manufacturer's pamphlet as one of the possible effects of the Hep B vaccine. All the medical establishment could suggest was that the vaccines should have been administered at different times, or in a different order, with this classic piece of advice which she wrote in her diary just after it was given to her:

> ***"If your baby collapses and stops breathing in response to the vaccination, what caused the reaction is not the point. He becomes another patient who needs to be resuscitated whatever the cause. When you immunize him next time, do it month by month and bring him in to hospital where it is safe for him. We can resuscitate him if we need to."***

Her faith in the medical profession was totally shattered. She characterizes their responses to her concerns as "insulting, patronizing, dismissive arrogance at worst, and at best a genuine concern that something was wrong, but an inability to pinpoint what was wrong, and the comment, 'There is nothing we can do'."

1 Centre for Adverse Reactions Monitoring, Dunedin.

70 How do you Define "Responsible"?

A man.

A woman.

A marriage relationship between the two begins.

A husband and a wife.

A child is conceived and eventually that child is born.

The relationship widens.

A mother and a father.

A family.

Nothing unusual about this sequence. It is part of our Creator's plan and purpose from the beginning.

With it comes awesome responsibility.

Now, at this point, there needs to be introduced a crunch question.

WHO "OWNS" THIS CHILD?

Do you look askance at this question?

"Surely," you may be saying, "the parents do."

The baby just born, ***is their child****.*

What this unique new life grows up to be, will be the expression of, among other things, what he or she has inherited from the parents.

As every parent knows (or should know), parenthood involves so many responsibilities and privileges.

So many decisions have to be made on their child's behalf, and although this may appear a daunting prospect, especially for first-time parents, usually they will want the best for their child(ren).

The problem is that there are those others who consider it their job to tell parents what to do.

"Parenthood is too complex in today's society," they will say.

Therefore it is inferred right from the beginning that parents need to be conditioned to be willing to share "responsibility" with others who are "professionals". They know best, don't they?!

And, if necessary, the "ownership" of a child can be given to someone else who will be able to exercise responsibility more responsibly!

"Much as we don't want to say this, you know," they say, saying it anyway, "If you won't cooperate, there are penalties you know . . ."

Every now and again we read in the newspapers about parents who make decisions on behalf of their children which result in their being delivered an ultimatum. If you don't comply then legal proceedings are commenced and then maybe a Court ruling is handed down which can be shattering for the family concerned.

A few years ago one such example really aroused my anger, and I wrote to the Commissioner for Children as follows:

> *Dear Sir,*
>
> *I am writing to you in connection with the ________ case which has been featuring in the news lately.*
>
> *My wife and I have been following this case (as reported in the media) very closely, and have listened to interviews with you on the radio. We are very concerned about what we read and hear.*
>
> *As loving and caring parents we wholeheartedly support the British Court of Appeal's decision. We believe very strongly that in the situation like ________, the parent's wishes and decisions should be respected.*
>
> *The medical experts can talk all they like about what* ***they***

can do, but it does not alter the fact that the child and the parents are on the receiving end. To subject a child to such major treatment with no guarantees of "success" long or short term, with all the pain, discomfort and ongoing treatments (with side-effects) **IS ABUSE**. Why can't the parents be allowed to enjoy their baby for as long as possible without the invasive treatments advocated by the medical people whose feathers seem to be so ruffled. There are other forms of treatments which may well be more appropriate for this situation, and which would allow the parents and child to make the most of what time they have together.

We are appalled at any suggestion that New Zealand authorities should try to interfere with the choice the parents of ________ have made and the decision of the British Court of Appeal.

Yours sincerely,

Peter Butler

The letter was also sent to other "appropriate" departments. The usual vague replies or acknowledgements were received and eventually the story ran its course in the media, and other news took its place, diverting people's attention and concerns away from the issues.

Hilary and I were not satisfied with the outcome, and always find similar cases so frustrating.

Why?

Because basically you can't win. The clobbering machine will get you.

Are we talking about parents' rights?

Or the child's rights?

Or someone else's rights?

Regulations enacted under the 1994 Health and Disability Commissioner Act (NZ) state that every person, child or adult, has the right to practise his or her religion and the right to refuse or withdraw from medical treatment. However, as a lecturer in medical law said, "Children do not have the same rights as adults".

For example, the Guardianship Act gives the court the power to act in the best interests of a child under its guardianship and it prevails over the other Acts. Loving, caring parents can be accused of being child abusers.

In New Zealand, unlike some other places in the world, it is not yet mandatory to have your child vaccinated. This does not please some medical people and some politicians. All sorts of schemes have been advocated to change this state of affairs including "no vaccination, no welfare benefits".

This book is about vaccinations and immunizations in particular, and how so many lives have been affected by adverse reactions to this vested-interest-driven procedure.

The right to exercise informed choice cannot be taken for granted. To retain it requires vigilance and being proactive consistently.

NOW.

"Tomorrow" may be too late.

Then what would loving caring parents do? If parents refused to vaccinate their child(ren) they could become child abusers and consequently punished according to the law.

If it were **YOU** what would **YOU** do?

Would it be a costly cop out or a costly opt out?

71 Sebastian's Story

Written by Sebastian's mother, Phoebe.

Life was going pretty smoothly for our family. Sebastian was looking forward to his twelfth birthday, NOT looking forward to his vaccinations MMR, Td, and OPV4 that were due, but it was something that had to be done.

We decided to celebrate the birthday first and deal with the horrible injections a bit later.

So a couple of weeks after Sebastian's birthday, the nasty deed was done. Everything went fine, there was no immediate adverse reaction, a bit of a sore arm but that wasn't so bad.

Then Sebastian started complaining of having heavy, tired legs and just not feeling right. I suggested he might be suffering from growing pains, but one morning he woke feeling miserable, with an earache as well, so I made an appointment with the doctor. Half an hour later Sebastian was diagnosed with having GBS (Guillain Barre Syndrome).

I had never heard of it before but with the explanation the doctor had given me, I realized it was serious and not just growing pains! He sent us home insisting that I contact him immediately if Sebastian deteriorated.

Later that night, about 9 pm, the doctor rang to see how Sebastian was doing. He had fallen a couple of times but otherwise seemed okay. The doctor suggested we should go to A&E straight away as the GBS was progressing, and the danger was that Sabastian might start to have trouble breathing.

In A&E they did lots of tests, blood test, lumbar puncture, etc, then sent us to the ward, where we stayed for a week.

In that week Sebastian deteriorated further. He was unable to stand, and swallowing became very difficult. He choked at times when drinking, and had no appetite really, but it would have been very hard for him to swallow any food anyway. He was very tired but often unable to sleep, having nightmares and unable to get comfortable. His breathing deteriorated, the nurses were doing peak flow measurements on him every couple of hours. If this dropped below a certain level he was to be admitted to ICU.

The paediatrician conferred with the neurologist and they decided to give him some units of IV plasma. Sebastian improved after he had this. He was swallowing and breathing better and he was able to stand, very wobbly, but he was standing. Fortunately we didn't have to go to ICU.

The doctors and staff were very helpful, but whenever I queried whether the vaccinations could be the cause of this they didn't deny it but they wouldn't confirm it either!

The hospital doctor did mention to me that there was a 15-year-old boy in the hospital ICU with GBS. He had also had a tetanus vaccine previous to his illness!

I asked the doctor to report Sebastian's adverse reaction. He said he would but I never really followed this up as I was busy dealing with Sebastian's illness.

A week later we returned home. The doctor thought that Sebastian would recover in a couple of months and gave us a follow-up appointment, but a couple of days after we got home, Sebastian got worse. He became unable to walk, wouldn't eat (he had lost a lot of weight) and was feeling very ill.

We visited an osteopath/naturopath that we had been going to. He prescribed high doses of Vitamin C and antioxidants. Sebastian's appetite returned but he was still unable to walk.

Regular visits to the hospital proved that his recovery was going to take longer than two months.

In the meantime, the osteopath suggested I contact Hilary, who sent me lots of interesting information. Also, I had been reading about the connection between GBS cases and the tetanus vaccine.

This made me confident that what I had suspected seemed correct. The medical staff never denied it but they wouldn't support me either.

Sebastian was in a wheelchair for eight months, needing a lot of help with daily living skills. Then just as he was starting to walk again, he broke his leg! This set him back about six weeks but then he progressed to crutches. It was a good feeling to give the wheelchair back to the hospital.

All in all it took Sebastian a long year to recover. He is now 19 and leading a normal life. We were very lucky that Sebastian's adverse reaction caused no permanent damage that we know of!

Our experience also gave me a chance to learn about the "other side" of vaccines.

No more "little pricks" for this family!

72 There are Some Things in Life that You Never Forget

Written by Sebastian's father, George.

There are also things that happen that change your life forever. Sebastian's GBS certainly did that for us. I remember going to see Sebastian for the first time at the hospital the day after he was admitted and being assured by the doctor that though his condition could get very serious, there was little to no chance of him dying. Though I was grateful for his openness and honesty at least to warn us of possible further complications, the thought of death was also very real to me. As Phoebe said, Sebastian's breathing was becoming more and more shallow.

I knew then and there that things were going to get rough for Sebastian in those next few hours and so we waited . . . I also well remember during this period how Phoebe and I spent much time talking about the whole thing and going through all the different scenarios. Yet each of us both felt very much at peace with it. As Christian believers this was all completely out of our control and totally in the hands of God, no matter what.

That became another life-changing moment. To believe in God was one thing, but to totally trust Him was something else.

After Sebastian's survival in the hospital, having him home again was great, except I don't recall being told that he was going to go from wobbly walking to no walking at all. Time for Sebastian must have really started to slow down, as his ability to move his arms and legs steadily got worse and worse to the point of paralysis. How horrible a time that was for him!

For us the task was simply to get on with it. We really never gave the work involved a second thought. Looking back on it, I wonder how many times that wheelchair got thrown into the boot each day, especially once Sebastian was able to go back to school. As he slowly recovered, there was the silly thing of learning to walk again and regaining his sense of balance. There were a lot more laughs too as he was regaining strength. The worry of a bad fall became less and less, and so life for Sebastian was becoming more normal.

Throughout that whole year, Phoebe and I had grown very close to each other. I think this was a result of both the emotional strain as well as the physical demands that were placed on us. As I mentioned earlier, this was to be another life-changing event. This trial really strengthened our marriage and relationship, even to this day.

Incredibly, I thought I had done rather well coping with this GBS for a year but it wasn't until a year or more later that whenever I talked about Sebastian's illness to someone else, my eyes would begin to well up with tears. I realized then just what we had ALL been through and perhaps how much emotion had been put aside during that time.

I know our family has changed and become more sensitive to the good of others. I know there is a time, a place and a purpose for not only nice things, but also for awful things in life to occur and when they do, we believe there is hope, and that good can come out of it all. Not just in terms of relationships, but also in terms of rethinking what we do in life, and how and why we make decisions.

73 The Point That Isn't Mentioned

It came from a website – one of those "things" on the computer.

What did?

A print-out, consisting of three pages on which there were 141 words, and 23 shapes, or drawings, in colour, leaving plenty of spare space on each page.

The whole lot could be read and looked at in less than a minute and a half.

The story is called, ***"Vaccines and the Immune system"****.*

Sounds exciting?! (Re-arrange tongue in cheek.)

As you won't have the pages in front of you, I'll try to explain them to you, and as I do so, let your imagination run riot. Get a picture in your mind. Doodle too, if you feel like it.

I think the back-room boys and girls in the graphics department must have taken the specifications of their new assignment very seriously.

First of all, they had to design some bad-guy characters called Germs. Gone are the images of the mid-twentieth century, when Bertie Germ reigned supreme, sneaking in and out of people's teeth with his hammer and chisels, or driving madly around a racetrack and spinning off, as the cars of Vitamins, Minerals, Fresh Air, Sunshine and Exercise squeezed him out.

Instead, some of his cousins take on new shapes for this 2005 presentation.

The green down-at-the-mouth quadrilateral is probably Rubey. The blue wide-eyed hexagon could be Meningo, while the red circle, which looks like it's been cut out with pinking shears, is probably Fluesy. Their nefarious activities have to be dealt with, of course. We can't have them running around unrestrained, can we?

So bring into the picture the Goodies.

Who are they?

The drawings and captions portray them as Antibodies – part of the special defence force equipped to deal with any invaders.

To do the job entrusted to them, they have to come to grips with Bertie Germ's gang of blackguards!

The drawings show them sort of cuddling up to the uninvited visitors. The trouble is they're the wrong shape for real closeness and smothering tactics, but eventually, with the use of an egg-timer, they manage a total embrace.

The nasties are framed! Contained! Whooppee!!

Now that the defence forces have taken the baddies' mug-shots, measured up the picture frames for future close encounters and refined techniques for disposing of types like Rubey, Fluesy and Meningo, the recording system has to be updated.

So, there's a nice drawing of a filing cabinet. Only two drawers though!

The next lot of pretty "pictures" shows some weaker-looking doubles of Bertie's cousins, looking snug and smug in their picture frames. They have actually lost their threatening scowls, as if they had been suddenly surrounded before they had had a chance to do anything they were supposed to do. Bewildered surprise you could call it!

According to the caption, this has happened because the Defence forces have a new "weapon" called Vax Ene.

Now, remember that everyone using the services of Vax Ene, will be safe and not get sick! (At this point you can cheer, or boo if you feel so inclined.)

Then follows a drawing of a smiling, orange Square, poking out its red tongue at you!

How rude!

The Square also looks as if it's trying to smoke a cigarette, or something. Maybe it's a straw. Could it be a thermometer?

Because the smiling Square is so photogenic the next drawing shows it in a picture frame – still poking its tongue out even though the "whatever" has gone.

Finally, on the third page, the face is removed and the frame is put into the filing cabinet to be used when the next red alert sounds.

That's the end of the story as presented on the website. Make of it what you will. Maybe I haven't done justice to the message. "Naughty boy", some are bound to say, but there are some omissions in the picture-story which CANNOT be left out.

We started off with the Baddies.

Then came the Goodies.

Vax Ene made a pointed entry.

As a Goodie or a Baddie?

Well, definitely not a Goodie, so neither word is really suitable.

We have to introduce another: the TERRORISTS!

Baddies which are badder.

Who are they?

Well they don't like getting any publicity, but information does leak out, you know. For example, have you heard of:

- For ma Lin
- Ali Minium
- Neo Mycin
- The Monkey "business"
- Yet Unknowns?

As with all terrorists, there are all sorts of comings and goings amongst their ranks. Name changes; dubious communiqués, and denials. But the good name of the new "weapon" must be protected at all costs.

Vax Ene is more than an enigma too.

"She" has invisible, unpredictable qualities which can have undesirable and far-reaching consequences for some of those in whom she takes up lodgings. Rarely does she do this through a natural entrance way. Rather, a dart-like approach is preferred. The dart usually receives its momentum from another "she" who will take great pains to assure the human "dwelling" about to be entered, that it won't hurt much. "Just a little prick. There now, it's all over . . ."

Ouch!! (And whatever goes with it!)

Is it all over though? Does it have that lovely fairytale ending:

"And they all lived happily ever after"*?*

This book wouldn't have been written if it did.

74 Vaccines: How Safe? How Toxic?

***"If they were willing to look at all the studies that were done with vaccines, they would find that they are, I think without question, the safest, best-tested thing we put into our bodies," says Offit. "I think they have a better safety record than vitamins"*[1]**

"The safest, best tested thing we put into our bodies." ?? Interesting statement don't you think, from a US vaccine expert. It seems Dr Offit wasn't at an FDA Scientific workshop in December 2002[2], convened to work out how to test vaccines for toxicity. Someone had done a review only to find that, apart from the pertussis tests mentioned previously in this book, there isn't that much testing done in terms of "toxicity". Why is that? And what do they mean by safety anyway?

The FDA definition[3] of safety, which is *"relative freedom from*

1 Dr Paul Offit, USA's most outspoken vaccine pusher. (CBS) *60 Minutes*, 20 October 2004 .

2 (Scientific) workshop on Non-Clinical safety evaluation of Preventive Vaccines: Center for Biologics Evaluation and Research, Held in Arlington, Virginia, Monday December 2, 2002. The transcript from tape recordings can be found http://www.fda.gov/cber/minutes/tox120202.htm . To enable easy use of quotes in this book, this transcript was downloaded, and put into a standard page set-up WORD document so that quotes could be ascribed page numbers. To get a sense that I have not misquoted anything, reading the whole laborious transcript would be useful, and give a much broader education than a short review.

3 FDA Code of Federal Regulation (21 CFR 600.3).

harmful effect to persons affected directly or indirectly by a product when prudently administered, taking into consideration the character of the product in relation to the condition of the recipient at the time."

Which can mean all things to all people depending on what they want to explain away.

The reason that this workshop was convened was that in the past, toxicity testing hasn't been done, because, as Dr Midthun says on page 4: *"Historically, the non-clinical safety assessment for preventive vaccines has often not included toxicity studies in animal models. This is because vaccines have not been viewed as inherently toxic, and vaccines are generally administered in limited dosages over months or even years"*

Dr Sutkowski follows that up on page 6 with this statement:

> *". . . As Dr. Midthun mentioned, the Office of Vaccines is giving consideration to whether or not, prior to proceeding into phase I clinical trials, there is going to be extra consideration given to whether or not non-clinical safety assessments will need to be supported by toxicity testing in animals."* And on page 10: *"For which product category type should toxicity testing be performed? And, how to best design appropriate toxicity tests for preventive vaccines".*

Later on page 23 when someone points out that since vaccines are given to newborns with fragile immune systems, shouldn't they be tested in juvenile animals to get some close approximation of similarity? Well, yes, says a Dr Verdier on page 23, but there is only one problem: *"I think today we need to get more information about the immune system of juvenile animal models. We are not yet ready to use these juvenile animals in toxicology."* And he also admits on page 17, that vaccines were considered safe *"ipso facto"*, seventy years ago, when the use of aluminium started, so few vaccines were given to babies, no one even thought to think about it.

And yes, on page 24 he agrees: *"To what extent this (juvenile animal models) can be used for toxicology and to assess the potential risk that we have there, I think that there is a whole bunch of work to be done there. And we know that for some adjuvants it's probably important to look at young animals*

as well, because we see different types of reactions. But the knowledge is still quite limited."

Dr Midthun[4] and others, admit that toxicity studies were never done on aluminium in vaccines or other potential toxicity issues for which they now have to formulate some guidelines. A bit late, don't you think?

A Mr Feder in the audience pipes up on page 69 to say: ***"I think this highlights one of the problems of vaccine toxicity. Very little is published. Having had to write a short review of alum toxicity recently, I was horrified to find how few publications there were on this. And I see a problem."***

None of this will come as a surprise now to Vancouver neuroscientist Chris Shaw, who was looking at the anthrax vaccine for something else[5], when he found that the aluminium hydroxide in the vaccine, which is the same as that in childhood vaccines, was causing symptoms associated with Parkinson's, amyotrophic lateral sclerosis (ALS or Lou Gehrig's disease) and Alzheimer's. In a 20 week study of mice, 38 per cent had statistically significant increases in anxiety and memory deficits and 20 per cent had an increase in allergy. When they killed the mice and looked at the brains, in a part that controls movement, 35 per cent of the cells were destroying themselves. Two comments he made stand out:

"No one in my lab wants to get vaccinated," he said. "This totally creeped us out. We weren't out there to poke holes in vaccines. But all of a sudden, oh my God – we've got neuron death!"

Then later when he said that he couldn't find any studies that looked further than immediately post vaccination, he said: ***"This is suspicious. Either this [link] is known by industry and it was never made public, or industry was never made to do these studies . . . I don't know which is scarier . . . if anyone has a study that shows something different . . . put it on the table. That's how you do science."***

In order to understand the "safety" of vaccines, you have to know several things, including how a baby's immune system works from

4 P. 37, scientific workshop transcript. P. 69, Dr Garcon admits very little is known about aluminium in vaccines.

5 Wooley, P. "Vaccine show sinister side" *The Georgia Straight*. Available from <http://www.straight.com/content.cfm?id=16717>

birth onwards, and what vaccines do biochemically in the body. That work has never been done. In Italy in 1998 big-wigs from vaccine companies and interested parties attended a meeting[6] where vaccine issues were discussed. On the final day there was a nearly two hour "Concluding Round-table" euphemistically called "How to Move the Field." R Rappuoli, the Head of Research of *Chiron Vaccines* when asking himself what knowledge had been gained about the functioning of the immune system in infants below the age of 6 months, said that his answer would have to be nothing. Professor Nossal, an immuno-pathologist from the University of Melbourne, remarked that in Japan 36% of children had atopies[7] and in Australia, 25% of children had asthma. He said that more intensive research was needed in the field of allergy and that "It is strange how little we know about immunity in the first 6 months of life".

The Sunday Times[8], UK recently revealed that severe allergic reactions had increased 146% in the last five years, and that epi-pen use had increased 122%. The article also reported a 2003 study which showed that admission of serious allergies had jumped dramatically over the previous decade. There are no grey areas with allergies in the UK. Children only get epi-pens after testing for high allergic sensitivity.

A lawyer friend of mine, tracked down the 1998 – 2004 information. What was found, but not printed in the article is that 1 in 53 children in the UK; in other words, around 1 in 20 UK families now have a child with a life-threatening allergy. Also, roughly 99.5% of cases are in children under 16. Given that there were significant changes to the immunization schedule in the UK in the early 1990s, with a greatly increased intake of toxic chemicals like thiomersal, aluminium hydroxide etc at a much earlier age, I think some questions need to be asked of these "safer than vitamin" biological substances doctors want to spread with liberal abandon.

Allergy increase in children is not just a UK problem either. The

6 "Protection of Newborns and Infants from Infectious Diseases. Interplay of Immunology and Biotechnology. A EU-US workshop, June 3–5, 1998, Siena, Italy.

7 Atopy = hypersensitivity to environmental allergens, principally asthma, allergies and atopic dermatitis, proven by IgE antibodies.

8 Foggo, D. 2006. "Number of children treated for nut allergies soars" *Sunday Times* (UK) April 2. Available from <http://www.timesonline.co.uk/article/0,,2087-2114328,00.html>

Grand Forks Herald[9] reported that: ***Physicians don't understand why food allergies are becoming more prevalent, though they have plenty of theories.*** " Two weeks after the *Times* article, the *Observer*[10] analysed the data finding a 54 per cent increase in severe allergy between 2003–2005 and a 610 per cent increase between 1995–2005.

We have a situation where the experts know very little about a baby's immune system up to six months. They haven't tested the toxicity of adjuvants and other compounds in vaccines, because they assumed there was none. We DO know that to have serious allergies, a person has to have high levels of IgE antibodies, and to have a Th2 skewed immune system. And we also know that aluminium-adjuranted injected vaccines don't activate the first defences (Th1) that infections normally trigger in the cellular immune system. Instead they activate the last defences of the humoral system, antibodies, ***which are preferentially Th2.*** That is the job that aluminium is designed to do.[11] But no-one has looked to see if the increasing numbers of vaccines, by skewing the baby's immune system to exactly the state it needs to be to provoke serious allergy, are implicated.

What do doctors know about how vaccines work? You saw the explanation in the previous chapter, but is that explanation correct? According to these vaccine researchers, the antibody theory has some holes, which it would if you haven't any idea how vaccines work in the first place:

> ***"Vaccines work simply by producing antibodies, right? Well, probably not. And this misconception coupled with basic ignorance of how they do work is stalling the urgent quest for an AIDS vaccine . . .***
>
> ***'I'm amazed by the amount of basic science we don't know,' Philippe Kourilsky, director of the Paris-based Pasteur Institute . . .***

9 Olsen, J. 2006. "Doctors see more food allergies, few remedies." February 23. http://www.grandforks.com/mld/grandforks/living/13938632.htm

10 Doward, J. 2006. "Big rise in patients with deadly allergies. Children are worst hit by rise in killer reactions". *Observer*, April 16. Available from <http://observer.guardian.co.uk/uk_news/story/0,,1754840,00.html>

11 Del Giudice. G. et al. 2002. "What are the limits of adjuvanticity?" *Vaccine*, Oct 15; 20 Suppl 1: S38–41. PMID: 11587808. S39 under "Immunological targeting".

The assumption that successful vaccines work by simply producing antibodies is almost certainly wrong, Neal Nathanson, director of the US Office of AIDS Research, warns. 'Hepatitis B vaccine is a good example. It's amazingly effective but no one knows how it works.'"

The whole article does media over-kill with ad nauseum phrases like *"highly successful"*, *"amazingly effective"*, as if they need to keep maximum hype to detract from the fact that they know very little about what vaccines DO in the body. Unfortunately, researchers have to admit what they don't know, if they want more money to figure it out. You mean, they really don't know how the immune system works?

You be the judge:

"It is known that in many instances, antigen-specific antibody titers do not correlate with protection. In addition, very little is known on parameters of cell-mediated immunity which could be considered as surrogates of protection."[12]

The Russians discovered a thing or two in the 1990s about how the body fights diphtheria as evidenced by information provided to me by an Israeli doctor of Russian origin, Dr Alexander Kotok.

Studies on children with diphtheria in Russia in the 1990s proved quite clearly that there was no difference in the course of diphtheria in the vaccinated and non-vaccinated.[13,14] Serious diphtheria was almost always seen in patients with pre-existing conditions like an immunodeficiency,[15] alcoholism, etc. Doctors found that the course

12 Del Guidice. G. et al. 2001. "What are the limits of adjuvanticity?" *Vaccine*, Oct 15; 20 Suppl 1: S38–41. PMID: 11587808.

13 Ivanova, V.V. et al. 2002. *Difteriia u detei* (Diphtheria in children). St Petersburg, p. 41. Ibid., p. 114: the last outbreak casts doubt the common opinion that toxic diphtheria is observed in the non-vaccinated children exclusively . . . According to the Research Institute for Children Infection's observations, there were 14.0% of the fully vaccinated, 42.4% of the partially vaccinated and 43.6% of the non-vaccinated among those children who fell ill with toxic diphtheria.

14 Nekrassova, L.S. et al. 2000. "Epidemic diphtheria in Ukraine, 1991–1997". *J Infect Dis*, February: 181: Suppl 1:S35–40. Among 5 - 14 year-old children who died from diphtheria, 24% had been fully immunized (according to the immunization schedule at this time) - Table 3, page 539.

15 Kuz'menko, L.G. and Ariziamova, V.V. 2004. "Nedostatochnost' produktsii protivodifteriinyh antitel u detei s timomegaliei pri immunizatsii vaktsinoi AKDS". (The insufficiency of the anti-diphtheria antibodies production after immunization with DPT vaccine). *Detskie infektsii* (Children infections), Vol. 2(7): 23–26. Thymomegalia is registered in every third child in some regions [of Russia]. In this paper the authors confirm that after DPT-immunization of the children with thymomegalia, the anti-

of diphtheria did not depend on the level of the antitoxin antibodies, but on the cellular TH1 immunity; i.e. interferon,[16] Patients who had serious problems with their body's ability to produce interferon fell victim to diphtheria regardless of their antitoxin antibody status.

Even more interesting was that in thymomegalia immunodeficient children, the DPT caused not only reactions but reduced immunity.[17] I wonder what they would find if they studied other immunodefiencies as well.

The only reason that the medical profession's basic ignorance about the immune system and vaccines hasn't been found out, is that parents don't know what doctors haven't studied. We assume that doctors wouldn't be doing something if they didn't know the basics.

American subscribers to Babytalk, woke up one morning in 2005[18] to read:

> ***"In fact, Dr Offit's studies show that in theory, healthy infants could safely get up to 100,000 vaccines at once."***

---

diphtheria antibodies are not being produced at all or in an insufficient quantity.

16 Ivanova V.V. et al. 2002. *Difteriia u detei* (Diphtheria in children). St Petersburg, p. 41: the factors of the specific cell immunoreactivity and non-specific mechanisms of defence are of significance as well. Page 43: The system of IF (interferon) has neither specialized cells, nor all the more organs, it exists in every cell, for every cell is able of becoming a victim of the antigen aggression, thus it has to possess its own system of recognizing and further eliminating of the foreign genetic information . . . By its importance the system of IF-genesis may be well compared with the immunity system in total, while by its universality it even surpasses the latter. Just this universality of IF makes it the most important factor of the non-specific resistance. There is the tight coordination between the systems of IF and immunity in the macroorganism. Pages 47–48 The findings confirmed that the severity of the disease depended upon the ability of the body to synthesize α- and γ-IF. "The represented clinical and experimental findings testify to the complicated interactions between the system of IF-genesis and diphtheritic toxin and confirm the important role of the system of non-specific resistance in creating immunity to diphtheria.

17 Adishcheva, N. I. 1996. Kliniko-immunologicheskie pokazateli vaktsinal'nogo protsessa AKDS u detei s uvelicheniem timusa I stepeni (Clinical-immunological characteristics of the vaccinal process in children with 1st grade thymomegalia. Abstract of PhD thesis. Tomsk pp. 2 and 24. It is known that DPT vaccination even in healthy children not only produces a specific immune response, but causes the allergic reorganization in the body, lowers the specific resistance . . . The children with modified reactivity from the high-risk groups react to DPT-vaccination by the long-term suppression of resistance, by developing postvaccinal complications, by defective immune response, by high morbidity . . . It was demonstrated the DPT-vaccinations (from the first to the third shot) in the most children with thymomegalia of the 1st grade by their first year of life caused the complicated course of the vaccinal process, namely allergic complications, acute respiratory diseases, the lack or inferior immune reaction to diphtheria or pertussis toxins and enlarging the thymus up to 2nd to 3rd grade. The result of the three shots was the factual absence of immunity to whooping cough, low anti-diphtheria and high anti-tetanus . . . immunity."

18 Howard, B. 2005. "10 vaccine myths – Busted". *Babytalk*.

There was considerable discussion on Internet boards as to what this astonishing statement meant, and whether he really meant that. There can be no doubt that Dr Paul Offit meant that, because he is the Henle Professor of the Immunologic and Infectious Diseases at the Children's Hospital of Philadelphia and made sure that this article was put onto his section of the University's website.[19]

You may ask who is this man who considers vaccines safer than vitamins, and babies capable of receiving 100,000 vaccines in one day? And where are these studies that back up such theory?

Dr Offit is the USA's most prominent provaccine advocate and has received hundreds of thousands of dollars in grant money from Merck Vaccines Division, holds a vaccine patent, and acts as a consultant to them. He is also a member of the CDC Advisory Committee on Immunization Practice. He has written a book on vaccines, which a friend of mine borrowed from her doctor to find inside, a letter inside, donating the book to the doctor saying, "Merck Vaccine Division is pleased to present you with a copy of the recent publication, 'What Every Parent Should Know About Vaccines,' . . . The authors designed the book to answer questions parents have about vaccines and to dispel "misinformation" about vaccines that sometimes appears in the public media."

Dr Offit's view of his ACIP[20] work is:

> ***"It provides no conflict for me," he insists. "I have simply been informed by the process, not corrupted by it. When I sat around that table, my sole intent was trying to make recommendations that best benefited the children in this country. It's offensive to say that physicians and public-health people are in the pocket of industry and thus are making decisions that they know are unsafe for children. It's just not the way it works." . . . "Science," says Offit, "is best left to scientists."***

Because parents bring up their children they have every right to research all issues and ask scientists questions like, "What does

19 Retrieved on 27 February, 2006 from <http://www.chop.edu/consumer/jsp/division/generic.jsp?id=81553>

20 Robert F. Kennedy Jr "Deadly immunity" June 16, 2005 Salon/Rolling stone Joint investigation. Available from <http://www.salon.com/news/feature/2005/06/16/thimerosal/print.html> Accessed 18 June, 2005 & 27 February, 2006.

mercury or aluminium in vaccines do in the body?" They are also entitled to honest answers . . . The medical establishment continues to say that mercury in vaccines has nothing to do with autism, and that it's quite safe. The problem is there are many studies from way before 1999 that show thiomersal had problems:

> ***"The present study[21] confirms the high frequency of sensitization to thimerosal in atopic children and suggest that vaccination can cause clinical symptoms in sensitized children."***

Of course the medical establishment concluded that that doesn't prevent those children from continuing to be vaccinated. If they hadn't said that, the study probably wouldn't have been published.

The first study showing thiomersal allergy and vaccination reactions in the UK was in 1988[22] which said, ***"individual cases of severe reactions to thiomersal demonstrate a need for vaccines with an alternative preservative."*** Even more forthright was a 1990 study[23] which pointed out that the reactions can be ***"very long lasting"***.

Twenty-three years ago Russian researchers[24] said that thiomersal was highly toxic and should not be used in children's vaccines.

Others can argue the toss as to whether thiomersal in vaccine causes immune dysfunction contributing to autism but the fact is that scientists know that thiomersal is immunosuppressive and provokes autoimmunity in mice.[25] The study showed that in terms of the immune system, thiomerosal (EtHg) leads to a much stronger immunostimulation and autoimmunity than organic mercury (MeHg),

---

21 Patrizi, A. et al. 1999. "Sensitization to thiomersal in atopic children". *Contact Dermatitis*, February: 40(2): 94–7. PMID: 10048654.

22 Cox, N.H et al. 1988. "Thiomersal allergy and vaccination reactions". *Contact Dermatitis*, April: 18(4): 229–33. PMID: 3378430.

23 Rietschel, R.L. et al. 1990. "Reactions to thimerosal in hepatitis B vaccines". *Dermatol Clin.*, January: 8(1): 161–4. PMID: 2137393.

24 Kravchenko, A.T. et al. 1983. *Zh Mikrobiol Epidemiol Immunobiol.*, Vol. (3), March, pp. 87–92. "The toxic action of preparations kills and damages the cells at the site of injection, thus inducing the formation of autoantigens whose effect on the body cannot be predicted. Thus thimerosal, commonly used as a preservative, has been found not only to render its primary toxic effect, but also to be capable of changing the properties of cells. This fact suggests that the use of thimerosal for the preservation of medical biological preparations, especially those intended for children, is inadmissible." PMID: 6845931.

25 Havarinasab, S. et al. 2005. "Immunosuppressive and autoimmune effects of thimerosal in mice". *Toxicology and Applied Pharmacology*, Vol. 204: 109–121.

but now, what possible relevance could mice have to babies?

Doctors like to brush aside worries about aluminium by talking about "70 years of use" and aluminium being very common. There's two problems with these sorts of dismissals. When you check the articles quoted you find the studies discussed hypothetical statements based on 1960 studies with single antigens on mice. In those days babies started a limited schedule at an age when the now-crowded primary neonatal schedule is finished. Furthermore, it is not possible to compare aluminium in food or water, to an injection. As one study says,[26] ***"Accumulation of aluminium in the body tends to occur when the gastrointestinal barrier is circumvented."***

Medical people also like to say there is no replacement candidate for aluminium. There is. It's called Inulin. What is inulin? Fructose with small amounts of glucose. Inulin has been extensively tested before and since 1991,[27] using many different candidate vaccines in mice, rats, rabbits, dogs, horses, monkeys and man. With the exception of small granulomas when very high doses are injected subcutaneously, inulin has none of the problems of aluminium. If you are someone who wants to have a vaccine, inulin adjuvant creates Th1 cellular immunity as well as Th2.[28]

Sometimes it seems the wheels of change suffer from the severe lack of an axle jack. Instead we read that some would like to revisit previously rejected Freund's incomplete adjuvant,[29] but in general all articles rave over aluminium considering it safe, very efficient at making the immune system take notice, which it is, but best of all, very cheap.[30] This same author dismisses many side effects saying, ***"Some side-effects seen after vaccination with adjuvanted vaccines, must, however be attributed to the vaccine preservatives, like thiomersal, betapropriolactone or formaldehyde or . . . to bacterial toxins from the antigen preparation."*** (p. 3665)

Theoretically the most interesting issue is that aluminium is only

26 Monteagudo, F.S. et al. 1989. "Recent developments in aluminium toxicology". *Med Toxicol Adverse Drug Exp*, Jan–Feb; 4(1): 1–16. PMID: 2651849.

27 Cooper, P.D. et al. 1991. "The adjuvanticity of Algammulin, a new vaccine adjuvant". *Vaccine*, Jun; 9(6): 408–15. PMID: 1887671. (In this study it was used with aluminium.)

28 Petrovsky, N. 2005. (In Press. Still!). "Novel human polysaccharide adjuvants with dual Th1 and Th2 potentiating activity". *Vaccine*, February 5.

29 Eidkhoff, T.C. et al. 2002. "Workshop summary. Aluminium in vaccines". *Vaccine*, May 31; 20 Suppl 3: S1–4. PMID: 12184358.

30 Lindblad, E.B. et al. 2004. "Aluminium compounds for use in vaccines". *Immunol Cell Biol*, Oct; 82(5): 497–505. PMID: 15479435.

of any "use" for the first shot of any series. It "wakes up" the immune system. After that, it's not needed in booster shots.[31] But it's given, because it's cheap and much less complicated to only have one set of bottles, rather than a primary dose, and aluminium free booster doses. Never mind that since 1965[32] it's been known that you can induce an encephalopathy and neurofibrillary tangles in the brains of animals by injecting aluminium salts. Or that since 1973[33] neurofibrillary degeneration after injection of aluminium can result in decline in learning and memory. So really, Vancouver neuroscientist Chris Shaw shouldn't have been too surprised to find that aluminium hydroxide injected as a vaccine into mice could do exactly this.

You have to understand what aluminium can do in a body to see the multi-facetted significance of aluminium. In the previous chapter, when the pretty coloured body was making antibodies, they missed out the bit where the nasty is handed to what we call an antigen presenting cell. Rather like a postie who is given a letter to deliver to where its supposed to go. These are called "dendritic" cells. Aluminium switches them on, and leaves them on.

In some people dendritic cells won't turn off. And when they don't, you can land up with something called Systemic lupus erythematosus (SLE). The problem with lupus is that the antigen presenting cells get switched on, stay on, and eventually abnormal autoimmune antibodies form. The scientists have no idea why that happens. It's clear an environmental trigger plays a role, but none of them are looking at aluminium, even though aluminium's function is to overstimulate antigen-presenting cells to force the immune system to respond to antigens it wouldn't otherwise take note of. That's why almost all vaccines contain aluminium.

However, aluminium also affects other cells called "macrophages", which become loaded with aluminium which disrupts their function. When those macrophages cross into the brain, they take the aluminium with them, which can demyelinate neurons, which could result in diverse disorders. Aluminium also makes the blood-brain barrier

31 Eidkhoff, T.C. et al. 2002. "Workshop summary: Aluminium in vaccines". *Vaccine*, May 31; 20 Suppl 3: S1–4. PMID: 12184358.

32 Klatzo, I. et al. 1965. "Experimental production of neurofibrillary degeneration". *J Neuropathol Exp Neurol*, Apr; 24: 187–99. PMID: 14280496.

33 Crapper, D.R. et al. 1973. "Aluminium induced neurofibrillary degeneration, brain electrical activity and alternations in acquisition and retention". May; 10(5); 935–45. PMID: 4736728.

weaker,[34] making the brain more accessible to other toxins. Aluminium hydroxide in vaccines is highly reactive and separates spontaneously. And since it is injected through the skin right into your tissue, it is instantly absorbed and enters the brain.[35,36,37]

The fact that thiomersal is immunosuppressive, and that injected aluminium has a high affinity for brain cells, has been known since 1980.[38]

In terms of research looking at what vaccines do in babies, the early research before 1970 wasn't reassuring. And for whatever reason, that work hasn't been repeated, even though babies are now getting so many more vaccines than 35 years ago. So why hasn't the research been repeated? And why don't doctors even know about the research that was done then?

A very interesting report published in 1969[39] showed very significant changes. For instance:

> ***"It is necessary to admit firstly that vaccination is always a trauma of considerable intensity . . . Satisfactory safety of vaccines on a mass level does not necessarily coincide with total safety on an individual level."***

Dr Del Campo found albumen decreases, heavy rise in the sedimentation rate, decreased transferring, retention in the tissues of various electrolytes, alkali reserve decreased conspicuously and for a rather long time. Serum glucose and serum cholesterol decreased, but lipemia increased steadily. Some enzymes showed an increase while others showed a decrease. Prothrombin time was lengthened. Changes in the EEG reading of the cerebral cortex of the brain were

---

34 Banks, W.A. et al. 1989. "Aluminium-induced neurotoxicity: alterations in membrane function at the blood-brain barrier". *Neurosci Biobehav Rev*, Spring; 13(1): 47–53. PMID: 2671833.

35 Redhead, et al. 1992. "Aluminum-adjuvanted vaccines transiently increase aluminium levels in murine brain tissue". *Pharmacology and Toxicology*, Vol. 70: 278–280. PMID: 1608913.

36 Yokel, 2000. "The toxicology of aluminium in the brain: a review". *Neurotoxicology*, October: 21(5): 813–25. PMID: 11130287. (Not related to vaccines, but essential reading.)

37 Verstraeten, et al. 1997. "Myelin is a preferential target of aluminium-mediated oxidative damage". *Archives of Biochemistry and Biophysics*, Vol. 344(2): 289–94. PMID: 9264541.

38 Zheng, W. 2001. "Neurotoxicology of the brain barrier system: new implications". *J Toxicol Clin Toxicol*, 39(7): 711–9. PMID: 11778669.

39 Del Campo, A. 1969. "Physiological changes of the vaccinated organism: a basis for the interpretation of the clinical complications due to prophylactic vaccines". *Prog Immunobiol Stand*, Vol. 3: 280–4. PMID: 5379945.

seen. There was in increased excretion of 11 cortico-costeroid, and rises in serum complement for an extended time. Phagocytic activity increased at a marked rate. He showed that properdin and lysozyme decreased, which explains the easy occurrence of secondary infections after vaccinations.

But he also stated that:

"every effort must be made to prevent individuals just vaccinated from being exposed to a new stress be this of a physical or infectious type while weakening of the natural defence and the disorder of the biochemical activities are still operating. Only in this way does it seem possible on the one hand to reduce the intensity and the duration of this post-vaccinal syndrome, and on the other to limit its consequences and the danger of the real clinical complications which arise from it."

And that was in the days when they only used a few vaccines. Safer than vitamins eh?

Furthermore, as was stated in a letter to the doctor about the testing of the Hep B vaccine in babies, not only had Merck not looked at the effect of the Hepatitis B vaccine on immune parameters, but that:

"Estimates of the frequency of various complaints following vaccination have usually been based on uncontrolled studies, i.e. there has been no parallel unvaccinated group in the study."[40]

Bearing in mind that the studying of a large group of people cannot assess the exact outcome for any individual, it's interesting to consider the following.

There are vast numbers of medical articles showing, for instance, high and unexpected duration of the IgE responses to DT boosters[41] in humans, which from animal studies[42] would indicate that allergies would worsen. There are an equally large number of more recent ones showing the opposite. It's always been the case with vaccines, that

40 Letter: Dr J.W. West to Dr D.F. Woolner; 20 September, 1988.

41 Mark, A. et al. 1997. "IgE and G antibodies two years after booster dose on an aluminium-adsorbed or a fluid DT in relation to atopy". *Pediatr Allergy Immunol*, May: 2: 83–87. PMID: 9617777.

42 Frick, O.L. et al. 1983. "IgE antibodies to pollens augmented in dogs by virus vaccines". *Am J Vet Res*, March: 44(3): 440–5. PMID: 6301317.

when something is hypothesized, you will get a downpour of studies pouring scorn on the hypothesis. It's become such a pattern now, that I usually look for information on who has funded any material before I minutely scrutinize the full body of the article.

However, it pays to think seriously about the positive studies, because regardless of the hail of negative studies, you have to consider that where there is smoke in the absence of knowledge, there may well be a lot more fire, in the absence of water.

There was some hope that the IgE production after pertussis vaccination would decrease with the new acellular vaccines, but that hasn't turned out to be so. In fact, the acellular pertussis vaccines provoke a lot more Pertussis Toxin-stimulated IgE than the so-called crude whole-cell vaccines.[43]

Bearing in mind the recent vaccine drive in Auckland with the BCG,[44] of a vaccine that's only marginally better than useless, it should be noted that the BCG increases sensitivity to house dust mites.[45]

Another study showed:[46]

> ***"The odds of having a history of asthma was twice as great among vaccinated subjects than among unvaccinated subjects (adjusted odds ratio, 2.00; 95% confidence interval, 0.59 to 6.74). The odds of having had any allergy-related respiratory symptom in the past 12 months was 63% greater among vaccinated subjects than unvaccinated subjects (adjusted odds ratio, 1.63; 95% confidence interval, 1.05 to 2.54). The associations between vaccination and subsequent allergies and symptoms were greatest among children aged 5 through 10 years."***

Almost as if the authors suffered an allergic reaction to their own findings, they conclude:

---

43 Nilsson, L. et al. 1998. "Pertussis IgE and atopic disease". *Allergy*, Vol. 53(12): 1195–1201. PMID: 9930597.

44 Mentjox, L. 2005. "Children at risk from TB". *The Aucklander*, 24 August: 7. (7500 shots a year).

45 Mommers, M. et al. 2004. "Infant immunization and the occurrence of atopic disease in Dutch and German children: a nested case-control study". *Pediatr Pulmonol*, October: 38(4): 329–34. PMID: 15334511

46 Hurwitz, E.L. and Morgenstern, H. 2000. "Effects of diphtheria-tetanus-pertussis or tetanus vaccination on allergies and allergy-related respiratory symptoms among children and adolescents in the United States". *J Manipulative Physiol Ther.*, Vol. 23(2): 81–90. (UCLA School of Public Health, Department of Epidemiology, Los Angeles, Calif 90095-1772, USA.) PMID: 10714532.

"CONCLUSIONS: DTP or tetanus vaccination appears to increase the risk of allergies and related respiratory symptoms in children and adolescents. Although it is unlikely that these results are entirely because of any sources of bias, the small number of unvaccinated subjects and the study design limit our ability to make firm causal inferences about the true magnitude of effect." (Underlining mine.)

A study in Sweden, however, didn't find an increase in allergies, but did find a positive association between whooping cough vaccine and asthma by 2½ years of age.[47]

As to all the other immunological pointers that are missing in this discussion, don't even get me started. The issue of how safe vaccines are won't be sorted out as long as medical people only want to play number crunching games like giving 10,000 kids a lolly. Looking at actual individual risk to real people seems to be much too dangerous. Perhaps something might be found that they would rather not see.

You be the judge. Are vaccines the safest, best tested thing you've had put in your body?

47 Nilsson, L. et al. 1998. "A randomized controlled trial of the effect of pertussis vaccines on atopic disease". *Arch Pediatr Adolesc Med*, August: 152(8): 734–8. PMID: 9701130.

75 A Challenge

Clubs.

Societies.

Associations.

Organizations for just about everything you can think of.

Many of them have been formed to protect some right or freedom.

Others are unashamedly militant as they look for opportunities to protest against some current issue.

They all have one thing in common. To succeed in their aims and objectives, they need people who will identify with the cause they represent. Very often the members of the organization give voluntarily of their time and energies. Sometimes the workload is spread pretty thinly.

Occasionally the shortage of volunteers reaches a crisis point.

Some years ago, Hilary was involved in this sort of situation. The workload was getting too much for a few and no one seemed available to be President or Secretary or Treasurer or a committee member. Should the society be allowed to disband or go into recess?

Was this going to be an occasion when I would have to spend time wiping tears away, defusing tensions and uttering soothing noises?!

Well, I probably did all those things and more.

I wrote a poem designed to be published in the society's newsletter.

Because this book requires a **response** *of some sort from those who read it, the following lines seem totally pertinent. Similar challenges will appear in the pages to come.*

FRONT-UP OR COP-OUT

Here is another book to read –
How much of its message will I heed?

I know it's taken hours of work;
Time which I am happier to shirk.

Maybe I shall write a letter,
But there're others who'd do it better.

I'll be bold and stick out my neck!
Or perhaps I'll mutter, "What the heck."

I've stored many "facts" in my head,
But what might be wrong, is what I dread.

Am I guilty of double-talk?
And do my decisions match my walk?

These pages now before my eyes
Could help me to answer many lies.

So many thoughts come to mind;
Ways to deal with them are hard to find.

Deep down inside I really know,
That it's hard to go against the flow.

If I postpone my read today,
Perhaps my waverings will go away.

Maybe just a skim-read would do.
That would make me feel more faithful too!

There's so much information stuff
Which bombards my ears. I've had enough!

I often ask myself, "What's right?
Do I walk by faith, fear or by sight?"

Within these lines a point I make
So other strategies to awake.

You are you, and I am me –
What do we really want to be?

The time has come to make **my** *choice.*
My decision boldly now I voice.

Strong convictions I will convey,
There's no need for any more delay.

At last I'll leave the rhyming line,
Plain prose my message will define.

Actions I'll take number at least nine.

- ❍ *I will question what I hear and read, testing it for the truth.*
- ❍ *I will start giving "I KNOW", rather than "I THINK" answers as soon as I can, and whenever possible.*
- ❍ *I will continually keep testing the confidence I have in my decision making.*
- ❍ *I will keep asking myself, "How firm is my commitment to the choices I make?"*
- ❍ *I will guard against becoming over-dependent on other*

people and systems to maintain my commitment.

- ❍ *I will try to eliminate double-standards and inconsistencies in my lifestyle.*
- ❍ *I will develop strategies against the pressure of such things as the "latest claims", "discoveries", advertising, smooth-talk, "persuasive arguments", "smoke-screens" and the like.*
- ❍ *I will learn how to focus on the real issues – to be able to distinguish the wood from the trees.*
- ❍ *Finally, I will ask, "Can I accept the responsibilities that my decisions place on me, as well as any consequences that might follow?"*
- ❍ *If I need to, I will work through it all again (and again, and again . . .) until I can.*
- ❍ ***If I can't reach such a position, then I should stay with the compliant majority and take what comes without complaint. (It's certainly an easier option, but that's a cop-out isn't it?)***

76 Informed Choice – the Key Concept

DELUDED OR INFORMED?

The Associate Professor of Otago University's School of Medicine, Glenn Buchan, worked up a head of steam:

> *"As the dreaded polio virus spreads from Nigeria through to other countries in Africa, we can at least take comfort that such things don't happen in New Zealand. Efforts to stamp out the virus there have been hampered by conspiracy theories that the vaccine contains a contraceptive that would render the population infertile.*
>
> *Luckily, we New Zealanders don't suffer from the same kind of delusions. But the same kind of rumour-mongering and subsequent poor health outcomes are part of the New Zealand scene as well." (New Zealand Herald, 24–25 July 2004, P. B15)*

Normally the first two paragraphs might not have interested me, but I had heard rumours from scientist friends in New Delhi about ructions that had gone on there relating to some Nigerian vaccine samples, but ignored it at the time. However, when the medical profession talks about the impact of delusions by rampant lunatic radicals, you can be sure something has got them riled up.

While awaiting a response from New Delhi, I researched polio in Africa which was said to be spreading out at a rate of knots from Nigeria causing cases in fully vaccinated countries which had previously professed to have eradicated polio. There were countless articles on the BBC website and on some medical sites about how all these countries, some of which had previously vaccinated children more than six times with oral polio vaccine, were going to have to coordinate yet MORE mass vaccination campaigns in February and March to try to halt the march of polio through their fully vaccinated countries. All because Nigeria had spoiled the tea-party. This story has now taken on a life of its own, with many variations and embellishments, depending on the needs of the embellisher. But most provaccine commentaries use a mouthful of potent words, like "conspiracy" and "antivaccination". Familiar emotive language was seen everywhere, as in one article telling about a wee boy in Burundi who hadn't travelled anywhere, but who had nonetheless been struck down by a Nigerian strain.

What amazed me in all these articles was that no one has asked the blatantly obvious question. Why were these over-vaccinated children still getting polio in the first place? Wouldn't you think that a vaccine worth its salt would, after six doses, stop a Nigerian strain not just in the middle of Burundi but right at the border of Cameroon? And isn't the reason the oral polio vaccine was used in developing countries not just to give personal immunity but to also stop the spread by providing communal immunity?

Even more interesting, if you believe this story, is that this virulent Nigerian polio virus silently infected millions of people, and multiple countries without striking anyone, until paralysis struck a boy in Burundi, who then made world headlines?

Systematically working through searches looking at every single African country, I then came across Uganda, where another concern about polio caught my attention.

A Ugandan by the name of Kihura Nkuba had spoken at the National Vaccine Information Center's Conference held from 7 to 9 November 2002, in Arlington Virginia. A transcript of his presentation is on the web in several places.[1]

It's the journey of an intelligent radio broadcaster with a pair of eyes and a brain, who had noticed that every time there was an oral

1 Nkuba, K. *Polio vaccine genocide in Uganda*, Available from <http://www.whale.to/a/nkuba.htm> Accessed on 18 September, 2005.

polio campaign, children would die in droves, and mothers would try to hide their children from the vaccination teams wherever possible.

As a pro-vaccine broadcaster, he hadn't thought anything of the deaths to begin with, but because they were doing routine polio campaigns in Uganda at the time, he started to notice anomalies. He took the trouble to look at which vaccines other countries gave to children, and stumbled across the American CDC (Atlanta) website, where he found that the USA no longer used the oral polio vaccine, because it could cause polio. Which started him thinking.

So he asked on his radio station, "Why, if it was good enough for USA to use the killed vaccine, was it NOT good enough for Uganda?" Next thing he knew, there were newspaper articles claiming that he had anti-government tendencies.

The more newspapers attacked him, the more he researched. He was given a Pasteur-Merieux Oral Polio vaccine package insert, which said that polio vaccine should never be used in families where there was either HIV or a history of HIV.

Uganda, like most African countries, is riddled with HIV.

So then he mused out loud to his radio listeners, "Why is it that the manufacturer's package insert and CDC website says this vaccine shouldn't be used where there is HIV, yet the Ugandan government is forcing many, many Oral Polio vaccine doses into our children?" He started wondering, then, if the connection between the deaths he had dismissed after the polio campaigns were related to the HIV/OPV issues.

The Ugandan president wrote to the Attorney-General, wanting Nkuba to be tried for sedition, which carries a death sentence. On investigation, however, the Attorney-General wrote back to the president saying that if they did bring Nkuba to trial, they would lose the case.

So they tried frightening all the advertisers away from his radio station to get him off air, and when that didn't work, they tried twice to debate with him on the air, but none of the experts knew anything. In one talkback, parents rang in asking intelligent questions which so upset the medical people that they literally ran out of the radio station.

Next, a big meeting was organized, including the UNICEF, WHO and the Ugandan government. Nkuba took with him a large document printed from the American CDC website, which they tried to say wasn't genuine. The meeting was adjourned on the understanding that it would be reconvened 24 hours later, after the government had confirmed with the CDC that the document was their information.

He's still waiting for that meeting to reconvene several years later.

All of this happened because he asked the very obvious question, "Why are you giving Oral Polio vaccine in African countries which have huge rates of HIV, when the very manufacturer's documents, and your advisers, the CDC, say that polio vaccine could result in a death sentence?"

It's a very basic question. Perhaps Rotary might like to explain exactly what is achieved through throwing millions of dollars at an Oral Polio Vaccination campaign in Africa, given to nations with widespread family histories of, or actual infection with, HIV?

My scientist contacts in New Delhi had directed me to a source which they stated was accurate,[2] which was this:

The JNI (Jama'atu Nasril Islam) in Nigeria had come across some documents that talked about population control, which they said had been declassified from the USA. That much is true. It is possible to speculate about what they thought it meant in terms of the great satan and events in Afghanistan, Iraq and Palestine, but this is not relevant to what happened next. The JNI went to the Nigerian Government and said to them, "Give us an assurance that all polio vaccines for our children are pure, then we will assure you that all Muslim children will be lined up. Every one of them. But first, we want scientific proof."

The Secretary-General of the Supreme Council of Sharia'a Implementation, Nafi'u Baba Ahmed clearly stated, right at the start, that the only reason that the council would reject the polio vaccine, would be relating to issues of purity.

Doctors were assembled, to take samples of the vaccine to India, because the Nigerian government had no facilities in Nigeria to test the vaccine, and provide the required assurances. The group first consulted with WHO, UNICEF, and the sponsors of the programme, USAID, and with NAFDAX, and all other stakeholders. The World Health Organization recommended that they use gas-chromatography/mass spectrum and radio-immuno assay to conduct the tests, because they were the most sensitive and state-of-the-art tests, and directed them to a suitable facility in New Delhi.

---

2 Retrieved on 18 September, 2005 from <http://www.taxtyranny.ca/images/HTML/Vaccines/29Vaccines.html>

The team arrived, and, working with Indian scientists who were experts in using the WHO-recommended technology, found that the vaccine samples were contaminated not only with toxic substances, but also with detectable estradiol. The testers didn't believe the results at first, and neither did the Indian scientists, so the tests were repeated many times, and each test written up in very careful detail, covering every laboratory procedure, every aspect of testing, and leaving no stone unturned.

The head of the delegation returned to Nigeria with a full and comprehensive report from India, and held a meeting where copies of the joint report with India were given to the government, WHO, UNICEF, all stakeholders, whoever wished to have it. The Federal Government team, while admitting that there were contaminants there, said there was no longer any cause for concern, because all that vaccine had been used up, and the new lots would be just fine. The government put out its own report[3] which has, according to the testers, been kept secret "because they know it's the same as ours."

The returning doctors wanted answers to two questions. The first was, "How did the estradiol get into the vaccine?" The second was, given that there had just been a criminal bust in Nigeria on a group of people illegally selling dangerous and useless drugs, and they had been put in jail for it, shouldn't such action be taken against the people who brought in a vaccine which was not pure and contained contaminants? Both questions remain unanswered.

In some northern states the fact that the oral polio vaccine was contaminated fuelled the original anti-American speculation, which had forced the question to be raised in the first place. Kano State Government, however, defused the issue, by getting rid of all the OPV that they had, which came from the lots in question (and had NOT been used up as alleged). They brought in new vaccine, and after the "clean" testing results were shown to all the community leaders, as promised, all the children in Kano State lined up, and the vaccine was administered to them.

Problems arose because other states didn't want to do that. Had all the other states done the same, what was a legitimate issue might not have provided ammunition to people who want to portray Muslims as

3 Raufu, A. 2004. "Traditional rulers in northern Nigeria call for halt to polio vaccination". *British Medical Journal* [Internet] Available from <http://bmj.bmjjournals.com/cgi/content/full/328/7435/306-d> Accessed on 18 September, 2005.

deluded conspiracist zealots, and to suggest that such species might also exist in their own country.

But for those who are into the art of propaganda creation, having some deluded scapegoat to blame is always much better than having to answer questions about the actual issue.

Perhaps I should take this opportunity to thank the pro-vaccinators in this case, for giving me an opportunity to educate myself more thoroughly on some thought provoking issues that I might not otherwise have studied.

For without their ire, I would not now be puzzling as to why, in one breath, the medical profession talks about Africa as the out-of-control face of a decimating AIDS tragedy that has reached pandemic proportions, but in the very next breath, thinks it's okay to give people in those same countries anywhere up to ten oral polio vaccine doses, or more which is contraindicated in such circumstances.

Or how it is that polio can then silently spread through all those African countries which had previously eradicated polio from their lands by using 5–10 doses of oral polio vaccine,[4] only to make headlines, by striking down a boy in Burundi before moving on?

If the oral polio vaccine works, it works. Surely the reason so many doses have been given in Africa is to create a large herd immunity barrier which will stop the spread of disease and tragedy in the face of any epidemic of any polio pathogen, no matter the country of origin. Why is it that when that barrier doesn't appear to work, no one asks any questions? What is it that Indian babies since 2004 have received 8 oral polio vaccines every year[5] and having already had 16, will get 8 more this year? Why is it that 18-month-old Shan-e-ali who had had 15 doses of OPV suddenly became paralysed from the waist down?[6] What are we not being told?

Recent events in America are even more revealing. In 1997, America swapped the oral polio vaccine for a new killed injectable Salk vaccine, to stop cases of vaccine-associated paralytic polio. In June 2005, an immunodeficient four-month-old Amish baby was admitted to a Minnesota hospital with pneumonia. As her case became more

4 Retrieved on 18 September, 2005 from <http://www.who.int/vaccines-access/financing/docs_bibliography/xingzhu.pdf> p. 41

5 Dugger, CW. 2006. "On the brink: polio a fragile immunity". *New York Times*. 20 March.

6 Jain, M. 2006. IBNLIVE "Only vaccination will not curb polio". 10 April, 10:43. from http://www.ibnlive.com/article.php?id=7992&section_id=3

complicated, she was sent to a second hospital, and then a third where she developed diarrhoea. In running a battery of tests, the hospital found a viral isolate from the oral polio vaccine. They then tested family contacts and found four more oral polio vaccine virus isolates. Though there were no symptoms of disease in any of these children, the *New York Times* headlines rang out, ***"5 Cases of Polio in Amish Group Raise New Fears."*[7] *"The girl is now a wellspring for polio, a modern-day Typhoid Mary who can pass it along to others . . ."***

Would someone like to figure out *who* in the second or third hospital passed the vaccine virus to the baby, who then passed it to her visiting family? Why is the real index case not being tracked down? Why aren't all the hospital staff and all the contacts that might have spread out from the real index case tested? Why is it always the unvaccinated and their communities who are labelled the "Typhoid Marys", and made pariahs? Without this immunodeficient child throwing up a viral isolate, no-one would ever have known that oral polio virus had spread through at least part of America. It was inferred by the media that the polio virus was only to be found in the Amish, but the facts suggest the Amish family was the end point, not the starting point. And this immunodeficient child didn't even have clinical polio. Yet again, moralizing about non-vaccinators was the most popular angle.

The American public was told that one in 200 cases of polio result in paralysis, but then they were told[8] that study of the virus from the child reveals it has been circulating for at least two years, which does not make this child a "typhoid Mary". If you look at older text books, and even talks by eminent polio experts, the rate of sub-clinical disease to actual infection is 1 in 1000. Why do figures change when the need changes? In this way the figures used resemble weapons of mass destruction. Only the Amish community and the other non-vaccinators were being fingered in the media.

Strangely, no one has pointed out that until the USA used the injectable vaccine, circulating oral polio vaccine in the community was the norm, and to spread the vaccine virus into the community

---

7 Harris, G. 2005. "5 cases of polio in Amish group raise new fears". *New York Times*, 8 November.

8 Bahta, L. et al. 2005. MMWR. "Polio virus infections in four unvaccinated children Minnesota, August–October, 2005". October 21; 54(41) 1053–5. PMID: 16237378. See under "Editorial note" on CDC website."

was precisely the reason it was used.[9,10] It wasn't considered dangerous then, yet now the fact an immunodeficient Amish child picked it up in a hospital is seen as an indictment on non-immunizers. And furthermore, even though we know that the injectable polio vaccine does NOT stop the spread of polio in the community, it would appear from what is being said that no attempt is being made by the medical community to look and see if anyone other than Amish are excreting virus. Do they honestly expect us to believe that the virus is now only circulating amongst the Amish? Will five Amish viral isolates also be written into the annals of history as examples of circulation of polio vaccine virus by the great unwashed?

But then, what about Africa where OPV spreads freely? It's apparently all right to allow the oral polio vaccine to be used and to spread the vaccine virus throughout the immunosuppressed and HIV communities. That doesn't seem to matter.

---

9 Retrieved on 18 September, 2005 from <http://www.sabin.org/vaccine_science_polio>.htm Inactivated polio vaccine (IPV) needs to be injected and works by producing protective antibodies in the blood (serum immunity) – thus preventing the spread of poliovirus to the central nervous system. However, it induces only very low levels of immunity to poliovirus locally, inside the gut. As a result, it provides individual protection against polio paralysis but, **unlike OPV, cannot prevent the spread of wild poliovirus** . . . IPV only induces serum immunity, not intestinal immunity. Thus, IPV vaccination can effectively protect the vaccinated individuals against paralysis, but does not readily protect all of them against infection with the wild virus. If vaccinated children are infected, they can become a source of infection by wild virus if their antibody levels are not high enough to stop virus excretion.

10 Liu, X., Levin, A., Makinen, M., and Day, J. 2003. *OPV vs IPV: Past and Future Choice of Vaccine in the Global Polio Eradication Program*, Available from <http://www.who.int/vaccines-access/financing/docs_bibliography/xingzhu.pdf> page 41. Details that IPV cannot stop the spread of either wild virus or OPV, which can cause polio in both vaccinated and unvaccinated people.

77 Chuckles or Chortles

I love stories which are allegorical – stories which are a type of parable – stories which have a deeper **hidden** meaning.

If you want them to, they can provide so much food for thought. Something to think about when you wake up in the early hours of the morning!

Not long ago, I spent many enjoyable hours writing such a story.

It was about The Great Divide.

About Mindset Mountains;

About the city of Orlsrite;

About Vista Boulevard and the systems and structures to be found along this stretch of real estate dedicated to the public well-being.

There were **goodies** and **baddies** too.

Ernest C. Kerr and Mai Aye Zopend.

Dick Tait, and Lucy Furr, the master of deceit and disguise.

Plenty of ordinary people living in the shadow of The Great Divide.

Pru Dent, Hope More, Vic Tory and Sam Heard.

There was mystery and intrigue such as Fogg Optics and Associate's scam to convince the populace that they all needed to wear contact lenses so that they could see **properly**.

The sinister activities of the Ministry of Conformity, Compliance and Control.

Commander (abbreviated to Com) Pugh Turr's role as National Director of the SIS (Systems Integrating Suspicions), so as to make it more effective in tracking down dissidents.

Yes, I got many a chuckle as the story came together.

You know, this book is an extension of The Great Divide!

Mindset Mountains are still an obstacle in the lives of so many people.

Ernest C. Kerrs can still find the answers they're looking for.

It was obvious that my original story had to be extended with a few more chapters!

The chuckles began to vibrate through my being again. Characters identified themselves.

Sharlot Sleaze,

Doctor Trusta Mee,

Polly Tishan,

"Weasel" Speek;

Mene Hertz,

The Wright family;

Hugh Mann and I.S.M.

Iddy Ott;

Robin Mune;

Pretty Good;

Ignor Factz.

*And of course Dick Tait and Com. Pugh Turr reappeared along with Wylie Fox. The conning schemes of Fogg Optics and their **special** contact lenses for distorted vision, make an appearance in Fall City to enhance among other things, subliminal messaging. A new subdivision has opened up called Whittle Downs. A huge vested interest appears in the form of Q-4 Health Pharmaceuticals.*

Oh yes, the wheels of imagination have produced more chapters. I'm sure others will follow.

*For me, one of the great **overwhelming** reasons for writing allegory* *is that it allows you to express real-life circumstances, situations, emotions and observations in ways which allow you to freely say what you want to say, without standing on flesh-and-blood corns, toes, feelings or whatever.*

I have just used the word **overwhelming** *deliberately.*

Do you ever feel overwhelmed by what is happening to you, or going on around you?

I do.

I can experience those feelings when I read this book.

But there is no need to be overwhelmed to the point of utter defeat.

In spite of **feelings**, *there are FACTS.*

Those facts need to be identified. The "I thinks", the maybes, the doubts and so on can be replaced with "I KNOWs". That makes all the difference.

Now where was I?

I know – "The Great Divide".

O.K. Orlsrite, Fall City and Lulling Sounds. Here I come again.

Look out Dick Tait of C.C.C.,

Lucy Furr,

Nurse Jabbin,

Fogg and Company,

Robin de Light,

Eileen Harder,

Digby Low,

Justice Maybe,

Sir Pent-Athol Blackadder and H.I.S.S.

Acton Sight . . .

Hmm. Better stop before I get completely carried away although I could tell you about the vaccination campaign to eradicate the terrible disease of antisystematosis using the vaccine Pluracydefex!

78 Reducing the Problem to Size

This conversation was between myself and a local principal.[1] A parent rang me, concerned that her child was paralytic with fear having been told that unless she was vaccinated NOW with the new MeNZB meningitis vaccine she would die. So I rang the school. The secretary couldn't help and passed me to the principal. I'll call him Mr Stevens.

HB. "Hello Mr Stevens. I'm ringing on behalf of a parent who wanted my advice about the meningitis talks given in your school."

Mr. S. "Yes . . ."

HB. "Can you tell me how you explain to the children what their risk are of catching meningococcal B disease, please?"

Mr. S. "What do you mean?"

HB. "Exactly that. How do you tell children what their chances of catching meningitis are?"

Mr. S. "Look, I really don't see what you mean. They could catch it anytime, that's why they are doing the campaign."

HB. "No, I mean the precise risk, not the theoretical risk."

Mr. S. "Look, I think you are . . ."

HB. "I don't think you understand. Let me explain."

1 Taken down in shorthand at the time, transcribed, and salient points used.

Mr S. "Please do, I've lost the plot here . . ."

HB. "This epidemic has been raging here for 14 years, correct?"

Mr S. "Right . . ."

HB. "How many cases of any type of meningitis have there been at your school in the last 14 years, Mr Stevens?"

Mr. S "Well I haven't quite been here 14 years . . . (seems to ask a question of the secretary who it appears has been there more than 14 years . . .) Well . . . None that we know of . . . but there could have been cases, and we weren't told."

HB. "But Mr Stevens, if there were cases, don't you think the Health Department would have been in here, swabbed the children's contacts, staff and given them antibiotics? And . . . don't you have a health register, and an absentee register?"

Mr. S. "Oh, right. Well, yes . . . I suppose they would, then . . ."

HB. "So can I go back to my original question? If you haven't had any cases in this school in 14 years, how would you explain to children what their actual risks are?"

Mr. S. (silence) . . .

HB. ". . . because right now, you are trying to persuade children that even though they have lived just fine for 14 years, and though you've had no cases in the school in that time, that . . . all of them will get sick and die . . . today . . . now . . . if they are not vaccinated immediately. Can you explain why you tell them that?"

Mr S. "As a school principal I endorse vaccination programmes. It's what we do."

HB. "My question has nothing to do with whether you endorse a programme or not. It's about giving children accurate, real information as to whether there has been a problem in your school district in the past, and might be in your school in the future."

Mr. S. "But they might go up to Auckland in the holidays and pick it up, and when they play sport there as well."

HB. "But they've been doing that for 14 years. With cases declining, what difference does it make to them now?"

Mr S. "Oh, are you one of those weird conspiracy people, like those strange people who tried to stop the vaccination programme in Nigeria?"

HB. "Are you talking about the oral polio vaccine provided to

Nigeria that had estradiol in it?"

Mr. S. "There wasn't anything in it!"

HB. "Have you asked the WHO for the report that Dr Kaita and the Indian vaccine testing team gave them?"

Mr. S. "Well, I'm with Rotary, and I think it's important to wipe out polio."

HB. "I also think it's important if you are going to use or 'push' vaccines, to offer safe vaccines without contaminants. But that wasn't why I rang. I had a very simple question, which you haven't answered."

Mr. S. "I will tell the children whatever it is that the Health Department thinks is appropriate."

79 A Different Perspective

A number of years ago I prepared the following article for a newsletter.

It still remains a very important "perspective" and sets out what I believe every person needs to consider before getting bogged down in the vaccination issue. A solid "foundation" has to be laid before **any** "building" can take place.

Here is the article with a few minor adjustments to update it.

> ". . . As parents, are Hilary and I united over those things that relate to the immunization debate? The simple answer is 'that a house which is divided against itself cannot stand'. It will destroy itself.
>
> It would be very difficult, were we not united, to survive in the lifestyle we have chosen.
>
> United in the cause, yes, but . . . we see things differently. Usually I keep to the shadows and say little outside of our home, but I have listened to countless hours of 'talk' in one form or another. I have read thousands of pages of printed matter, and am sometimes called upon to offer advice, opinion, and smooth my owl's ruffled feathers!

The time has come when I feel constrained to offer another perspective for wider circulation – a perspective which needs to be considered because it raises issues which are rarely, if ever, specifically and bluntly set out for very personal consideration before any crisis situation arises.

Vaccination, of course, relates to the topic of health. Anything to do with health, whether we like it or not, confronts us with birth and death, and everything in between. Disease, sickness, and especially death are not welcomed. Are we going to face up to how we handle these inescapable matters, or are we going to run away from them? A solid belief basis or "foundation" THAT WE CAN CONFIDENTLY COMMIT OUR LIVES TO *is essential. How often do people ask the question, "What if something goes wrong?" A question that has to be answered* **whichever** *way we finally decide to go.*

Carefully consider the issue I am writing about, when it is simply and clearly stated as a question:

To vaccinate or not to vaccinate? *(and other health-related questions could be substituted.)*

A choice is offered. There is no compulsion in this country – yet. But a DECISION *has to be made.*

A decision **not** *to vaccinate will mean that you have to go against the flow of the majority. The costs of "being different" have to be worked through point by point, e.g. pressures from the Health Department, doctors, family, friends, school, etc. Plus the "What if?" question mentioned above. Very strong convictions are necessary, and maybe a pretty thick skin!*

- *Time has to be found to make this decision.*
- *Ask, look and listen.*
- *Question everything, but keep the issues simple.*
- *Too much information can often be counter-productive and lead to confusion.*
- *Not all decisions will be based on medical literature.*

- *For some, the "spiritual" component of one's being will be more important.*

Readers having got this far, may say, "What's new? We've heard this before!"

But have you really ***"heard"*** *it? Or have you only "heard" it as you* **want** *to hear it?*

Let me put to you some questions to be answered at a personal level:

1) *Are you willing NOW to face up to the possible consequences of any sickness or disease especially as it may affect your children, whether you vaccinate or not?*

2) *If something goes wrong, e.g. life-threatening "complications", side-effects, brain damage or even death, do you have a "faith" which will see you through the crisis, however long it may be?*

3) *Continuing good health is what everyone wants, but how are you going to achieve it? Who are you going to listen to? Are you confused by the many voices of the so-called experts who seem to say so many different and "new" things – almost on a daily basis?*

4) *Do you have convictions that will not be compromised whatever strategies, pressures and arguments are brought to bear on you? Are you able to verbalize them simply with confidence and clarity? This is important. If you are not convinced yourself, how can you convince others?*

5) *When faced with the choice to vaccinate or not to vaccinate, are you prepared to acknowledge that you HAVE to make* ***a decision****?*

6) *What is that decision to be based on? For example, pressure and/or smooth talk of health "professionals"; your "gut*

feeling"; a "faith" (that won't let you down!); human wisdom?

7) When you make your decision, are you prepared to accept responsibility for it, **whatever the outcome?** Or will you want to look around for scapegoats if something goes wrong – someone or something to blame?

8) If you are unwilling to make a well-informed decision then you have to allow someone else to make it for you. If you delegate your responsibility to another person, are you prepared to accept the outcomes without apportioning blame if they are not what you want?

Working through searching questions such as those you have just read will not be easy, and that is why you need to face the life-and-death issues (and everything in between!) for they will **not** go away, no matter how much you try to dodge them. Decisions have to be made, because they can't be dodged either.

On both sides of the vaccination debate you will have to deal with people – either face to face, or by considering their points of view, persuasions, arguments, recommendations or whatever, expressed in a variety of ways and often very "convincingly". Remember however, that people and human wisdom are certainly not infallible.

I am totally convinced that the points I have focused on need to be dealt with BEFORE any in-depth study introduces red herrings, and people become bogged down in medical terminology, and with the dubious promises and guarantees of **vested interests** – yes, on BOTH sides of the fence!

I know where I stand, and I know what my convictions are based on. Without such a foundation I would have every reason to be scared stiff. Whether to vaccinate or not is an important question to be resolved, but this other matter of

> *convictions is even more important, because it must provide an answer for life's uncertainties."*

This is page 478! There are less than 20 pages to go before "Just a little Prick" comes to an end and you weigh up the effects of all these little pricks.

Personalize all the questions asked and the stories told.

Will you be the same person when you finish this book as you were when you started?

Will you be more, or less, convinced?

Do you still hold to nice, pat answers?

Do you ***really*** *believe them or are they just straws to clutch at?*

Are you trusting "someone" or "something" because you can't, or won't, trust yourself?

The little pricks these questions represent may well evoke another anguished "OUCH!"

The back cover of this book remains the challenge.

80 Nice, Pat Answers?

***People are better at estimating their own risk of an illness if they stick to personal experience rather than number crunching, say researchers.*[1]**

People like simple, nice, pat answers. I might even become a millionaire if I was given a few thousand dollars for every time someone enclosed an ordinary-sized self-addressed stamped envelope and asked me to fit into that all the information I have on vaccines.

For years, I've been tempted to have some sort of standard letter that says, "We've a spare bed, so why not hire a photocopier, stay a few weeks, copy it all, then use a small removal truck to take it all home?"

This book was written to show you that there might be very good reasons to slow down and consider all your health decisions more thoroughly. I wanted to allow people to tell their stories, to illustrate what the consequences can be when a decision is more or less made for you, not by you, and to focus on some of the pressures parents face if they ask too many questions. This book is to start people talking and thinking about why they do what they do. Not just about the issue of

1 "People warned off sickness stats". 2005. Available from <http://news.bbc.co.uk/1/hi/health/4748349.stm> Accessed on 18 September, 2005.

immunization, but about where we are 'going' as parents in all areas of life. What do you want the future to be, and what do you want your part to be in making those decisions? How do you make your decisions? When should we let others make decisions for us, when is that appropriate, and when is it not?

To make choices we need information. Not just in the form of a small, colourful, smart-looking glossy pamphlet which tells you, "Be wise, Immunize" and which leaves out much of the relevant information that any intelligent, thinking parent needs to make an informed choice.

Until recently, the medical profession has told everyone that the 'problem people' who don't vaccinate are the ones who are unable to get their children to the doctors to have the vaccines. That is, the people who don't have doctors, transport, or the means to do "the right thing".

What they aren't telling you is that the problem isn't really those people at all. The problem is intelligent, thinking parents who decide not to immunize, and ***who can explain why they don't want to.***

Two recent medical studies, on opposite sides of the world, looked at how people make choices about immunization. The first study, done in Israel, looked at the Hepatitis B vaccine.[2] The second study, done in the USA, wanted to see what might convince parents to vaccinate their children against the flu.[3] Both articles came to the same conclusion. The parents who didn't vaccinate were intelligent educated people who had looked at all the facts and had said, "No".

Doctors are trying to figure out how to re-educate parents who might not like the possibility[4] of vaccinating under-fives against the flu, because doctors want to prevent flu in the elderly. The parents who believed that children with influenza would get seriously ill and land up in hospital, and that the vaccine would have no side-effects, were the keenest on the idea.

Another two studies on different ethnic groups of parents in Holland

2 Maayan-Metzger, A. et al. 2005. "To vaccinate or not to vaccinate – that is the question: why are some mothers opposed to giving their infants hepatitis B vaccine?" *Vaccine,* (Israel) Vol. 23: 1941–8. PMID: 15734066.

3 Humiston, S.G. et al. 2005. "Parent opinions about universal influenza vaccination for infants and toddlers". *Archives of Pediatrics and Adolescent Medicine*, Feb; 159(2): 108–12. PMID: 15699302.

4 Humiston, S.G. et al. 2005. "Parent opinions about universal influenza vaccination for infants and toddlers". *Archives of Pediatrics and Adolescent Medicine*, Feb; 159(2): 108–12. PMID: 15699302.

were similarly interesting. The first study[5] showed:

> ***"a higher prevalence of non-compliers with influenza and pneumococcal vaccination among highly educated elderly persons as well. Because the average educational level has been increasing over the last decades, it might be assumed that more and more persons will adopt a critical attitude towards vaccinations."***

The second study[6] showed that:

> ***"Generally, people largely overestimated the risk of contracting the disease and the risk of dying after contracting the disease. Dutch parents were best informed, least worried, had the most critical attitude toward the campaign, and the lowest vaccination level compared to other parents."***

Researchers blamed the lack of direct experience of diseases for this, which is rubbish, as I know plenty of Dutch parents who have experienced diseases for which there are immunizations.

There were also some astonishing admissions in this study. Parents of many ethnic backgrounds were given a brochure to read AFTER their child had been vaccinated against Meningococcal C, and before a five- to ten-minute interview.

Most Moroccan and Antilles parents didn't read the brochure, because to them the issue was *self-evident*. These parents were the ones who also overestimated the risk of catching the disease and dying from it, and who worried more about the disease. The Dutch parents who were better educated knew more about the actual risks and were, therefore, less worried. Ironically the team admitted it would be hard for parents to learn the real risks because the Meningitis C brochure used the words 'small chance' and didn't mention an exact risk figure. It was interesting to see that those who did vaccinate but were critical of the programme, were the educated parents.

The researchers acknowledged that there might be problems with their study because it didn't include parents who had refused

5 Hak, E. et al. 2005. "Negative attitude of highly educated parents and health care workers towards future vaccinations in the Dutch childhood vaccination program". *Vaccine*, Vol. 23: 3103–7.

6 Timmermans, et al. 2005. "Attitudes and risk perception of parents of different ethnic backgrounds regarding meningococcal C vaccination". *Vaccine*, Vol. 23: 3329–35. DRM.

vaccination. This was an exploratory study and future studies were proposed that would include parents who refuse to vaccinate. These studies would attempt to find out what their worries were so that they could address them when designing new materials.

The Hepatitis B group[7] interviewed Israel mothers who don't vaccinate. The staggering thing about the study was the tone of intellectual hate and venom that seemed to spill off the pages with their use of adjectives. Even worse was that the parents had no idea they were part of a study.[8]

The ***"prevent"*** group (those who chose not to vaccinate, but who, in the minds of the researchers, were mothers who prevented administration, or refused to administer . . .) were more likely to breastfeed for longer, expressed a more natural and less conventional approach to medicine and felt that home delivery was preferable to giving birth in hospital. And, horrors, a fifth of the ***prevent*** mothers worked in a field related to medicine!

The ***prevent*** group also had a higher level of education and income than the ***comply*** group who couldn't really give many reasons as to why they complied. Most just vaccinated. Even though the researchers had not asked any *prevent* women where they got their information from, they nevertheless came up with the astonishing statement: ***"We can assume, however, that many visited the anti-vaccination websites."***

A classic sentence in discussing the ***prevent*** group was: ***"This rejection requires more determination and willingness to defy a common procedure"***, and right at the end, after discussing how dangerous Hepatitis B is, they say, ***"We feel it is important to try to overcome the trend . . ."***

In 2005 a popular USA magazine[9] interviewed Phil Smith, an epidemiologist/statistician with the CDC who said that until recently, CDC annual poll results were divided into two groups: up-to-date kids, and those who were not up-to-date or under-vaccinated. Totally

7 Maayan-Metzger, A. et al. 2005. "To vaccinate or not to vaccinate – that is the question: why are some mothers opposed to giving their infants hepatitis B vaccine?" *Vaccine*, (Israel) Vol. 23: 1941–8. PMID: 15734066.

8 Maayan-Metzger, A. et al. 2005. "Keep in mind that women did not know the purpose of the survey." *Vaccine*, (Israel) Vol. 23: p. 1944. PMID: 15734066.

9 2005. *Brain, Child* (the magazine for thinking mothers) Winter: See Smith P.J. et al. 2004. "Children who receive no vaccines: who are they and where do they live?" *Pediatrics*, Jul; 114(1): 187–95. PMID 15231927. Use the link and go to the site. Download full text and read it all. Says the same as *Brain, Child* but more comprehensive.

unvaccinated children were categorized as "under-vaccinated", but they had no idea whether they were unvaccinated by choice or not. So Phil Smith decided to look at the under-vaccinated group, and what he discovered stunned him. The article says:

> ***"Unlike the mothers of under-vaccinated children – mothers who tend to be young, black, single, not educated beyond high school, and living in poverty in urban areas – mothers whose children have never received any shots generally are white, married, in their thirties, holding a bachelor's degree, and living in a suburban household that earns more than $75,000 a year. They have flexibility and resources, yet have opted not to vaccinate."***

While some parents had religious or medical exemptions, many of the parents had concerns about vaccine safety.

> ***"'They are definitely thinking parents, and that's a good thing,'. . . Armed with the new demographic data, Smith says that the campaign to reach parents of no-dose kids will likely look a lot different than that used to reach parents of under-vaccinated kids."***

He went on to say that to change these people's minds would be an uphill battle, because it appeared that what doctors say had little or no influence on the decision making as to whether or not to vaccinate. Smith admitted:

> ***"They are also 'unlikely to be persuaded to change their decision'."***

Why will the campaigns to reach the intelligent educated people look a lot different? Because only the parents of under-vaccinated children can be more easily emotionally blackmailed with fear-laden messages, and won't require good solid factual information? Will the results of such studies be non-stop TV infomercials to attempt to dumb down intelligent, thinking parents?

On the other hand, the intelligent parents will probably be able to recite the Atlanta CDC website by heart and will also know all the medical articles which presents the side of the coin that CDC doesn't.

How do you find out what you need to know, to make a really informed choice? How do you assess that information? If you are told you should vaccinate because these diseases aren't around since the introduction of vaccines, on what basis do you accept that argument? Have you researched it?

The most common comment made to me when researching the issue was that as a mother I couldn't possibly understand the issues involved. The attitude was, as Dr Paul Offit says, "Science should be left to scientists."

Vaccines are not 100% safe.

We are no longer talking about just a few vaccines like the ones people who are now 50 first received when they were about 6 months old. (In my case, at three years of age) We're talking about a huge raft of vaccines now, with far more waiting in the wings to be incorporated in schedules every year until you die. How else are vaccinationists going to cram a potential total of 400 vaccines into a person's life? Where is there a guarantee that this increasing raft of vaccines aren't creating new problems which are hard to fix? A 1998 article[10] said: ***"In the early era of vaccine development, empiricism was the rule and it still is in many instances."*** Empiricism may be all very useful, occasionally. But assumption upon assumption can lead to fallacy on fallacy. These words,[11] in the light of history, bear careful consideration:

> ***"But we warn you that you will hear from all kinds of experts today. Those same experts told you to support the Swine Flu Programme, and I think it's worth noting the quote here that we've found, which is from someone who studies experts. He says, 'An expert is a person who avoids the small errors while sweeping on to the grand fallacy'."***

My first duty in life was, and is, to the health of my child. I knew, and this knowledge was proved right over time, that even my younger son, whose immune system isn't quite right, would get through the commoner diseases if I looked after him correctly, and found the knowledge I needed to do that.

In 1982, any information was very hard to find, and there was no

10 Halloran, M.E. et al. 1998. "Population biology, evolution, and immunology of vaccination and vaccination programs". Feb; 315(2): 76–86. PMID: 9472906.

11 Committee on Labour and Human Resources. 1985. "To amend the Public Health Service Act to provide for the compensation of children and others who have sustained vaccine related injuries". S.827, June 18, p. 39; Mr Jeff Schwartz (lawyer) to Senator Hawkins.

cooperation from the medical profession to find it either. There was no internet in those days, and working out where information was, was plain hard work, and cost lots of shoe leather.

Never be scared to go to a nearby medical library. Your taxes pay to run it, and you have every right to be there. Yes, they will prevent you from seeing anything on line, and they may charge you twice as much to make photocopies as they charge medical users. But if you have the time, then going to a medical library like I did, is still the best way to gather the information you need, because then you can never be accused of "mouse-hunting",[12] or of being tainted by lay-people who write books!

That is why this book has been written solely based on what I did. It includes only a tiny proportion of the information that I have gathered and would have liked to have shared, but the focus of the book is to give the reader a sense of what has been said and done by the medical profession, in this country in the past, and that the past does matter. The medical profession wants you to believe that if we don't vaccinate we will go back to the "bad old days". However, that is an assumption which isn't always correct, but you aren't given the information to show you that. Furthermore it assumes that there is only one solution to any "epidemic" problem.

There is a saying that he who does not know history will repeat it. If you know the medical profession's inconsistencies and misinformation of the past 25 years, you can ask yourself, "Can I really trust this new pamphlet today? What did they say about this in the past?" Finding the answers to the second question will sometimes give you the answers to the first.

You also need to know exactly how the medical profession, the media and the conformed majority out there are likely to view you, and treat you, should you cop the wrong end of whichever choice you make.

While parents of vaccinated children who catch the diseases get treated really well by the medical profession, if you choose not to vaccinate, the events related in this book tell you what you might experience. You may feel the need to take that into account, because how well you can stand up to that type of pressure depends on how good a backbone you have. Conversely if you vaccinate and everything turns

12 "Mouse-hunting" a term used to describe people who make decisions solely based on internet websites or abstracts of medical articles found on internet.

to custard, how you are treated is a lottery, depending on that medical person's ethics, empathy, logic, conditioning and philosophy.

When somebody says to me that I should use all vaccines, because vaccines have wiped out diseases previously, I don't bother to argue. I just say, "What's your point?" and follow up that with another question: "How vaccinated are you?" Most adults these days are more than grossly under-vaccinated in comparison with their children, and often fail to appreciate the fact that they are walking proof that they don't owe their current existence to vaccines that didn't exist when they were children, and neither did their ancestors.

Until 1950, most children were rarely vaccinated, yet all the death rates for common diseases, with the exception of polio, were declining in developed countries because of the work of public health, and improvements in areas such as nutrition, sanitation, hygiene, drainage and safe water supplies. Specific medical interventions, as MacKinlay's articles show (see chapter entitled "Other Sinbinned Voices in the Wilderness"), had little to do with the decline of the death rate in infectious diseases, and I understand his frustration that *public health* has been hijacked by technocentric, simple ideas which far from being a solution, barely scratch the surface of the current health problems facing society today.

Even in parts of Africa today, *public health is what really has been the key.* A study was done in South Africa looking at trends in admission and mortality rates.[13] The researchers found that diseases for which there were vaccines had decreased but that others for which there weren't vaccines, had similarly decreased. They put the latter down to better living conditions, while attributing the decrease in the other diseases to the vaccines. I can imagine how hard it would be for them to have faced up to the fact that just maybe, had there been no

13 Jeen, P.M et al. 1998. Infectious diseases at the paediatric isolation units of Clairwood and King Edward VIII hospitals, Durban". *SAMJ*, July: 88(7): 867–872. "Although the more extensive immunization programme is the most likely reason for the substantial epidemiological changes in paediatric infectious diseases over the past decade described above it is clear that the prevalence of other non-vaccine-preventable diseases has also declined over this same period. Causes of this latter phenomenon are not clearly understood. It seems to us that a gradual amelioration in living conditions of the poor over the past decade or so, is the most likely basis for the overall reduction in infectious diseases such as typhoid, varicella and mumps . . . the trend in typhoid fever seen here and nationally exemplifies this phenomenon. Similarly cholera occurred as a brief epidemic in the mid 1980's and has since virtually disappeared . . . This study demonstrates fundamental improvements in the prevalence and outcome of both vaccine-preventable and non-vaccine preventable diseases . . ."

vaccines, those diseases might have fallen as well, as they did in the rest of the world, which is presumably why they dared not venture there.

How is it that so many New Zealand parents don't even realize that there is a choice regarding vaccinations?

It's because practice nurses and doctors have conveyed vaccine information in such a way that parents are made to believe vaccination is something you just do, and so they are left feeling that they have no choice about vaccines.

Whether to vaccinate or not *IS* a matter of choice, *NOT* a matter of compliance.

The medical profession talk about how they entrust their cars to mechanics without casting doubt on the mechanics' knowledge or abilities, so we should likewise entrust our children to them without question.

There's one big difference. If a mechanic stuffs up, especially if your car is still under warranty, you expect them to fix whatever problem they have caused, and that could be repeated until the fault is corrected, even if they have to provide you with a new car!

When the medical profession gets it badly wrong with a vaccinated child, you can't send the doctors off to get multiple replacement parts, or buy a new child for you. Neither vaccines nor medical treatment of any sort, come with any warranties worth the paper they are written on.

The medical profession trade on the fact that they are doctors, and that people assume doctors know everything there is to know about health matters. Most doctors don't have any difficulty with using graphic portrayals of the dire consequences of 'failure to vaccinate' using videos, photographs and other visuals that tug at the heart strings. Some would call this emotional blackmail or fear mongering.

Here is a recent example:[14]

A child is shown a video[15] in school which shows footage of near fatal meningococcal septicaemia so graphic that some children vomited on the floor. Next, they are handed an information sheet[16] showing a Polynesian holding a large photo of a blackened child with wires in ICU to reinforce the subconscious message of the video that this

14 relates to Chapter 76.
15 This video was shown in many schools during the 2004 meningitis campaign.
16 Meningococcal B immunization, Ministry of Health, Printed April 2004, code MVA0601.

could happen to them. There is a biro which says *"Meningococcal B – be wise, immunize"* to create the subconscious message that if you don't vaccinate you are unwise, and will end up sick and possibly die. Then on the front of the consent form[17] next to pictures of a pen is the statement to Parents and Guardians: *"This is all it takes to help protect them. Give your consent for Meningococcal B immunization at school"* which means that you should use the pen to sign the consent because that is "all" you can do. Subconsciously that can read that there is nothing else you can do to protect your child.

So the information that the medical profession describes as "realistic", is aimed at creating pressure and fear on everyone at school, and to force children to pressure parents (who saw similar messages on television) to submit to vaccination without looking at either the reality of relative risk, or the motives behind the worst case scenario message.

The Health Department justify these strategies as a way of conveying to children what could happen to them. Was the information you as parents, and the children were given, fair, unbiased and factual?

Consider this. Had this book contained all the cases of vaccine damage I have had contact with over the years, in New Zealand alone, you would have at least five volumes in front of you, not one. Listening to the medical profession discuss serious vaccine damage in public, I have only ever heard them admit to one case, and that is easy for them, because that case involved a vaccine we don't use now. Vaccine damage, and the selective omission of key factual *incidence and epidemiological data* is never talked about. That is why I'm talking about it. As we saw on TV after the MeNZB campaign, and as I know from telephone calls from the local area, there were many nasty side effects from the Meningitis B vaccine some of which involved hospitalization for a week . . . which the medical profession considered good value, since they say there have been no permanent consequences. So a side effect is better than dying of the disease. Was your child any more likely to get meningococcal disease than in any of the previous years they were exposed and didn't get it? You couldn't assess that, since the demographic data on which to judge that risk for yourself wasn't shown to you as part of the information provided with the school campaign. Looking back we can also see that the

17 Ministry of Health, Printed April 2004, code MVS0101.

numbers of meningitis cases of all types has not decreased as a result of the 2004–2005 campaign. Neither have the deaths. If anything the downward trend for deaths has stopped.

Some, amongst those who assume they are responsible for the nation's health also believe that ***"it's dead stupid not to"*** vaccinate. That ***"by not vaccinating children, parents are withholding a necessity of life"*** and that anyone who doesn't vaccinate, or puts out information to the contrary is a quack. That "the media and anti-lobby need to be more accountable for their actions." That parents should ***"think hard about vaccination"*** before making a decision.[18]

The implication of the last of these statements, then, is that if you think hard you WILL vaccinate. And anyone who doesn't is both stupid and a criminal. That concept of thinking is not my concept of thinking.

The observations from studies done overseas on the issue of choice is that usually it is parents who DON'T think the issues through thoroughly, who just go with the flow of the emotional messages and vaccinate.

So let's presume that you are an intelligent, thinking parent, who has read this book because you want to make an informed choice. Let's presume that perhaps you have some time on your hands. What might you do next?

In a democratic world where we are supposedly taught at school, how to find information, use logic and thinking skills, how to analyse what is truth and what is not, I'm not going to tell you what to do with your decision making as a parent. That's your right.

If you want and need to vaccinate your children, you should do so.

But you and I should not be forced into a policy of all or nothing and neither should anyone be bullied into having vaccines they don't want. The point is, people should be able to have all the vaccines, or pick just a few, or none at all, as a matter of course, and informed choice.

The purpose of *Just a Little Prick* is to show that vaccines are not just a little prick. And that you are not told everything. Can you accept the following?:

"Pamphlet authors should determine the key points that the

18 Fox, R. 2004. *Otago Daily Times*, 12 July. Quoting Dr Glen Buchan. Available from <http://www.odt.co.nz/?issue=2004/12July> click on "local interest".

> ***patient (or parent) needs to know to achieve the behavioural objectives. Non-essential concepts can then be deleted. The key is to write for the desired health behaviour, rather than for high-level knowledge."***[19]

What do you think the authors mean by *non-essential concepts*? Is this a strategy to deny you essential information so necessary for an informed choice? While this quote relates to vaccine brochures, the same tactics seem to apply to any medical drug for which there is a patent. How many drug users find out at a later stage that they are victims of some condition of which they were unaware, because they were denied access to "non-essential concepts"?

The quote below applies to any vaccine campaign at any point in history, not just the SV-40 polio controversy about which it was written:

> ***". . . any possible doubts, whether or not well founded, about the safety of the vaccine, cannot be allowed to exist in view of the need to assure that the vaccine will continue to be used to the maximum extent consistent with the nation's public health objectives."***[20]

True informed consent requires a lot more information than the Health Department in this country supplies. No matter what the medical issue is, or whether you think it's straightforward or not (that pin and screw put in to keep fractured bones together should be left in there, right?) check it out. Learn where to find information, and how to use medical libraries. You can also use medical search engines like Pubmed on the Internet. Register on Medscape, search and study the full-content on free on-line medical journals. You owe it to yourself, your children and your whole family to make carefully considered informed choices on all health issues.[21]

People who take responsibility for their own health choices, who think through the broader implications of health, and make careful decisions on everything without capitulating to coercion or bullying of any kind, will reap the benefits in the long term.

---

19 Davis, T.C. et al. 1996. "Parent comprehension of polio vaccine information pamphlets". *Pediatrics*, June; 6(7): 804–10. p. 809. PMID: 8657518.

20 1984. *USA Federal Register*, Vol. 49(107): 23007.

21 Don't be scared to ask your doctor questions and if you think you'll forget, give them a written list.

81 As Far as I Can Go

This is Hilary's book.

With all the wealth of information that has come from her research and contacts with other people, what lies between these covers is but a drop in the bucket. There is just so much that she would like to say and needs to say.

I have contributed short "bits and pieces" to provide a little light relief between the more lengthy chapters which, let's face it, require a fair bit of concentration! In many of these "in betweens" there is more than meets the eye during a casual read. There are some rather subtle links that can be made, and finding them may be determined by whether or not you are a "between the lines" and "between the chapters" reader.

I too have a lot that I could say. But I can't say it – not in this book. It is more than just another perspective.

In so many areas of life there are the Great Divides. The more controversial the issues, the greater the Divides.

The uniqueness of each individual has been mentioned elsewhere in this book. We are all different in so many ways. Eventually we have to take sides, or remain neutral.

Taking sides is divisive. That's a fact of life. It always has been and always will be. We can accept another's viewpoint and still remain friends. Or we can allow that difference to produce stand offs, confrontational relationships, and in the extreme, war is declared.

I have strong views and convictions which I will not compromise, but I hope they will never cause me to be disrespectful to someone else, or to dismiss them as an irritant (or worse) and therefore on the list to be "eliminated" by fair means or foul.

The Great Divides are really Mindset Mountains.

The Great Divides will shrink, or disappear altogether, when mindsets are dealt with and changed.

This could be called a "conversion" experience. History records many of these – for better or for worse.

Yes, I've touched on this back further.

How do you convert a person to your way of thinking and to your way of living?

There are all sorts of ways ranging from very suspect motives to a genuine change of heart – a "become a totally new person" experience.

I have used the word "totally" here. If we use the analogy of sailing a yacht, progress in a particular direction is maintained by constant adjustments to the helm to compensate for the effects of the wind in the sails. Sometimes the wind is helpful, sometimes it has to be overruled. Most of us will make minor adjustments to our thinking as time goes by. I did, in terms of allowing myself or my older children, to have a few vaccinations in the past. As my knowledge base increased, and my observations revealed things I could not agree with, I changed. Course corrections were made

However a total lifestyle change which affects ***every*** *area of my lifestyle, is a complete turn around – an about face. This involves radical new thinking, which leads to a conscious act of the will to live differently whatever the consequences. As the boom comes swinging round, you certainly have to change position! To spell this out in more detail would be to take advantage of those who read this book. I am not prepared to do this, much as I would love to, because I believe it* *is the difference between "seeing" and not being able to. There are so many I KNOWs that others may be crying out for. For still others there would be a completely different reaction. Another Great Divide would be created.*

So I will continue to look for the opportunities to be in the right place at the right time, and to share my perspectives with any who ***want*** *to sit down and have a talk – and a cuppa maybe.*

I hope Pete's ponderings have not been too imponderable. I've enjoyed sharing them and maybe you'll understand Hilary and me a little better – just ordinary human beings like you.

Postscript . . . or the Last Straw!

Hilary and I often share our perspectives with each other and strange as it may seem these exchanges have intensified as "Just a Little Prick" enters the home straight, and heads for the prize of the finished product.

"Chop this out . . ."

"Perhaps this should go in . . ."

"We can't cover everything in one book though."

*"**As Far as I Can Go**", was supposed to contain the last words of wisdom for the book.*

Until . . .

"Would you like to write another page," said Hilary, as we nestled up to each other while we kept an eye on the saucepans steaming away on the stove.

A few soothing noises from me, and then the question, "What about?"

"Have a look at what I've just put on the table," she said very quietly.

Reluctantly I left the warmth of our closeness, and sat down to read the pages before me. Only two pages! Shouldn't take long.

It was a BBC News item[1]: "Vaccines at birth a possibility", while a little further down the page there was a quote from Dr Ofer Levy, a lead researcher from Harvard Medical School:

> "We believe we have found the holy grail of neonatal immunology."

Did this warrant another page or two?

After nearly 500 pages already?

As I read on, the implications of the article hit us. Instead of having to wait two, four or six months before babies are vaccinated, the discovery of a molecule called Toll-like receptor 8, which could stimulate a baby's immune system, would then open up the way for the immediate start of vaccination schedules, hardly an enjoyable welcoming present to this strange new world of bright lights, loud noises and painful jabs.

And although that little body won't understand, there may be some added words of encouragement, "Never mind little fella. Just think how lucky you are. We've got plenty more little pricks to come. We've given you a great start to life."

The news report also quotes Prof. Adam Finn from Bristol University as saying that it was too early to say whether this research could and would change vaccination.

Well, we're getting in early by drawing your attention to this very sobering piece of news. By the way, remember that piece of bedtime reading in Chapter 9 – about Th1 and Th2 cytokines? The researchers in the BBC article talk about an evolutionary factor inactivating the baby's immune system during pregnancy so as to prevent it from attacking its mother's. You might like to check that out, because they seem to have got it wrong, which doesn't inspire confidence.

We wonder what else they might have got wrong.

And do you remember in Chapter 74 the quote from Dr Paul Offit, that in theory, healthy infants could safely get up to 100,000 vaccines at once?!

---

1 BBC News 2006. "Vaccines at birth a possibility" 25 April from http://news.bbc.co.uk/go/pr/fr/-/1/hi/health/4939996.stm 03:58:17 GMT

If at all possible vested interests will capitalize to the full any opportunity to begin vaccinations at birth.

Why is lack of immune response in the newly born seen as a weakness? With breastfeeding to give natural protection on top of maternal antibodies at birth, is there need for yet more interference?

This is the last straw for us, and it just had to be a "stop press" item.

Made in United States
North Haven, CT
06 September 2026

18154005R00271